PHYSIOLOGY
OF
DOMESTIC
ANIMALS

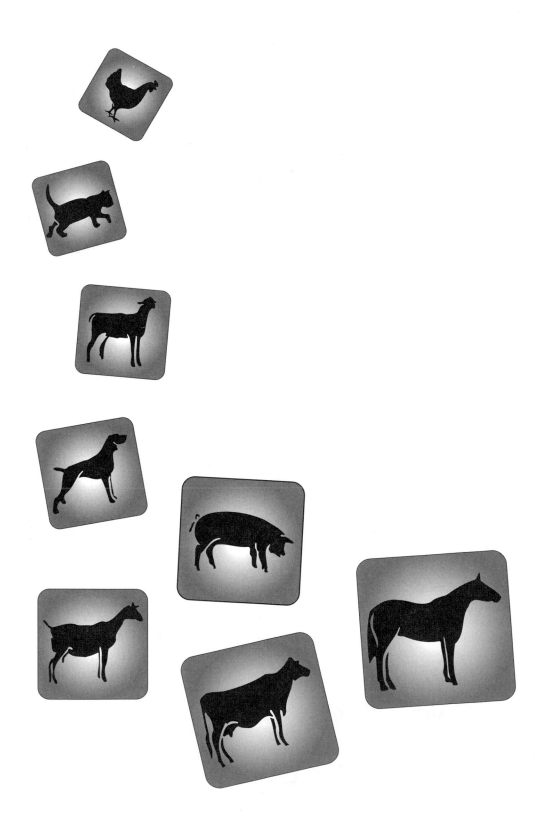

PHYSIOLOGY
OF
DOMESTIC
ANIMALS

second edition

William O. Reece, D.V.M., Ph.D.

*Department of Veterinary Physiology
and Pharmacology
College of Veterinary Medicine
Iowa State University of Science and Technology, Ames, Iowa*

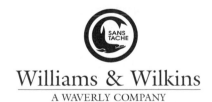

Williams & Wilkins
A WAVERLY COMPANY

BALTIMORE • PHILADELPHIA • LONDON • PARIS • BANGKOK
BUENOS AIRES • HONG KONG • MUNICH • SYDNEY • TOKYO • WROCLAW

Editor: Carroll Cann
Managing Editor: Susan Hunsberger
Production Coordinator: Cindy Park
Copy Editor: Kathy Gilbert
Designer: Maria Karkucinski
Composition: Mario Fernández, Donna Smith
Digitized Illustrations: All Systems Color
Manufacturing: Edwards Brothers

351 West Camden Street
Baltimore, Maryland 21201-2436 USA

Rose Tree Corporate Center
1400 North Providence Road
Building II, Suite 5025
Media, Pennsylvania 19063-2043 USA

Accurate indications, adverse reactions and dosage schedule for drugs are provided
in this book, but it is possible that they may change. The reader is urged to review
the package information data of the manufacturers of the medications mentioned.

Printed in the United States of America

First Edition,

Library of Congress Cataloging-in-Publication Data

Reece, William O.
  Physiology of domestic animals / William O. Reece.—2nd ed.
    p. cm.
  Includes bibliographical references and index.
  ISBN 0-683-07240-4
  1. Veterinary physiology. I. Title.
  [DNLM: 1. Animals, Domestic—physiology. 2. Animals, Domestic—anatomy &
histology. SF 768 R322p 1996]
SF768.R44 1996
636.089'2—DC20
DNLM/DLC
for Library of Congress   96-18088
                                                                               CIP

*The publishers have made every effort to trace the copyright holders for borrowed materials.
If they have inadvertently overlooked any, they will be pleased to make the necessary arrangements at the first opportunity.*

To purchase additional copies of this book, call our customer service department at
(800) 638-0672 or fax orders to **(800) 447-8438**. For other book services, including
chapter reprints and large quantity sales, ask for the Special Sales department.

Canadian customers should call **(800) 268-4178**, or fax **(905) 470-6780**. For all other
class originating outside of the United States, please call **(410) 528-4223** or fax us at
(410) 528-8550.

Visit Williams & Wilkins on the Internet: **http://www.wwilkins.com** or contact our
customer service department at **custserv@wwilkins.com**. Williams & Wilkins customer service representatives are available from 8:30 am to 6:00 pm, EST, Monday
through Friday, for telephone access.

                                                                          98 99
                                                            3 4 5 6 7 8 9 10

TO MY WIFE
Shirley

AND OUR CHILDREN
Mary
Kathy
Barbara
Sara
Anna
Susan
William O., II

Preface

I have been encouraged by the widespread use of the first edition and also by the favorable student and publisher comments. Accordingly, I have been privileged to bring forth a second edition whereupon improvements can be made that are based upon experience with the first edition. In other words, I have been given a second chance.

This textbook continues to be directed to undergraduate students desiring a basic understanding of domestic animal physiology. It assumes a basic background in biology and a strong interest by the student in obtaining a greater understanding of the purpose and function of the animal systems. The functional studies are always preceded or presented in concert with a review of the essential anatomy. The book will continue to be of particular interest to preveterinary students, veterinary technology students, and animal science and animal ecology majors because of its survey of the systems presentation. This approach has provided excellent preparation and appreciation for courses that follow which may have either an application of or greater depth in a particular system. Veterinary students have found the book to be useful as a bridge to other books required for greater depth of understanding required in veterinary courses.

My belief in the liberal use of illustrations continues and many of those used previously have been replaced with newly created ones that have eliminated extraneous detail and are more directed to the text reference.

Many beginning students need assistance in their study of textbook information. We are now providing that assistance in the form of study aids and self-evaluation questions at the end of each chapter. These will direct students into the text for better utilization of their study time.

A new chapter has been added with a presentation on the skeleton. This was not included with the previous edition because of the constraints of time for its preparation. The skeleton is an important component of physiology and is supportive to other systems. It is fitting for it to be included in a survey course.

Another new addition to the textbook is the inclusion of avian physiology in those chapters where their physiology is decidedly different. This has been done for the chapters on the kidney, respiration, digestion, and male and female reproduction. Also, tables that present physiologic data now include a column for the chicken. Chickens and turkeys are important components of the agricultural industry and veterinary profession. As before, a bibliography supports each chapter and provides a resource for more detailed information.

It has always been my objective to provide pleasant reading for students in order for them to achieve greater understanding of the science of animal function.

Ames, Iowa   *William O. Reece*

Acknowledgments

Textbook writing requires not only attention to detail by the author but also a large number of pretty nice people that are willing to work in one's behalf. My indebtedness and thanks are extended as follows to these people:

Ms. Vern Hoyt is our talented Department of Veterinary Physiology and Pharmacology secretary who typed the manuscript. Her superior computer skills allowed for a fast turnover for my beginning manuscript changes and additions all the way to their final form that was submitted to the publisher and for the corrections that followed.

Ms. Linda Erickson, Vern's office manager, provided a friendly environment for Vern to be productive and assisted with administrative duties as needed.

Dr. Richard Engen, Chairman, Department of Veterinary Physiology and Pharmacology, Iowa State University, consented to diversion of staff time and other resources to this project.

Mr. William Wiese and Ms. Linda Meetz, Veterinary Medical Library, Iowa State University, provided friendly and helpful library services in order to expedite reference searches.

Mr. Steve Hade, biomedical illustrator, provided nearly 100 new illustrations for this edition while at the same time he pursued graduate studies in biomedical illustration at the University of Illinois, Chicago campus.

Many publishers and authors gave permission to use their excellent illustrations. This is an unselfish act and their only reward is the credit given to their illustrations in the legends.

Mr. Carroll C. Cann, Executive Editor, Williams & Wilkins, has always been helpful through his administrative skills, encouragement, positive attitude, and friendliness. Ms. Susan Hunsberger, Managing Editor, has been equally supportive and friendly. Ms. Kathleen Gilbert was the Book Project Editor. Her word-for-word review of the manuscript, coupled with corrections and friendly suggestions, has helped fulfill my objective of providing pleasant reading for the student. Ms. Cindy Park, Production Coordinator, coordinated production activities that allowed for the book's completion in a timely manner. Ms. Diane Harnish, Marketing Manager, coupled her enthusiasm for the book with her marketing skills to achieve its commercial success. Many others, not known to me, also contributed their skills to the complex art of a published book. Carroll Cann has a great team and I appreciate the effort provided by each member.

The Biomedical Communications Section, College of Veterinary Medicine, Iowa State University, Mr. Stephen Pendry, Manager, provided artistic and photographic assistance. Ms. Donna Erickson channeled her artistic talent to the computer for the generation of several new illustrations. Mr. Charles Benn and Mr. James Fosse used their photographic skills for the provision of borrowed illustrations. Ms. Donna Wilson, friendly receptionist, kept the records for the eventual success of their activities.

My wife, Shirley, endured my absence on many evenings and weekends and was therefore willing to forego more enjoyable activities. In addition, she was an important advisor as well as an incentive for me to complete the book and to dedicate it to her and our seven children.

Above all, I thank God for this community of people and for giving my life its direction.

Contents

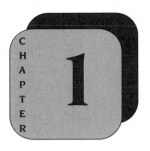

Nervous System

In its broad aspects, the nervous system enables the animal to adjust itself or its parts to changes in the external or internal environment. The nervous system acts as a control system.

STRUCTURE AND FUNCTION

Structure

Neuron

The neuron (nerve cell) is the anatomic and physiologic unit of the nervous system. It consists of the cell body and all its processes, the dendrites, and the axon (Fig. 1.1). Mammalian neurons can be bipolar (one axon and one dendrite) or multipolar (many branching dendrites and one axon). A nerve cell process is a dendrite if it conducts impulses toward the cell body and it is an axon if it conducts impulses away from the cell body. The axon (and its myelin covering, if present) is called a nerve fiber. The part of the cell membrane that covers the axon is known as the axolemma. In a myelinated axon, the axolemma is surrounded by a myelin sheath (neurilemma) that is interrupted at regularly-spaced intervals by myelin-free gaps, called nodes (of Ranvier).

A group of nerve cell bodies within the brain or spinal cord is referred to as a nucleus, and a group of nerve cell bodies outside the brain or spinal cord is called a ganglion. A bundle of neuron fibers within the brain or spinal cord is known as a tract, and a bundle of neuron fibers outside the brain or spinal cord is called a nerve.

Synapse

Continuity from one neuron to the next is provided by the synapse (Fig. 1.2). There is no physical contact of neurons at the synapse. A space exists between the neurons, and impulses from one neuron to the next are transmitted by chemical means through this space. Three notable characteristics of the synapse are (1) one-way conduction (direction), (2) facilitation (repeated impulses provide for easier subsequent transmission), and (3) greater fati-

1

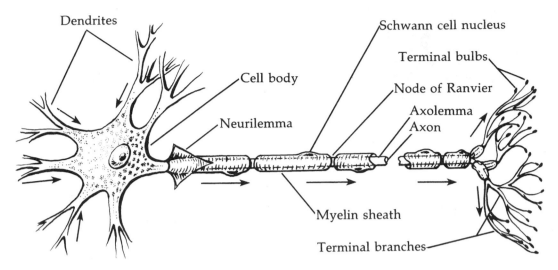

Figure 1.1. The neuron. Arrows indicate the direction of impulse conduction. In this myelinated nerve fiber in a peripheral nerve are shown the neurilemma (sheath of Schwann), axolemma (plasma membrane of axon), and internodal areas (nodes of Ranvier). (The axon is shown as discontinuous to allow for variable length.)

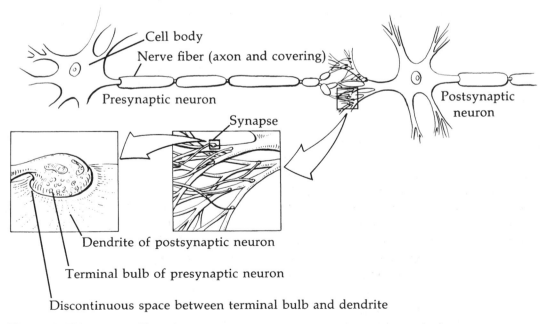

Figure 1.2. The synapse. The enlargements progress in the direction of the arrows.

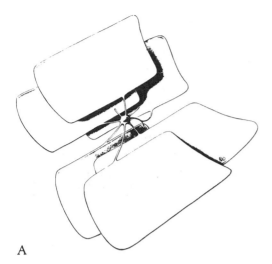

A

Figure 1.3. An oligodendrocyte (myelin-forming cell) of the central nervous system. **A.** The cell with its cytoplasmic extensions unwrapped. **B.** Cytoplasmic extensions wrapped around several axons. **C.** Cross section of a wrapped nerve fiber (NF). From Bunge RP. Structure and function of neuroglia: some recent observations. In: Schmitt FO, ed. The neurosciences: second study program. New York: Rockefeller University Press, 1970.

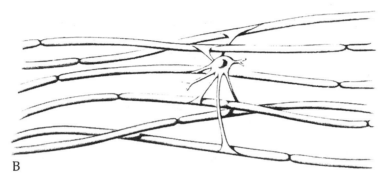

B

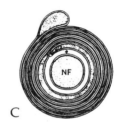

C

gability than the neuron (allows for repetitive impulses to fade).

Myelin Sheaths

Myelin is a white lipid (sphingomyelin) substance that forms a sheath around nerve fibers and serves as an electrical insulator. It is formed by oligodendrocytes in the central nervous system (CNS) and by Schwann cells in the peripheral nervous system (PNS). Both cells are components of the neuroglia, which is a special type of interstitial (between neurons) connective tissue in the nervous system.

Nerve fibers within the gray matter of the CNS are not myelinated, and its white glistening appearance outside the gray matter, as shown by the white matter and peripheral nerves, is provided by the myelin that envelops the nerve fibers. Not all nerve fibers outside the gray matter are myelinated, but because of the closeness of unmyelinated fibers to myelinated fibers, they tend to be invaginated (pressed) into the myelin substance. Even when this occurs, however, unmyelinated fibers are uninsulated because they maintain a direct association with extracellular fluid throughout their length.

The Schwann cell cytoplasm (which contains the myelin) is wrapped around a nerve fiber many times, and the outer layer, the neurilemma, contains the cell nucleus (Fig. 1.1). The cytoplasm of the oligodendrocyte is different from that of the Schwann cell because several extensions exist, each of which forms a wrapping around a nerve fiber (Fig. 1.3). One

Figure 1.4. The node of Ranvier as it would appear in the vertebrate central nervous system (CNS) and peripheral nervous system (PNS). Note the greater intimacy of the CNS node with extracellular fluid (ECF). From Bunge RP. Structure and function of neuroglia: some recent observations. In Schmitt FO, ed. The neurosciences: second study program. New York: Rockefeller University Press, 1970.

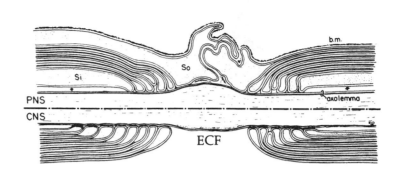

cell, therefore, provides a sheath at several locations.

Interruptions of the myelin sheath that occur along the length of a fiber are called the nodes of Ranvier. These nodes are the junctions of adjacent wrappings, either of the cytoplasmic extensions of oligodendrocytes or of Schwann cells. At these points, the nerve fiber plasma membrane (axolemma) is exposed directly to extracellular fluid. The exposure is more intimate in the CNS (Fig. 1.4). Whereas the sheathed portion of the nerve fiber is insulated, the nodes are uninsulated. Depolarization occurs at the nodes (see the following section), and the function of the myelin sheaths will become more apparent when nerve conduction is discussed.

Organization

For descriptive purposes, the various parts of the nervous system can be differentiated according to the following scheme:
1. Central nervous system
    a. Brain
    b. Spinal cord
2. Peripheral nervous system
    a. Cranial nerves
    b. Spinal nerves
    c. Autonomic nerves
    d. Ganglia

The CNS not only contains components of transmission, but also provides for those functions associated with computers, such as memory, a central processing unit for problem-solving, and input-output capability (sensations resulting from sensory input). The PNS functions in the transmission of nerve impulses.

The gross divisions of the brain are the cerebrum, cerebellum, and brain stem. An organizational scheme (Fig. 1.5) shows additional subdivisions. Another scheme (Fig. 1.6) is also commonly used; it has different names for the various parts. The relative locations of the various subdivisions to each other according to the first scheme are shown in Figure 1.7.

The Brain

CEREBRAL HEMISPHERES. The right and left cerebral hemispheres are large structures that make up most of the cerebrum (Fig. 1.8). Each hemisphere is composed of a covering of gray matter, the cerebral cortex, a central mass of white matter, the medullary substance (made up of nerve fibers), and the basal ganglia (Fig. 1.7).

The cerebral cortex has the following characteristics:
1. Acquired late in vertebrate evolution

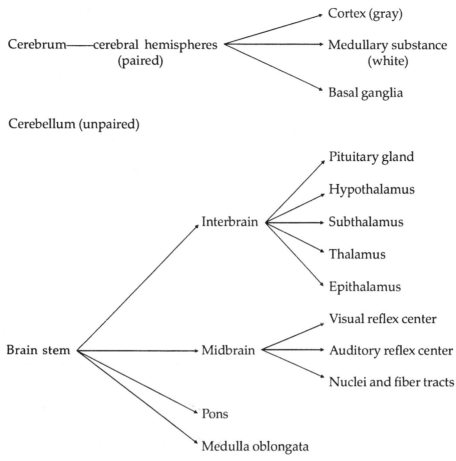

Figure 1.5. Subdivisions of the brain according to the major divisions: the cerebrum, cerebellum, and brain stem.

2. Concerned with those nervous reactions that result in consciousness
3. Regarded as the seat of the highest type of nervous correlation (association)
4. Marked by a high degree of educability (especially in humans)
5. Possesses a motor area:
   a. Impulses from these areas in one hemisphere cause muscle movements on the opposite (contralateral) side of the body
   b. Size of motor area and number and complexity of skeletal muscle movements of which an animal is capable are directly related
6. Contains sensory areas, or centers, into which sensory fibers discharge

The sensory areas are (1) the somesthetic or body sense area, which receives impulses from the skin concerned with touch, warmth, cold, and pain localization, impulses concerned with taste, and impulses from muscles, tendons, and joints, (2) the visual area (sight), (3) the auditory area (hearing), and (4) the olfactory area (smell).

The white matter is composed of myelinated nerve fibers situated beneath the cerebral cortex. These include association fibers, which establish connection between the different parts of the cortex, commissural fibers, which connect the two hemispheres, and projection fibers, which connect the cerebral cortex with other parts of the brain and spinal cord.

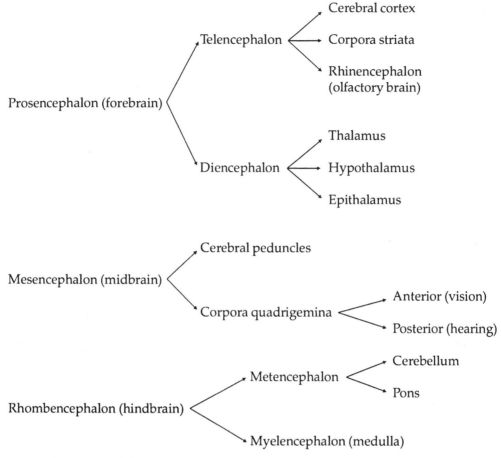

Figure 1.6. Subdivisions of the brain according to the major divisions: the prosencephalon, mesencephalon, and rhombencephalon.

Figure 1.7. Relative locations of brain subdivisions to each other. BG, basal ganglion; E, epithalamus; T, thalamus; H, hypothalamus; P, pituitary gland; M, midbrain; CER, cerebellum.

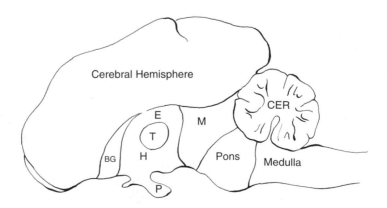

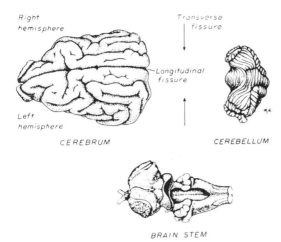

Right hemisphere

Transverse fissure

Longitudinal fissure

Left hemisphere

CEREBRUM   CEREBELLUM

BRAIN STEM

Figure 1.8. Gross subdivisions of the brain of the dog. In: Evans HE. Miller's anatomy of the dog. 3rd ed. Philadelphia: WB Saunders, 1993.

The basal ganglia (Fig. 1.7) lie deep within the cerebral hemispheres. They are composed of separate, large pools of neurons organized for the control of complex semi-voluntary movements, such as walking and running. In birds, the cerebral cortex is poorly developed, but the basal ganglia are highly developed. Because of this contrast, the basal ganglia perform nearly all the motor functions, even the voluntary movements, in much the same manner as the motor area of the human cortex controls voluntary movement. In the cat and, to a lesser extent, in the dog, removal of the cerebral cortex prevents many sophisticated motor functions. Because of the basal ganglia, however, this does not interfere with the ability to walk, eat, fight, and even participate in sexual activity.

CEREBELLUM. The cerebellum (Figs. 1.7 and 1.8) is not concerned with consciousness or sensation, as is the cerebral cortex. Because of its motor function, the cerebral cortex can start a limb or body part in motion, but once in motion, inertial forces would tend to keep it in motion until opposing forces stopped it. The cerebral cortex is not organized to mobilize the opposing force. The cerebellum, however,

can make automatic adjustments to prevent the distortion of inertia and momentum. To accomplish this, the cerebellum receives impulses (1) from the proprioceptive receptors (located in the internal mass of the body) found in all joints, muscles, and pressure areas (e.g., foot pads), (2) from the equilibrium apparatus of the inner ear, (3) from the visual cortex, and (4) directly from the motor cortex of all motor impulses being sent to muscles (Fig. 1.9). Whereas the motor area of a cerebral hemisphere exerts its effect on the contralateral side of the body, the effect of one side of the cerebellum is exerted on the same (ipsilateral) side of the body. Thus, the cerebellum acts as a "collecting house" for all information regarding the instantaneous physical status of the body.

BRAIN STEM. The brain stem is composed of the interbrain cranially followed caudally (in order) by the midbrain, pons, and medulla oblongata (Figs. 1.7 and 1.8). The cerebral hemispheres and cerebellum arise from the brain stem. In addition to the many fiber tracts that ascend and descend between the spinal cord and the cerebrum and cerebellum, the brain stem is the origin of all the cranial nerves except for the optic, olfactory, and acoustic nerves (special senses). The cells of origin for the latter lie outside the skull.

From below upward, the interbrain is comprised of the hypothalamus, thalamus, and epithalamus (Fig. 1.7). The hypothalamus contains the hypophysis or pituitary gland, which is an endocrine organ. Associated with the hypothalamus is a complex sensing and neurosecretory function. Also, the hypothalamus assumes a major role in the integration of functions carried out by the autonomic nervous system. For these functions, the anterior and middle portions contain parasympathetic components and the posterior portion contains sympathetic components. The thalamus contains many nuclei and is truly a relay center. Impulses from all areas of the

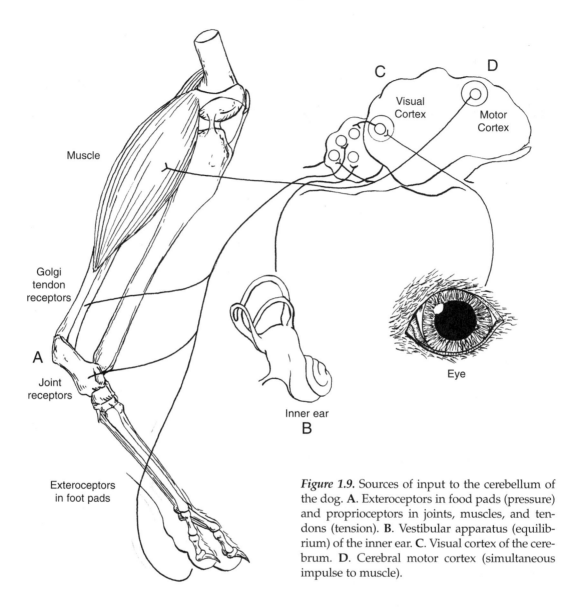

Muscle

Golgi
tendon
receptors

A

Joint
receptors

Exteroceptors
in foot pads

Inner ear
B

C

Visual
Cortex

D

Motor
Cortex

Eye

Figure 1.9. Sources of input to the cerebellum of the dog. **A**. Exteroceptors in food pads (pressure) and proprioceptors in joints, muscles, and tendons (tension). **B**. Vestibular apparatus (equilibrium) of the inner ear. **C**. Visual cortex of the cerebrum. **D**. Cerebral motor cortex (simultaneous impulse to muscle).

body are transmitted to the thalamus for transfer to the cerebral cortex. Other nuclei in the thalamus are associated with the relay of impulses within the brain. The epithalamus contains an olfactory (smell) correlation center and the pineal gland. The latter is a neurosecretory organ that regulates gonadal hormones and certain daily rhythms.

The midbrain (Fig. 1.7) contains the auditory and visual reflex centers, the nuclei of two cranial nerves, and several descending tracts.

The medulla and pons (Fig. 1.7) contain many ascending and descending pathways, the sensory and motor nuclei for all the cranial nerves originating in the brain stem (except the two located in the midbrain), and a large part of the central mechanism of the postural reflexes (e.g., hopping, righting, placing). There are also several reflex centers associated with the

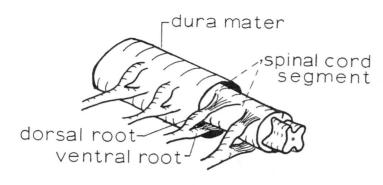

dura mater

spinal cord segment

dorsal root
ventral root

Figure 1.10. Structure of the spinal cord of the dog, showing a spinal cord segment. From Breazile JE. Textbook of veterinary physiology. Philadelphia: Lea & Febiger, 1971.

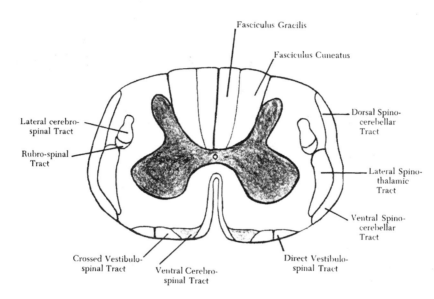

Fasciculus Gracilis

Fasciculus Cuneatus

Lateral cerebro-spinal Tract

Rubro-spinal Tract

Dorsal Spinocerebellar Tract

Lateral Spinothalamic Tract

Ventral Spinocerebellar Tract

Crossed Vestibulo-spinal Tract

Ventral Cerebro-spinal Tract

Direct Vestibulo-spinal Tract

Figure 1.11. Cross section of the spinal cord showing approximate location of some spinal tracts. From McGrath JT. Neurologic examination of the dog. 2nd ed. Philadelphia: Lea & Febiger, 1960.

regulation of important visceral functions such as heart rate, blood vessel muscle tone (vasomotor tone), respiration, and motor and secretory activities of the digestive tract.

Spinal Cord

The spinal cord is the caudal continuation of the medulla. Segmentation (association with the vertebral segments) is noticeable, with each segment giving rise to a pair of spinal nerves. The spinal cord receives sensory afferent fibers by way of the dorsal roots of the spinal nerves and gives off efferent motor fibers to the ventral roots of the spinal nerves (Fig. 1.10).

The centrally located gray matter (which resembles a capital H and is sometimes called the gray H) consists primarily of nerve cell bodies and their processes. The peripherally arranged white matter, which has a white appearance because of its myelin ensheathment, is composed of many distinct tracts (Fig. 1.11). The tracts connect the brain stem and higher centers with the spinal nerves. Different sensory and motor tracts are segregated in the cord. Proprioceptive (referring to the sensing of position of limbs or other body parts with-

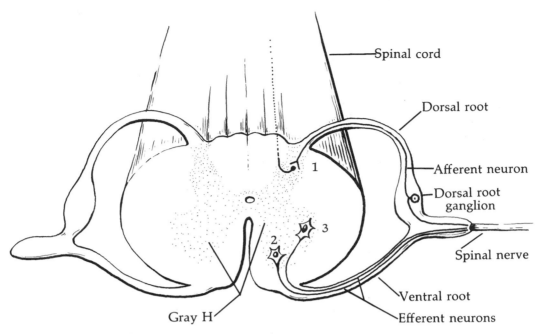

Figure 1.12. Cross section of the spinal cord of the dog. Located within the gray matter are 1, nerve cell bodies for sensory neurons, 2, somatic motor neurons, and 3, autonomic motor neurons.

out the use of vision) impulses from muscles, tendons, and joints have well-defined tracts, as do sensory impulses for pain, temperature, and touch. Similarly, impulses associated with certain motor functions descend in definite tracts. Many of the tracts are named according to the structures they connect. For example, the ventral spinocerebellar tract carries impulses from the spinal cord to the cerebellum. The lateral spinothalamic tract carries impulses from the spinal cord to the thalamus. The cells of origin for sensory impulses to the brain or to other parts of the spinal cord are located in the dorsal horns of the gray H, and the cells of origin of motor impulses to the spinal nerves are located in the ventral horns of the gray H. The cells of origin of the autonomic motor impulses arising from the spinal cord are the lateral masses of the ventral horns (intermediate location) of the gray H (Fig. 1.12).

As the spinal cord descends and proceeds caudally, its cross-sectional area decreases. This is because the cranial parts not only have tracts with fibers from the caudal portions, but also contain fibers associated with the cranial aspects of the body. Finally, at the caudal extremity, the tracts terminate and the spinal nerves fan outward and backward, giving the appearance of a broom or a horse's tail. Accordingly, the terminal part of the spinal cord, meninges, and nerves is called the cauda equina (Fig. 1.13).

Spinal Nerves

The spinal nerves are those that arise from the spinal cord and emerge from the vertebrae. In the dog, for example, there are 7 cervical, 13 thoracic, 7 lumbar, 3 sacral, and an average of 20 caudal vertebrae. With the exception of the cervical and caudal nerves, there is a pair of spinal nerves (one right and one left) that emerges

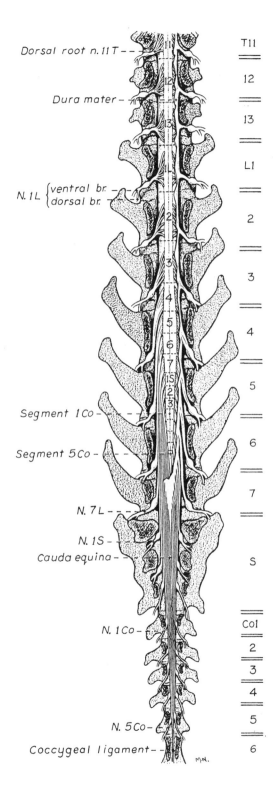

behind the vertebrae of the same serial number and name. In this plan, the first pair of thoracic nerves emerges through the intervertebral foramina located between the T1 and T2 vertebrae, and the last pair of thoracic nerves emerges through the intervertebral foramina between the T13 and L1 vertebrae (Fig. 1.14B,C). There are the same number of pairs of thoracic, lumbar, and sacral nerves as there are similar vertebrae. Instead of seven pairs of cervical nerves (corresponding with seven cervical vertebrae), however, there are eight pairs. The first pair of cervical nerves emerges through the foramina in the C1 vertebra, and the second pair emerges between the C1 and C2 vertebrae (Fig. 1.14A). Usually there are fewer pairs of caudal nerves than there are caudal vertebrae.

A spinal nerve is composed of a dorsal and ventral root and its branches. The dorsal root enters the dorsal portion of the spinal cord. It carries afferent (sensory) impulses from the periphery toward the spinal cord (Fig. 1.15). The nerve cell bodies of the neurons comprising the dorsal root are located in the dorsal root ganglion (DRG). This is visible as an enlarged part of the dorsal root close to the point where the dorsal and ventral roots join to form the spinal nerve proper. These neurons are embryologically bipolar, but the two processes later fuse near the cell body into one process, so that it appears to be T-shaped. One branch of the process becomes a peripheral afferent nerve fiber and the other branch passes into the CNS by way of the dorsal root. Although both branches are anatomically axons, the peripheral branch is physiologically a dendrite. This type of neuron has been called a pseudounipolar cell. Nerve impulses apparently pass from

Figure 1.13. Caudal extremity of the spinal cord showing the cauda equina. From Fletcher TF. Spinal cord and meninges. In: Evans HE, Christensen GC, eds. Miller's anatomy of the dog. 2nd ed. Philadelphia: WB Saunders, 1979.

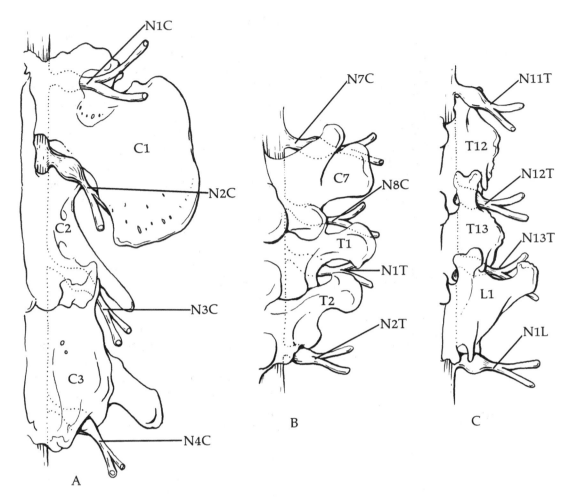

Figure 1.14. Association of spinal nerves with vertebrae in the dog. Only the right half of the spinal cord, vertebrae, and spinal nerve pair is shown. **A.** C1 to C3 vertebrae. **B.** C7, T1, and T2 vertebrae. **C.** T12, T13, and L1 vertebrae. C = cervical; T = thoracic; L = lumbar; N = nerve.

the peripheral branch to the central branch without entering the cell body.

The ventral root emerges from the ventral portion of the spinal cord. It carries efferent (motor) impulses from the spinal cord to striated muscle fibers (Fig. 1.15). Near the intervertebral foramen, the dorsal root joins with the ventral root to form the main part of the spinal nerve. The spinal nerve proper is classified as a mixed nerve because it contains both sensory and motor fibers. After the spinal nerve emerges from

the intervertebral foramen, it divides into a dorsal branch and a ventral branch; these supply innervation to structures dorsal and ventral to the transverse processes of the vertebrae, respectively (Fig. 1.16). The spinal nerves generally supply sensory and motor fibers to the region of the body in the area where they emerge from the spinal cord, but this is not the case for the appendages. They are innervated by the ventral branches of several spinal nerves and, near the limb they supply, the nerves

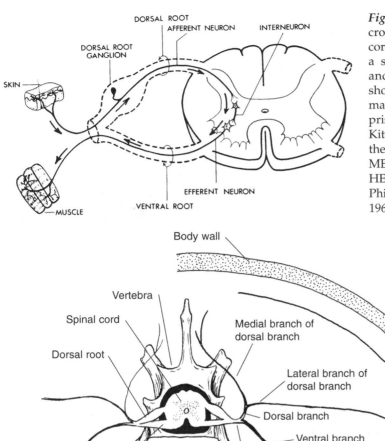

DORSAL ROOT
AFFERENT NEURON

INTERNEURON

DORSAL ROOT
GANGLION

SKIN

MUSCLE

EFFERENT NEURON

VENTRAL ROOT

Figure 1.15. Diagrammatic cross section of the spinal cord showing components of a spinal nerve. The afferent and efferent nerve fibers shown are only a part of the many nerve fibers that comprise a spinal nerve. From Kitchell RL. Introduction to the nervous system. In: Miller ME, Christensen GC, Evans HE, eds. Anatomy of the dog. Philadelphia: WB Saunders, 1964.

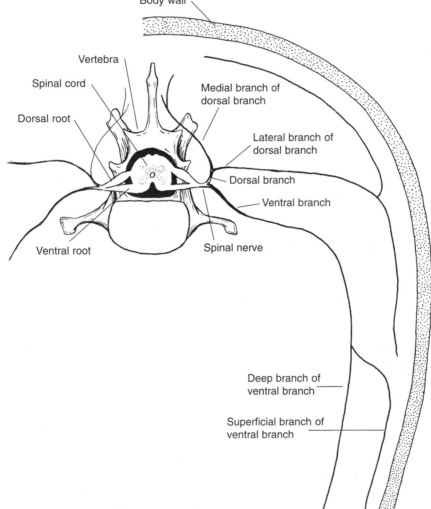

Body wall

Vertebra

Spinal cord

Dorsal root

Medial branch of
dorsal branch

Lateral branch of
dorsal branch

Dorsal branch

Ventral branch

Ventral root

Spinal nerve

Deep branch of
ventral branch

Superficial branch of
ventral branch

Figure 1.16. A spinal nerve and its location relative to its branches, roots, spinal cord, and vertebra.

Figure 1.17. Brachial plexus of the horse. It is formed by the contributions of the last three cervical and first two thoracic spinal nerves to supply the forelimbs. C = cervical; T = thoracic. The corresponding numbers refer to their respective spinal nerve.

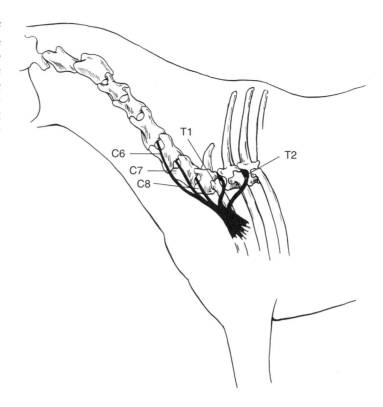

join together in braidlike arrangements known as plexuses. Each forelimb is supplied by nerves that arise from the brachial plexus (Fig. 1.17) and each hind limb is supplied by nerves that arise from the lumbosacral plexus.

CRANIAL NERVES. There are 12 pairs of cranial nerves, with a right and left nerve comprising each pair. The cranial nerves usually supply innervation to structures in the head and neck. The vagus nerve is an exception. In addition to its sensory and motor supply to the pharynx and larynx, it also supplies parasympathetic fibers to visceral structures in the thorax and abdomen (Fig. 1.18). These nerves have no dorsal or ventral roots and emerge through foramina in the skull (Fig. 1.19). Some cranial nerves are strictly sensory (afferent), some are strictly motor (efferent), and some are mixed (both sensory and motor). The cranial nerves are designated both by number and by name. The cranial nerves are listed

by number, name, type, and distribution in Table 1.1.

AUTONOMIC NERVES. The autonomic nerves are those parts of the peripheral nervous system that innervate smooth muscle, cardiac muscle, and glands. The autonomic nervous system has sympathetic and parasympathetic divisions. Most organs receive both sympathetic and parasympathetic innervation. The effect of sympathetic stimulation is generally opposite to that of parasympathetic stimulation. Accordingly, they can be considered as antagonistic to each other. To visualize their respective function in regard to an organ, the so-called "fight, fright, or flight" concept can be considered. Those actions that would be considered favorable in a fighting, frightening, or retreating situation can be attributed to sympathetic activity, whereas those actions associated with restful or tranquil situations can be attributed to the parasympathetics. A comparison of their respective

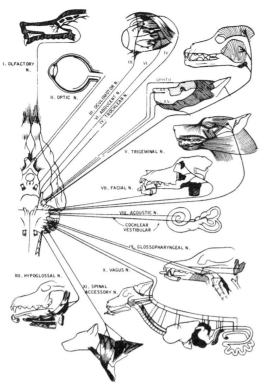

Figure 1.18. Origin and major distribution of cranial nerves in the dog. From Oliver JE, Hoerlein BF, Mayhew JG. Veterinary neurology. Philadelphia: WB Saunders, 1987.

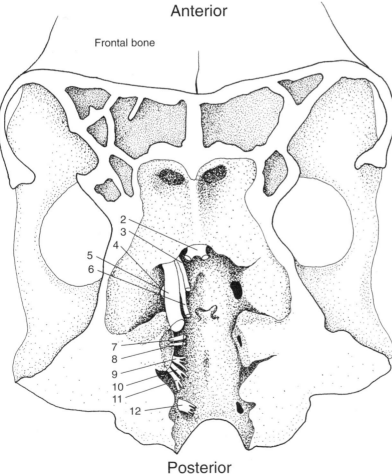

Anterior

Frontal bone

Posterior

Figure 1.19. Floor of bovine cranial cavity showing the exit locations of cranial nerves. The roots of the cranial nerves are shown on the left side. The roots emerge through foramina (openings); some foramina are visible on the right side. 2, optic nerve; 3, oculomotor nerve; 4, trochlear nerve; 5, trigeminal nerve; 6, abducens nerve; 7, facial nerve; 8, vestibulocochlear nerve; 9, glossopharyngeal nerve; 10, vagus nerve; 11, spinal accessory nerve; 12, hypoglossal nerve.

TABLE 1.1. Cranial Nerves

No.	Name	Type	Distribution
I	Olfactory	Sensory	Nasal mucous membrane (sense of smell)
II	Optic	Sensory	Retina of eye (sight)
III	Oculomotor	Motor	Most muscles of eye
			Parasympathetic to ciliary muscle and circular muscle of iris
IV	Trochlear	Motor	Dorsal oblique muscle of eye
V	Trigeminal	Mixed	Sensory—to eye and face; motor—to muscles of mastication
VI	Abducens	Motor	Retractor and lateral muscles of eye
VII	Facial	Mixed	Sensory—region of ear and taste to cranial two-thirds of tongue; motor—to muscles of facial expression; parasympathetic—to mandibular and sublingual salivary glands
VIII	Vestibulocochlear	Sensory	Cochlea (hearing); semicircular canals (equilibrium)
IX	Glossopharyngeal	Mixed	Sensory—to pharynx and taste to caudal third of tongue; motor—muscle of pharynx; parasympathetic—to parotid salivary glands
X	Vagus	Mixed	Sensory—to pharynx and larynx; motor—to muscles of larynx; parasympathetic—to visceral structures in the thorax and abdomen
XI	Spinal accessory	Motor	Motor—to muscles of shoulder and neck
XII	Hypoglossal	Motor	Motor—to muscles of tongue

Modified from Frandson RD, Spurgeon TL. Anatomy and physiology of farm animals. 5th ed. Philadelphia: Lea & Febiger, 1992:157.

actions for various organs is presented in Table 1.2.

The cells of origin for the sympathetic nerves are located in the thoracic and lumbar segments of the spinal cord, and the cells of origin of the parasympathetic nerves are located in the brain and sacral segments of the spinal cord—hence, the term for their origin is noted as craniosacral for the parasympathetics, as opposed to thoracolumbar for the sympathetics (Fig. 1.20). For both sympathetic and parasympathetic activity, two neurons are associated with the transmission of impulses from the cells of origin in the spinal cord or brain to the organ innervated. The cells of origin for the second neuron are located in ganglia. The first neuron is called preganglionic and the second neuron is called postganglionic. The preganglionic neuron for a sympathetic nerve traverses the ventral root of a thoracic or lumbar spinal nerve, enters the spinal nerve proper, and soon branches from it. It either synapses in a ganglion of the same vertebral segment (vertebral ganglion located close to each intervertebral space, with a ganglion on each side of each vertebra), or it can continue over a considerable distance to another vertebral ganglion, where it synapses. The synapse might not occur in a vertebral ganglion at all, however, but might continue to some paired ganglia that are ventral to the vertebral ganglia; these are called prevertebral or collateral ganglia. The prevertebral ganglia are fewer in number and are located more regionally. They include the celiac ganglia (distribution to stomach, liver, pancreas, kidney, adrenal), the cranial mesenteric ganglia (small intestine and upper colon), and caudal mesenteric ganglia (lower colon and neck of the

TABLE 1.2.   Actions of Autonomic Stimulation

Organ/Structure	Sympathetic Action	Parasympathetic Action
Eye		
Muscles of iris	Contraction of radial muscle (dilates pupil)	Contraction of circular muscle (constricts pupil)
Heart		
S-A node	Increase in heart rate	Decrease in heart rate
A-V node	Increase in conduction velocity	Decrease in conduction velocity
Muscle	Increase in force of contraction	Decrease in force of contraction
Intestines		
Muscle	Decreased	Increased
Secretions	Decreased	Increased
Lungs		
Bronchi	Dilatation	Constriction
Kidney	Afferent arteriole constriction and renin secretion	None
Urinary bladder		
Bladder wall	None	Contraction
Sphincter	Contraction	Relaxation
Penis	Ejaculation	Erection
Piloerector muscles	Contraction	None
Salivary glands	Mucus secretion	Serous secretion

bladder). The postganglionic fiber leaves the vertebral or prevertebral ganglion and proceeds to the organ supplied, usually by way of a blood vessel to that organ. It can also leave the vertebral ganglion, reenter a spinal nerve, and be distributed with the branchings of the spinal nerve. The interconnections among various levels of vertebral ganglia (by preganglionic fibers and postganglionic sympathetic fibers) form paired nerve trunks that pass along each side of the vertebral column from the region of the head as far back as the caudal end of the sacrum. The main paired trunk is known as the sympathetic trunk (Fig. 1.20).

The preganglionic neurons of the parasympathetic division are distributed to ganglia near the organs supplied before they synapse with the postganglionic neuron. Accordingly, the preganglionic fibers are relatively longer and the postganglionic fibers are relatively shorter compared with the preganglionic and postganglionic fibers

of the sympathetic division. The parasympathetic preganglionic fibers that arise from nerve cell bodies in the brain are distributed to their respective organs in common with one of four cranial nerves (III, VII, IX, or X). The first three supply regions of the head and the last, cranial nerve X (the vagus nerve), supplies the heart and lungs in the thorax and nearly all the abdominal viscera. The parasympathetic preganglionic fibers that arise from nerve cell bodies in the sacral portion of the spinal cord supply the last part of the digestive tract and most of the urogenital system. These fibers emerge from the ventral roots of their respective segments and are distributed to the ganglia near the organs supplied by the pelvic nerve.

Autonomic reflexes involve afferent transmission of impulses away from the structures supplied to the spinal cord and then back again as an efferent impulse. The receptive nerve endings for autonomic reflexes are located in most of the struc-

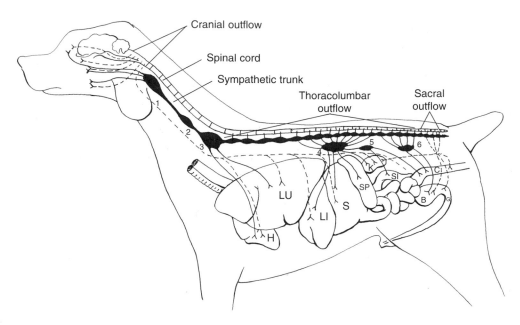

Figure 1.20. Diagrammatic representation of the efferent autonomic nervous system of the dog. The lines showing sympathetic outflow (thoracolumbar) are solid; lines for parasympathetic outflow (craniosacral) are broken. Numbers indicate sympathetic ganglia. 1, cranial cervical; 2, middle cervical; 3, stellate; 4, celiac; 5, cranial mesenteric; 6, caudal mesenteric. LU = lung; H = heart; LI = liver; S = stomach; SI = small intestine; SP = spleen; K = kidney; C = colon; B = urinary bladder; G = genitalia.

tures (viscera) supplied by autonomic innervation. A single neuron transmits the impulse to the central nervous system through much the same route as the autonomic efferent fibers except for the spinal segments, which enter the cord through the dorsal root. These impulses do not reach the conscious level, but form the afferent side of many autonomic reflexes that control such functions as blood pressure, heart rate, and the activity of the digestive and urogenital systems.

THE NERVE IMPULSE AND ITS TRANSMISSION

Mechanisms of Transmission

Resting Membrane Potential

The word "potential" is used in regard to nerve cells as it is in the study of electricity, in which it refers to relative electrical charges between two points in a field or circuit. For the neuron, the two points are the inside and outside of the confines of the cell membrane (Fig. 1.21). A measured potential is relatively small, however, and its units are in millivolts rather than volts. In a resting neuron, the potential between the two sides of the membrane is called the resting potential. The resting membrane potential results from the unequal distribution of sodium ions (Na^+) and potassium ions (K^+) on the outside and inside of the neuron. The active transport of Na^+ to the outside keeps the concentration of Na^+ low on the inside of the neuron. This is coupled with the transport of K^+ into the neuron. If their rates of transport were equal to each other, electrical neutrality between the inside and outside of the membrane would be maintained. However, the outward active transport of Na^+ occurs at a faster rate than the inward active transport of K^+, and thus an electronegativity is maintained on the inside of the membrane and an electropositivity is maintained on the outside (Fig. 1.22). The membrane is therefore polarized. The resting membrane potential has been measured as about -70 millivolts (mV). It does not exceed -70 mV because, at this level, the electrical gradient is sufficient to cause Na^+ diffusion inward to balance the rate of outward active transport.

Depolarization, Repolarization, and the Nerve Impulse

Chemical or physical stimulation of a neuron increases the permeability of the membrane for Na^+ at the point of stimula-

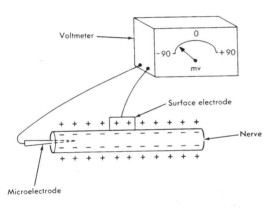

Voltmeter

Surface electrode

Nerve

Microelectrode

Figure 1.21. Measurement of the membrane potential of a nerve fiber using microelectrodes. From Langley LL, Ph.D. The physiology of man. 4th ed. © 1971 by Litton Educational Publishing, Inc. Reprinted by permission of Wadsworth, Inc.

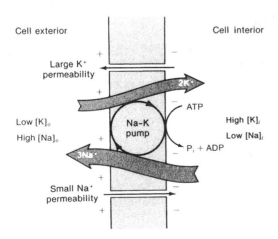

Cell exterior   Cell interior

Large K^+ permeability

Low $[K]_o$
High $[Na]_o$

Na-K pump

ATP

P_i + ADP

High $[K]_i$
Low $[Na]_i$

Small Na^+ permeability

tion and, because there is a high concentration of Na^+ on the outside of the membrane in the extracellular fluid, Na^+ rushes inward. This reverses the membrane potential at the point of stimulation, so the membrane now becomes positive on the inside and negative on the outside; this is depolarization. The inflow of Na^+ soon stops and the permeability of the membrane for K^+ increases; the K^+ then flows outward because it has a higher concentration inside the neuron than outside. The outflow of K^+ reestablishes the resting membrane potential at the point of stimulation; this is repolarization. Measurement of the membrane potential during membrane depolarization and repolarization and its continuous recording on a moving chart is shown in Figure 1.23.

When a microregion of a nerve fiber is stimulated and subsequently depolarized, a current flow occurs from the point of depolarization to the adjoining microregions. Current flow occurs because a positive charge now exists inside the membrane at the point of initial depolarization; because of the negative charge inside the membrane, beyond the point of stimulation, the positive charges (ions) flow toward the negatively charged portion. In addition, the outer aspect of the fiber membrane (which has become negatively charged at the point of depolarization)

Figure 1.22. Establishment of a resting membrane potential by active transport of 3 Na^+ outward coupled with the transport of 2 K^+ inward. The uneven distribution results in the electronegativity within the fiber. From Eckert R, Randall D, Augustine G. Animal physiology: mechanisms and adaptations. 3rd ed. © 1978, 1983, 1988 by WH Freeman and Co. Reprinted by permission.

Figure 1.23. Recording of a membrane potential during depolarization and repolarization of a nerve fiber microregion. The interior of the fiber becomes positive during depolarization. From Breazile JE. Textbook of veterinary physiology. Philadelphia: Lea & Febiger, 1971.

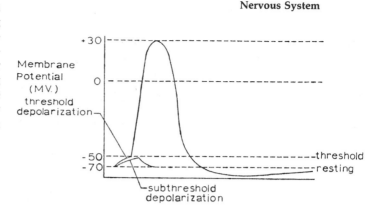

attracts positive ions to it from the charged membrane farther ahead. Because of these two events, the interior of the fiber just beyond the depolarized region becomes somewhat more positively charged and the exterior of the fiber just beyond the depolarized region becomes less positively charged. Accordingly, an electrical current flows outward through the fiber membrane from the interior (that gained positive charges) to the exterior (where positive charges were drawn away). The passage of current out through the membrane, just beyond the site where depolarization has occurred, causes this region of the membrane to become depolarized in turn (because current flow increases permeability to Na^+), just as the membrane did at the site of the stimulus. The process of depolarization followed by current flow is repeated throughout the length of the nerve fiber and accounts for the nerve impulse (Fig. 1.24).

Action Potential

Action potentials are changes in the resting membrane potential that are actively propagated along the membrane of the cell. The application of a stimulus to a nerve cell membrane diminishes the resting membrane potential (zero direction). When the membrane potential reaches a critical value (usually 8 to 12 mV lower than the resting level), an action potential occurs. The membrane potential at which an action potential is produced is referred to as the threshold. Not all stimuli can depolarize the membrane to threshold.

During an action potential, depolarization can change the membrane potential from -70 mV to about +30 mV. During repolarization there is a return to the resting membrane potential of –70 mV. The recording shown in Figure 1.23 represents an action potential. The nerve fiber cannot be stimulated again until repolarization is nearly complete; this is known as the refractory period. When an action potential has been initiated, the nerve fiber is said to "fire." If the stimulus is strong enough to initiate an action potential, the entire fiber will fire. This is known as the "all-or-none" principle for nerve fibers. There is no such thing as a weak impulse. If the stimulus is strong enough to initiate depolarization, the impulse will be conducted with action potentials of normal magnitude. Depolarization and repolarization proceed from one microregion to the adjoining microregion until the entire fiber has been traversed.

Saltatory Conduction

In myelinated fibers, the depolarization and repolarization processes are the same, but the action potentials occur from one node of Ranvier to the next instead of the

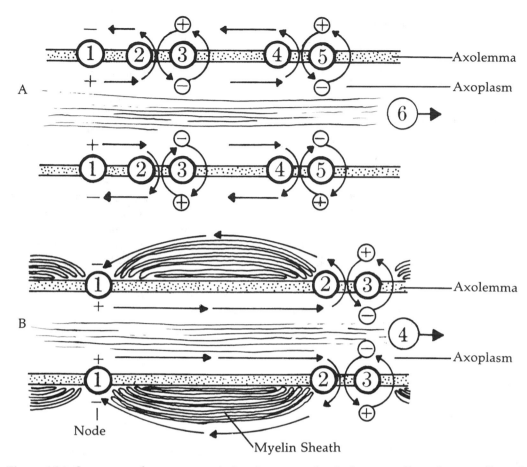

Figure 1.24. Summary of neurotransmission in mammals. **A.** In unmyelinated nerve fiber, the sequence of events is as follows: 1, depolarization at point of stimulation has occurred (now negative outside and positive inside); 2, current flow; 3, depolarization of adjacent region begins (will become negative outside and positive inside); 4, current flow; 5, depolarization begins (will become negative outside and positive inside); 6, repetition of current flow and depolarization, and impulse travels to end of nerve fiber. **B.** In myelinated nerve fiber the sequence is as follows: 1, depolarization; 2, current flow; 3, depolarization; 4, saltatory conduction to end of nerve fiber.

entire area of the membrane. This process of impulse transmission is referred to as saltatory conduction (saltation refers to an abrupt movement, such as dancing or leaping). The axolemma is in intimate association with the extracellular fluid at the nodes of Ranvier, and the remainder of the membrane is relatively insulated from the extracellular fluid. Thus, current flow sufficient to increase membrane permeability leaps from one node of Ranvier to the next, rather than being dissipated at the adjoin-

ing microregion. Two functions are served by saltatory conduction. First, impulse transmission is accelerated; second, less membrane is depolarized and repolarized, hence reducing the energy requirement for "recharging" the membrane.

Transmission Velocity

The larger the diameter of the fiber and the thicker the myelin sheath, the faster the transmission of the impulse. The fastest transmission is about 100 m/s and the slowest is about 0.5 m/s. Large myelinated fibers can transmit about 2500 impulses/s, contrasted to about 250 impulses/s for small unmyelinated fibers.

Neurotransmitters

A nerve impulse causes an effect at a synapse or at the structure being innervated. Axons terminate by branching; the branches terminate with a structure known as a presynaptic terminal bulb at the synapse and with other similar, modified structures at the organs innervated (Fig. 1.2). These terminations have vesicles containing chemical substances that are liberated when the impulse arrives. The chemical substance then diffuses to the membrane of the postsynaptic neuron or structure and

influences the permeability of the membrane for sodium ion.

Peripheral Neurotransmitters

The neurotransmitters of the peripheral nervous system are excitatory in nature—that is, they increase the permeability of the affected membrane for sodium ions. This substance is acetylcholine (ACh) for the spinal and cranial nerves. ACh is also the preganglionic and postganglionic terminal neurotransmitter for the parasympathetic division of the autonomic nervous system (Fig. 1.25). This division of the autonomic nervous system is therefore sometimes referred to as the cholinergic system. The preganglionic terminal neurotransmitter of the sympathetic division is also ACh, but the postganglionic terminal secretion is

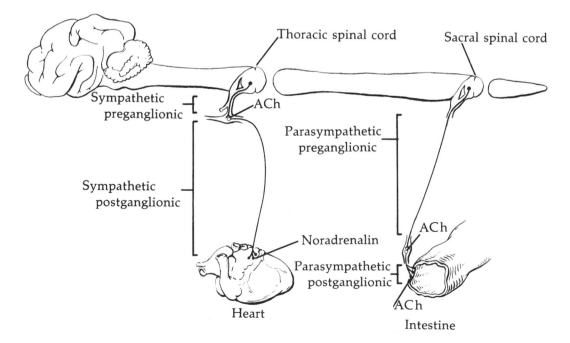

Figure 1.25. The neurotransmitters acetylcholine (ACh) and norepinephrine (noradrenalin) associated with the autonomic nervous system of mammals.

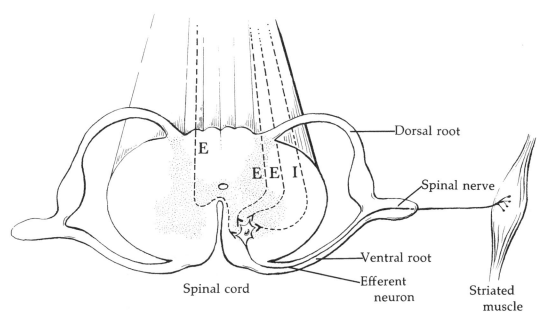

Figure 1.26. Neuron going to striated muscle. This represents the final common pathway. To fire, a greater amount of excitatory (E) neurotransmitter must be released than inhibitory (I) neurotransmitter.

norepinephrine. Another name for norepinephrine is noradrenaline, so the sympathetic division is often referred to as the adrenergic system.

Central Neurotransmitters

In the central nervous system, there are not only excitatory but also inhibitory transmitters. In addition to ACh and norepinephrine, which are present in peripheral neurons, other excitatory transmitters are probably found in the central nervous system. At least two inhibitory transmitters are recognized within the brain and spinal cord: gamma-aminobutyric acid (GABA) and glycine, which is a simple amino acid. Inhibitory transmitters appear to decrease the permeability of the affected membrane for sodium ions.

Final Common Pathway

In the central nervous system, the branches of many axons most likely impinge on a particular neuron. This neu-

ron could be the last in a series and could represent the final common pathway. Neurons that impinged on it might have been stimulated and, depending on the nature of their presynaptic terminal (excitatory or inhibitory), the effect of the final common pathway will have been determined by the predominance of excitatory or inhibitory presynaptic terminals that were stimulated. If the resultant of all excitatory and inhibitory effects is above the threshold for an action potential (start of depolarization), the neuron fires (Fig. 1.26).

Neuron Placement

CONVERGING CIRCUIT. Within the central nervous system are several schemes of neuron placement (circuits) that allow for different patterns of activity. The circuit described above, in which several neurons impinge on one neuron, is known as a converging circuit (Fig. 1.27A). It allows impulses from many different sources to cause some response or provide a sensation.

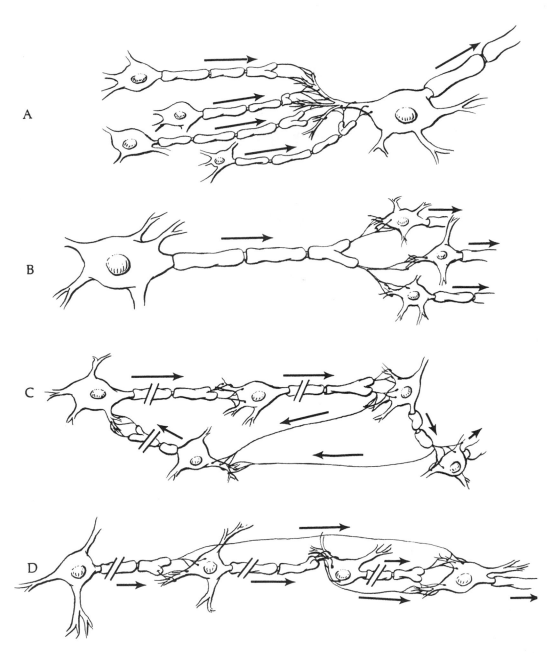

Figure 1.27. Examples of neuron placement within the central nervous system of mammals. **A.** Converging circuit. **B.** Diverging circuit. **C.** Reverberating circuit. **D.** Parallel circuit.

DIVERGING CIRCUIT. A diverging circuit is one in which the axon branches of one neuron impinge on two or more neurons, and each of these in turn impinge on two or more neurons (Fig. 1.27B). This type of cir-

cuit allows for amplification of impulses and is found in the control of skeletal muscles.

REVERBERATING CIRCUIT. A reverberating circuit is one in which each neuron in a series sends a branch back to the beginning neuron, so that a volley of impulses is received at the final neuron (Fig. 1.27C). This type is associated with rhythmic activities, and the volley continues until the synapses fatigue.

PARALLEL CIRCUIT. A parallel circuit contains a number of neurons in series, with each neuron supplying a branch to the final neuron (Fig. 1.27D). Because there is a delay of transmission at the synapse, a volley of stimuli reaches the final neuron. Unlike the reverberating circuit, the impulses then stop. This type provides reinforcement to a single stimulus.

SIMPLE CIRCUITS. Many complex neuron connections are possible, but neuron connections can also be direct and simple. In this regard, the neurons associated with the special senses might involve no more than two neurons for their projection to the cerebral cortex. A minimum of three neurons is required to transmit a nerve impulse from the periphery by way of a spinal nerve to the cerebral cortex (Fig. 1.28).

REFLEXES

A reflex is defined as an automatic or unconscious response of an effector organ (muscle or gland) to an appropriate stimulus. The reflex involves a chain of at least two neurons: (1) an afferent, sensory, or receptor neuron, and (2) an efferent, motor, or effector neuron. Usually, however, one or more connector neurons or interneurons are between the receptor and effector neurons.

Spinal Reflex

A reflex can involve parts of the brain and autonomic nervous system, but the simplest reflex is the spinal reflex. An example of a spinal reflex is the knee jerk reflex (Fig. 1.29), which is a stretch reflex. The reflex is elicited by striking the middle patellar ligament. This ligament, located at the knee, is the tendon of insertion for the quadriceps femoris and transmits its action to extend the tibia. Striking the middle patellar ligament stretches the quadriceps muscle, which in turn stimulates muscle spindles (receptors for muscle sense). An impulse is transmitted by way of the dorsal root of the appropriate spinal nerve to the applicable motor neuron in the ventral horn of the gray H, and then to muscle fibers of the quadriceps muscle, causing it to contract. The purpose of the reflex is to oppose stretch of the muscle. Because this

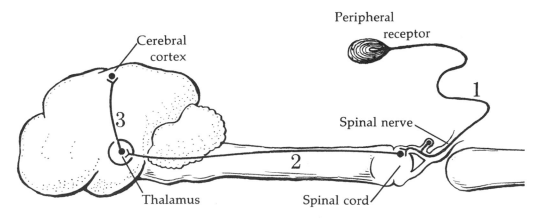

Figure 1.28. A neuron circuit from periphery to cerebral cortex. A minimum of three neurons is required. 1, afferent neuron in a mixed spinal nerve; 2, neuron ascending in a spinal cord tract to the thalamus; 3, final neuron in the circuit that transmits the impulse to the cerebral cortex.

reflex involves an intact and functioning spinal cord at a certain level of segmentation, the soundness of the cord at that level can be determined by this reflex action. Absence of the knee jerk reflex can help to confirm suspicion of damage or injury to the cord at that level. This reflex is a postural reflex because it aids in maintaining a standing position.

Somatic and Visceral Reflexes

If the effector organs are composed of striated muscle, then the reflex is somatic. If the effector organs are either smooth or cardiac muscle, or glands, then the reflex is visceral. Visceral reflexes regulate visceral functions and are transmitted by the autonomic nervous system (by visceral afferent fibers and preganglionic and postganglionic efferent fibers of the sympathetic or parasympathetic division).

Reflex Centers

Reflex centers are located throughout the central nervous system. They are involved with the integration of more complex reflexes. The simplest reflexes are those associated with the spinal cord and the more complex are carried out through reflex centers in the brain. Some of these centers are located in the medulla oblongata and include reflex centers for the control of heart action, vessel diameter, respiration, swallowing, vomiting, coughing, and sneezing. The cerebellum contains most of the reflex centers associated with locomotion and posture. The hypothalamus contains reflex centers associated with temperature regulation, and the midbrain contains visual and auditory reflexes, which can bring about constriction or dilatation of the pupils and evoke a startle reaction to loud noises.

Postural Reflexes and Reactions

The postural reflexes and reactions aid in maintaining an upright position. Responses that involve the cerebral cortex are more

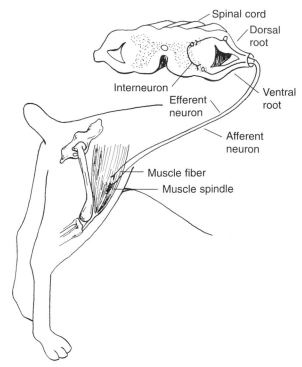

Figure 1.29. The stretch reflex. Stretch of muscle stimulates the muscle spindle. The impulse travels to the spinal cord by way of an afferent neuron. Transmission of the impulse to an efferent neuron may be direct or by way of an interneuron as shown. Stimulation of an efferent neuron to striated muscle counteracts stretch by causing contraction.

properly called reactions than reflexes. Muscle tonus (tone) is that state of muscle tension that enables an animal to assume and remain in the erect attitude. The stretch reflex, previously described, is the fundamental element of muscle tone. The following are examples of postural reflexes and reactions:

1. Standing reflex—pushing down on the back of a dog causes muscle movements that compensate for and resist the displacement
2. Attitudinal reflexes—displacement of one part of the body is followed by postural changes in other parts (e.g., lifting the head of a horse is followed by postural changes in the rear quarters so that a new attitude is assumed)

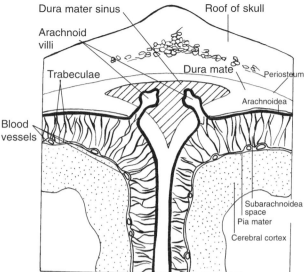

Figure 1.30. Cerebral meninges and arachnoid villi. The meninges consist of the dura mater, arachnoidea, and pia mater. The subarachnoid space contains cerebrospinal fluid. The arachnoid villi project into the dural sinus (blood sinus) and provide for an outlet for cerebrospinal fluid.

3. Righting reflex—dropping an inverted cat is followed by its landing in the upright position
4. Hopping reaction—pushing a supported dog with three limbs elevated results in a placement correction of the intact leg to act as a rigid pillar

The spinal cord of domestic animals constitutes a greater proportion of the total central nervous system (brain and spinal cord) than in humans. This reflects the fact that more of the total CNS activity in animals is accomplished by reflex than by cerebral activity. There is approximately 10 times more spinal cord activity in dogs than in humans.

THE MENINGES AND CEREBROSPINAL FLUID

Meninges of the Brain

The meninges are the coverings of the brain and spinal cord. From without inward they are the dura mater, arachnoidea, and pia mater, respectively (Fig. 1.30). In the skull, the outer aspect of the dura mater is fused intimately with the inner periosteum of the calvaria (brain case). Between the cerebral hemispheres and between the cerebrum and cerebellum there is a separation of the outer and inner aspects of the dura mater to form venous sinuses. These blood collection areas are continued as veins that return blood to the heart from the brain. The only space between the inner aspect of the dura mater and the arachnoidea is that which is sufficient for blood vessels. The arachnoidea has projections (trabeculae) from its inner aspect to the most intimate covering of the brain, the pia mater. The trabeculae give the appearance of a spider's web—hence the name arachnoidea (after the class name for spiders, Arachnida). The space between the arachnoidea and the pia mater is significant and is known as the subarachnoid space. There are projections from the subarachnoid space into the dura mater sinuses, the arachnoid granulations, or the arachnoid villi. The subarachnoid space contains cerebrospinal fluid and the arachnoid granulations allow for the resorption of this fluid back into the blood. The pia mater follows all the grooves and fissures of the brain surface. It forms a sheath around blood vessels and follows them into the substance of the brain (Fig. 1.31). The perivascular spaces thus formed extend as far as the arterioles and venules, but not onto the capillaries. The inner aspects of the brain are therefore in communication with cerebrospinal fluid (this might serve a "lymphatic" function because there are no lymph vessels in the brain). The meninges (and cerebrospinal fluid) continue for a short distance onto the cranial and spinal nerves. The vestibular (auditory) branch of the vestibulocochlear nerve (cranial nerve VIII), because of its closeness to the exterior of the body, subjects the meninges to some hazard if the inner ear becomes inflamed.

Meninges of the Spinal Cord

The meninges of the spinal cord are continuous with the meninges of the brain. The outer aspect of the dura mater is not fused with the vertebral canal (the hole through the vertebrae within which the spinal cord transcends) and an epidural (outside the dura mater) space exists, which contains fat (Fig. 1.32). The epidural space at the sacrocaudal location is used for the injection of local anesthetics in cattle. Spinal nerve projections are present in this location; when anesthetized, sensory and motor loss occurs in certain areas, which is advantageous for medical or surgical treatment. For example, a prolapsed uterus (uterus that has everted through the vagina) can be replaced in the cow without the straining that would otherwise occur.

Ventricles of the Brain

The four ventricles of the brain are cavities or hollowed-out spaces within the sub-

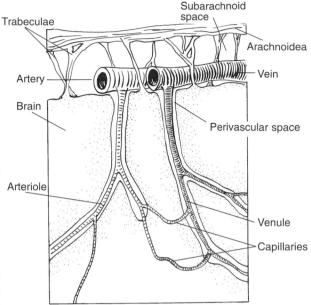

Figure 1.31. The perivascular space—the space lined by pia mater that follows blood vessels into the brain substance. The space is filled with cerebrospinal fluid and communicates with the subarachnoid space. It extends only to the level of the capillaries and serves a lymphatic function.

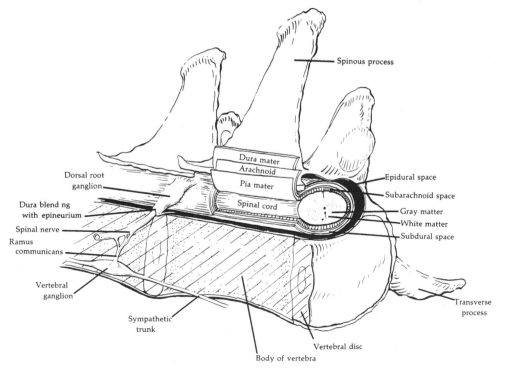

Figure 1.32. The meninges of the spinal cord. Only half of the vertebra is shown to indicate the extension of dura onto the spinal nerves. Note the presence of an epidural space.

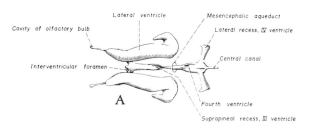

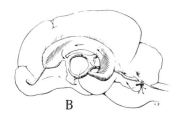

Figure 1.33. The canine brain ventricles. **A.** Dorsal view of ventricles without brain substance. **B.** Lateral view of ventricles which shows their location within the brain. **C.** Lateral view of ventricles without brain substance. From deLahunta A. Veterinary neuroanatomy and clinical neurology. 2nd ed. Philadelphia: WB Saunders, 1983.

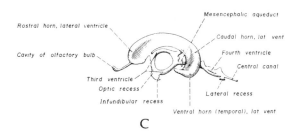

stance of the brain (Figs. 1.33 and 1.34). The lateral ventricles are paired cavities within each right and left cerebral hemisphere. They are continuous with the single third ventricle through the interventricular foramen. The third ventricle is located within the interbrain and is continuous with the fourth ventricle through the cerebral aqueduct (mesencephalic aqueduct). The fourth ventricle is located beneath the cerebellum and above the medulla oblongata. It communicates in turn with the subarachnoid space through the three foramina of Magendie (single) and Luschka (paired). The fourth ventricle is continued caudad as the central canal of the spinal cord. Each of the four ventricles has a structure, known as the choroid plexus, projecting into it. The choroid plexus is a tuft of capillaries that secretes cerebrospinal fluid.

Circulation and Function of Cerebrospinal Fluid

Cerebrospinal fluid formed by the choroid plexuses flows through the cavities of the lateral and third ventricles, through the cerebral aqueduct and fourth ventricle, and finally through the foramina of Luschka and Magendie to enter the subarachnoid space of the brain and spinal cord. Cerebrospinal fluid also enters the central canal of the spinal cord from the fourth ventricle. Cerebrospinal fluid then leaves the subarachnoid space of the brain through specialized structures (arachnoid granulations or villi) in which the subarachnoid space invaginates into the cerebral venous sinuses (the dural sinuses) (Fig. 1.30). The relationship of the subarachnoid space with the venous sinuses is such that valvular structures prevent the backflow of

Dural Sinus

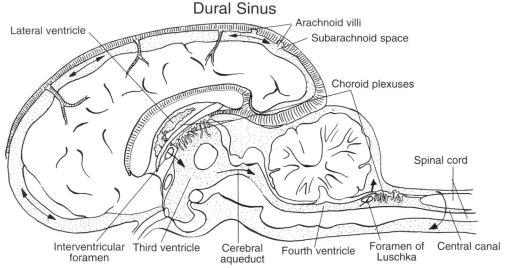

Figure 1.34. Pathway of cerebrospinal fluid flow from choroid plexuses to the arachnoid villi that protrude into the dural sinuses. The interventricular foramina are openings from each of the two lateral ventricles (one in each cerebral hemisphere). The choroid plexuses produce the cerebrospinal fluid (stippled). The two foramina of Luschka (one shown) and the foramen of Magendie (not shown) provide an exit from the sites of formation to the subarachnoid space of the brain and spinal cord. Cerebrospinal fluid circulates caudally through the central canal of the spinal cord.

blood into the subarachnoid space, but allow the forward flow of cerebrospinal fluid into the cerebral sinuses. Therefore, a higher pressure must exist within the subarachnoid space than within the venous system. The normal pressure of cerebrospinal fluid ranges from 8 to 12 mm Hg, whereas the pressure within the dural sinuses ranges from 1 to 8 mm Hg.

Cerebrospinal fluid is produced continually (0.1 to 0.3 mL/min). If the pathway for flow from the choroid plexuses to the venous sinuses is occluded, the cerebrospinal fluid pressure increases and hydrocephalus can result. Cerebrospinal fluid that accompanies the meninges for a short distance onto the cranial and spinal nerves can enter lymphatics at that level and be returned to the blood. This is particularly an important outflow for cerebrospinal fluid that surrounds the spinal cord. In the horse and in sheep, cerebrospinal fluid that enters the central canal has an exit at the caudal extremity via the

terminal ventricle. The terminal ventricle then communicates with the subarachnoid space of the spinal cord. A similar arrangement is likely present in other animals.

The cerebrospinal fluid is thin and watery; it is derived from blood plasma by a secretion process. Except for a few lymphocytes, the normal cellular elements of the blood are absent. In cases of injury or inflammation of the meninges, the number of cellular elements of blood can increase.

The principal function of the cerebrospinal fluid is provision of a watery cushion for the brain and spinal cord. Displacement of the brain is therefore minimized when rapid directional changes occur in the head. The "lymphatic" function (see previous section) serves the brain and spinal cord for the return of protein that leaks from the capillaries. When blood volume in the brain increases, the volume of cerebrospinal fluid decreases, thereby keeping the volume of cranial contents constant. Determining the pressure of the cerebrospinal fluid can be helpful (e.g., in the neurologic examination of an animal), and is usually about 10 mm Hg.

CENTRAL NERVOUS SYSTEM METABOLISM

The central nervous system receives its energy principally from carbohydrates, of which glucose is an important source. Unlike many tissues of the body, which require insulin for facilitated diffusion of glucose across cell membranes, the CNS receives glucose by simple diffusion, and insulin is not required. This is advantageous for the animal when insulin is lacking or in short supply, because it enables CNS function to continue when other systems fail.

The relatively high rate of metabolism of the CNS compared with that of other tissues can be shown by noting its oxygen consumption. Although the CNS constitutes only 2% of body mass, it consumes approximately 20% of the total oxygen supplied to the body. Also, the metabolic rate of gray matter is three to four times higher than that of white matter.

Blood-Brain Barrier

Many substances in the blood do not readily enter the cells of the CNS, a limitation referred to as the blood-brain barrier. The capillaries of the CNS have tight junctions between their endothelial cells rather than slit pores, which limit the diffusion of substances from capillaries. Lipid-soluble substances, however, such as oxygen and carbon dioxide, readily diffuse. Transport for most substances is provided for by CNS connective tissue cells, known as astrocytes, that are interposed between the capillaries and CNS cells. Astrocytes are selective as to the materials they transport—hence, the blood-brain barrier. Because it is an important center for monitoring blood con-

stituents, there is no blood-brain barrier in the hypothalamus.

A barrier also exists between the cells of the choroid plexus (tufts of capillaries that project into brain ventricles) and the cerebrospinal fluid that is provided for by the choroid plexus cells. A barrier probably exists between the cerebrospinal fluid and pia mater for certain substances, but most substances usually diffuse readily between the CSF and the brain. Drugs in the blood might have no effect on the brain, but when placed directly into the CSF, they can have a profound effect.

Blood Requirement

The CNS must have a continuous supply of blood for normal functioning. Other tissues can be deprived of a blood supply for extended periods and recover to normal function when blood supply resumes. Five to 10 minutes of little or no blood to the brain injures higher brain cells (in the cerebrum) so that no recovery occurs. Respiratory and cardiovascular centers (in the medulla) are more resistant to anoxia (no oxygen), and revival has occurred after 10 minutes without blood. The tolerance of an adult brain to anoxia is much lower than the tolerance of a newborn brain.

STUDY AIDS—NERVOUS SYSTEM

Structure and Function

1. What is a nerve fiber?
2. What is a nerve?
3. What is a tract?
4. What is a nucleus?
5. What is a ganglion?
6. Sketch a neuron.
7. What are the components of a synapse?
8. What are characteristics of a synapse?
9. How do myelin sheaths of the CNS and PNS differ?
10. What is the difference between neurilemma and axolemma?

11. At what location does the axolemma have contact with extracellular fluid in myelinated nerve fibers?
12. What are the three gross subdivisions of the brain?
13. What are the subdivisions of the brain stem?
14. Is the hypothalamus a subdivision of the cerebrum, cerebellum, or brain stem?
15. List major characteristics of the cerebral hemispheres, cerebellum, and brain stem.
16. What are the five groups of vertebrae in order from their cranial location to their caudal location?
17. What is the vertebral formula for the dog?
18. How are the spinal nerves numbered in relation to the vertebrae?
19. What is the cauda equina?
20. Which root of a spinal nerve does an afferent fiber traverse? An efferent fiber?
21. What are the relative locations of nerve cell bodies and tracts within the spinal cord?
22. What is a spinal cord segment?
23. Are motor neurons located dorsally or ventrally in the gray matter of the spinal cord?
24. What is the general distribution of a spinal nerve?
25. What is a nerve plexus?
26. How many pairs of cranial nerves are there?
27. What is the general distribution of the cranial nerves?
28. Which one of the cranial nerves supplies parasympathetic fibers to visceral structures in the thorax and abdomen?
29. Are all spinal nerves mixed nerves?
30. Are all cranial nerves mixed nerves?
31. What tissues are innervated by autonomic nerves?
32. Which division of the autonomics is associated with "fight, fright, and flight"?
33. Where are the cells of origin for the sympathetic and parasympathetic neurons?
34. How do autonomic neurons get their structures innervated?
35. Study Table 1.2.

The Nerve Impulse and Its Transmission

1. What is the function of the Na^+-K^+ pump in the axolemma?
2. What is the approximate value of the resting membrane potential?
3. What is the polarity of a resting neuron membrane?
4. What accomplishes depolarization?
5. What accomplishes repolarization?
6. What is threshold?
7. What is an action potential?
8. What is a refractory period?
9. What is meant by a nerve fiber being "fired"?
10. What is the "all-or-none" principle for nerve fibers?
11. Describe the sequence of events associated with neurotransmission in mammals.
12. How does neurotransmission differ in myelinated fibers?
13. What are two functions of saltatory conduction?
14. What kind of nerve fiber has the fastest impulse transmission?
15. What is the purpose of a neurotransmitter?
16. What neurotransmitters are associated with the autonomic nervous system and where are they located?
17. What is the nature of the central neurotransmitters?
18. Describe the "final common pathway" concept.
19. Differentiate between the different types of neuron circuits.
20. What is the minimum number of neurons required for the transmission of a nerve impulse from the periphery by way of a spinal nerve to the cerebral cortex?

Reflexes

1. What are the names of the neurons that may be involved with a reflex?
2. Describe the stretch reflex.
3. What is the purpose of the stretch reflex?

4. Why is the stretch reflex considered a postural reflex?
5. Differentiate between somatic and visceral reflexes.
6. How are visceral reflexes transmitted?
7. List functions of reflex centers located in the 1) medulla oblongata, 2) cerebellum, 3) hypothalamus, and 4) midbrain.
8. What is meant by muscle tone?
9. What is the basic element of muscle tone?
10. Describe standing, attitudinal, and righting reflexes.

The Meninges and Cerebrospinal Fluid

1. Visualize the relative location of the meningeal layers to each other, to the skull and brain, and to the vertebral canal and spinal cord.
2. What are the arachnoid villi extensions of and what do they extend into?
3. What is an epidural injection?
4. Is cerebrospinal fluid circulated within the epidural space?
5. Which meningeal layer forms the lining of the perivascular spaces and what is its extent?
6. What fluid fills the perivascular space?
7. Visualize the location of the brain ventricles.
8. What structures within the ventricles produce cerebrospinal fluid?
9. Describe the circulation of the cerebrospinal fluid?
10. What could cause the cerebrospinal fluid pressure to rise?
11. What are functions of cerebrospinal fluid?
12. Are blood cells present in cerebrospinal fluid?

Central Nervous System Metabolism

1. What is the principal energy source for the CNS? How does it get into brain cells?
2. What percent of the body's oxygen requirement is used by the CNS?

3. What is meant by the blood-brain barrier?
4. What cells transport substances between the blood and brain tissue?
5. Is there a CSF-brain barrier?
6. What are some maximum limits of oxygen deprivation to the CNS before injury occurs?

SELF-EVALUATION— NERVOUS SYSTEM

1. The myelin sheaths of nerve fibers in the central nervous system are cytoplasmic extensions of:
   a. Schwann cells
   b. oligodendrocytes
2. Nerve fiber is another name for:
   a. nerve
   b. neuron
   c. axon
   d. dendrite
3. Which one of the following statements about the neuronal synapse is FALSE?
   a. one-way conduction (axon to dendrite or soma)
   b. transmission by chemical means
   c. physical contact of one neuron with the next
   d. fatigue more readily than the neuron
4. The autonomic divisions having cell origins in the cranial and sacral (craniosacral) regions of the spinal cord and the thoracic and lumbar (thoracolumbar) regions are the _____ and _____, respectively.
   a. sympathetic; parasympathetic
   b. parasympathetic; sympathetic
5. A stimulus increases the permeability of the neuron for the sodium ion.
   a. true
   b. false
6. If a stimulus lowers the resting membrane potential of −80 mV to −70 mV and the threshold for an action potential is −65 mV, the nerve fiber will "fire".
   a. true
   b. false

7. Which one of the following contains the respective neurotransmitters for postganglionic sympathetic and parasympathetic neurons?
   a. acetylcholine, norepinephrine
   b. acetylcholine, acetylcholine
   c. norepinephrine, acetylcholine
   d. norepinephrine, norepinephrine

8. Afferent nerve fibers enter the spinal cord via the _____ root and efferent nerve fibers leave via the _____ root.
   a. dorsal; ventral
   b. ventral; dorsal
   c. dorsal; dorsal
   d. ventral; ventral

9. Muscle tone:
   a. is a state of complete muscle relaxation
   b. is a state of muscle tension (contraction) that enables an animal to assume and remain in an erect position
   c. refers to the sound made by contracting muscle
   d. is an autonomic nervous system function

10. Parasympathetic stimulation increases intestinal muscle and secretory activity.
    a. true
    b. false

11. Which one of the following best describes the function of the hypothalamus?
    a. important in equilibrium
    b. large pools of neurons for performing complex semivoluntary movement (walking and running)
    c. central mechanism for most postural reflexes (hopping, righting, placing)
    d. senses need for anterior pituitary hormones, forms posterior pituitary hormones, integration of autonomic nervous system functions

12. Which one of the following is an appropriate function for the cerebellum?
    a. modulate (adjust; tone down) motor activity
    b. provides for consciousness

c. relay center to cerebral cortex
   d. site of production of several hormones

13. Which one of the following statements about myelin sheaths is TRUE?
    a. the myelin sheath is formed by the cell body of the neuron of which it is a part
    b. there is no chance for extracellular fluid to be in contact with the nerve fiber throughout its length when a nerve fiber is myelinated
    c. unmyelinated fibers may be nearly surrounded by myelin from adjacent myelinated fibers but can maintain a direct association with extracellular fluid throughout their length
    d. nodes of Ranvier are the lymphatic structures of the nervous system

14. Parasympathetic stimulation to the heart would decrease its activity.
    a. true
    b. false

15. The phenomenon of saltatory conduction is associated with:
    a. the flow of cerebrospinal fluid
    b. unmyelinated nerve fibers
    c. myelinated nerve fibers
    d. nerve impulse transmission at a synapse

16. When a resting membrane potential of –85 mV is being measured in a nerve fiber at a particular point and the threshold for firing is –70 mV, which one of the following is FALSE?
    a. there is a high concentration of Na^+ on the outside and a low concentration of Na^+ on the inside
    b. there is a relative impermeability of the fiber for diffusion of Na^+
    c. there is no current flow at that point
    d. a stimulus that would decrease the resting membrane potential (from –85 to –80) would cause the nerve to "fire"

17. Repolarization of a nerve fiber:
    a. is accomplished by Na$^+$ being actively transported from the inside to the outside
    b. is accomplished by diffusion of K$^+$ from the inside of the fiber to the outside
18. Which one of the following statements about impulse transmission velocity is FALSE?
    a. fastest impulse transmission in the body would be a small diameter, nonmyelinated fiber
    b. when faster impulse transmission is required, less space is required for the fiber if it is myelinated rather than if its diameter is increased
19. Cerebrospinal fluid pressure:
    a. would increase if there was resistance to venous blood flow from the head
    b. would decrease if there was resistance to venous blood flow from the head
    c. is independent of any change in venous blood pressure
20. Acetylcholine is an excitatory neurotransmitter and accordingly increases the permeability of the nerve fiber membrane for Na$^+$.
    a. true
    b. false
21. Which division of the autonomic nervous system is referred to as the cholinergic system?
    a. sympathetic
    b. parasympathetic
22. A muscle spindle is best described as:
    a. a reflex center located in the spinal cord for the purpose of muscle control
    b. the point on a bone over which a muscle passes
    c. a specialized receptor for maintaining muscle tone which when stretched causes contraction of the muscle in which it is located
    d. a specialized receptor found in tendons which when stimulated causes the muscle of the tendon to be relaxed

23. The ability of a cat to land on its feet when dropped from a position of its feet in a skyward direction is known as:
    a. an attitudinal reflex
    b. hopscotch
    c. a righting reflex
    d. a placing reflex
24. Which one of the following statements about pain is FALSE?
    a. pain is a protective mechanism
    b. the cornea of the eye is an insensitive structure
    c. diversion of attention reduces pain perception
    d. referred pain is that which is perceived as coming from an exterior part of the body but is actually coming from the viscera
25. Cerebrospinal fluid is produced:
    a. by the choroid plexus in cavities (ventricles) within the brain
    b. by the ciliary processes in the posterior chamber of the eye
    c. as a neurosecretion by neurons in the hypothalamus
    d. by the nerve cell bodies in the cerebrum and spinal cord
26. Lifting the head of a horse in a standing position permits greater activity of the hind legs (attitudinal reflex).
    a. true
    b. false
27. Which one of the following brain structures is a subdivision of the brain stem, contains the pituitary gland, and assumes a major role in the integration of functions carried out by the autonomic nervous system?
    a. basal ganglia
    b. cerebral cortex
    c. hypothalamus
    d. thalamus

28. A myelin sheath on a peripheral nerve fiber:
    a. is uninterrupted throughout its length
    b. is produced by the neuron of which it is a part
    c. prevents contact of the nerve fiber with extracellular fluid throughout its length
    d. increases the velocity of impulse conduction

29. The vagus nerve (X cranial nerve) supplies autonomic fibers to visceral structures in the thorax and abdomen. Which division of the autonomics has fibers in this nerve?
    a. sympathetic
    b. parasympathetic

30. Sympathetic stimulation to the bronchi (air passages) of the lungs would result in:
    a. a decrease of their diameter
    b. an increase of their diameter

31. A stimulus applied to a neuron causes depolarization of the membrane. This means that the membrane:
    a. becomes positive on the outside because of the outflow of Na^+
    b. becomes positive on the inside and negative on the outside because Na^+ flows inward
    c. will not be able to propagate a nerve impulse

32. A stimulus of sufficient strength to cause an action potential means that the magnitude of depolarization was sufficient to:
    a. demyelinate the fiber
    b. incite a riot
    c. reach threshold
    d. raise or lower the threshold

33. The period of time when a nerve fiber cannot be caused to "fire" is known as:
    a. repolarization
    b. saltatory conduction
    c. leakage
    d. the refractory period

34. How many neurons are associated with the transmission of an autonomic impulse from its cell of origin (in brain or spinal cord) to its organ of influence?
    a. one
    b. two
    c. three
    d. too numerous to count

35. Which division of the autonomic nervous system is known as the adrenergic nervous system (postganglionic neuron secretes norepinephrine)?
    a. sympathetic
    b. parasympathetic

36. Which reflex is the fundamental element of muscle tone?
    a. stretch
    b. attitudinal
    c. righting
    d. crossed extensor

37. Which one of the following does NOT apply to cerebrospinal fluid?
    a. provides a watery cushion for the brain and spinal cord
    b. assists in maintaining volume of cranial contents constant
    c. contains numerous blood cells
    d. secreted by choroid plexus and returned to blood via arachnoid villi

38. The blood-brain barrier:
    a. exists for all substances in the blood
    b. applies to all areas of the brain
    c. excludes transport of some substances from blood to brain and permits transport of others

39. Brain injury occurs when it is deprived of blood for (select the most appropriate time interval):
    a. seconds
    b. minutes
    c. hours
    d. days

SUGGESTED READINGS

Bunge RP. Structure and function of neuroglia: Some recent observations. In: Schmitt FO, ed. The neurosciences: second study program. New York: Rockefeller University Press, 1970:782–797.

deLahunta A. Veterinary neuroanatomy and clinical neurology. 2nd ed. Philadelphia: WB Saunders, 1983.

Eckert R, Randall D, Augustine G. Animal physiology: mechanisms and adaptations. 3rd ed. New York: WH Freeman, 1988.

Fletcher TF. Spinal cord and meninges. In: Evans HE, ed. Miller's anatomy of the dog. 3rd ed. Philadelphia: WB Saunders, 1993:800—828.

Frandson RD, Spurgeon TL. Anatomy and physiology of farm animals. 5th ed. Philadelphia, Lea & Febiger, 1992.

Iggo A, Klemm WR. Nerves, junctions, and reflexes. In: Swenson MJ, Reece WO, eds. Dukes' physiology of domestic animals. 11th ed. Ithaca: Cornell University Press, 1993:771–786.

Kitchell RL. Introduction to the nervous system. In: Evans HE, ed. Miller's anatomy of the dog. 3rd ed. Philadelphia: WB Saunders, 1993:758–775.

Klemm WR. Design and basic functions of the nervous system. In: Swenson MJ, Reece WO, eds. Dukes' physiology of domestic animals. 11th ed. Ithaca: Cornell University Press, 1993:751–770.

Langley LL. Physiology of man. 4th ed. New York: Van Nostrand Reinhold, 1971.

Langley LL, Telford IR, Christensen JB. Dynamic anatomy and physiology. 3rd ed. New York: McGraw-Hill, 1969.

McGrath JT. Neurologic examination of the dog. 2nd ed. Philadelphia: Lea & Febiger, 1960.

Meyer H. The brain. In: Evans HE, Christensen GC, eds. Miller's anatomy of the dog. 2nd ed. Philadelphia: WB Saunders, 1979:842–902.

Oliver JE, Hoerlein BF, Mayhew JG, eds. Veterinary neurology. Philadelphia: WB Saunders, 1987.

Popesco P. Atlas of topographical anatomy of the domestic animals, vols. 1 and 2. 4th ed. Philadelphia: WB Saunders, 1985.

Ranson SW, Clark SL. The anatomy of the nervous system. 10th ed. Philadelphia: WB Saunders, 1959.

Robertshaw D. Visceromotor (autonomic) control. In: Swenson MJ, Reece WO, eds. Dukes' physiology of domestic animals. 11th ed. Ithaca: Cornell University Press, 1993:874–885.

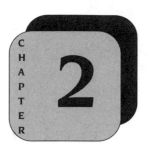

The Sensory Organs

Sensations result from stimuli that initiate afferent impulses, which eventually reach a conscious level in the cerebral cortex. Sensations include pain, cold, heat, touch, pressure, and a group known as the special senses—sight, hearing, taste, smell, and orientation in space. All sensations involve receptor organs; the simplest are bare nerve endings and the most complex are those associated with the special senses. Several receptor organs are shown in Figure 2.1.

SENSORY RECEPTORS AND THEIR FUNCTIONS

Classification of Sensory Receptors

The three principal groups of sensory receptors are the exteroceptors, interoceptors, and proprioceptors. The exteroceptors detect stimuli near the outer surface of the body and include those from the skin that respond to cold, warmth, touch, and pressure. The special receptor organs for hearing and vision are also classified as exteroceptors. The interoceptors detect stimuli from inside the body and include receptors for taste, smell, and those within the viscera that respond to pH, distention and spasm (as in the bowel), and flow (as in the urethra). The proprioceptors are inside the body, as are the interoceptors, but they signal conditions deep within the body to the central nervous system. Proprioceptors are located in skeletal muscles, tendons, ligaments, and joint capsules. Examples of proprioceptors are muscle spindles, Golgi tendon organs, and joint receptors. Muscle spindles and Golgi tendon organs are sensitive to stretching and reflexively prevent undue stretch of muscles, tendons, and ligaments. Muscle spindles also provide for muscle tone so that purposeful contraction is more effective and helps to prevent collapse of standing animals as a result of the force of gravity. Joint receptors are sensitive to the position or angle of joints and provide for a sense of body position.

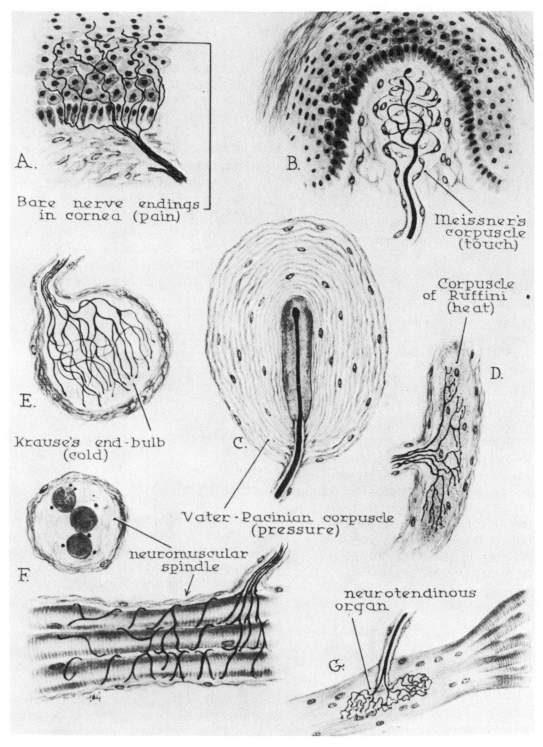

Figure labels within the illustration:

A. Bare nerve endings in cornea (pain)

B. Meissner's corpuscle (touch)

Corpuscle of Ruffini (heat) •

D.

E. Krause's end-bulb (cold)

C. Vater-Pacinian corpuscle (pressure)

F. neuromuscular spindle

G. neurotendinous organ

Figure 2.1. Receptors associated with sensations. Receptors that signal changes occurring near the surface of the body are known as exteroceptors (*A–E*). Receptors that are sensitive to the degree to which muscles are contracted (*F*) and tendons are tensed (*G*) are known as proprioceptors. From Ham AW. Histology. 7th ed. Philadelphia: JB Lippincott, 1974.

Because of the need for rapid transmission of proprioceptive impulses, the proprioceptive fibers have the heaviest myelination of all peripheral nerve fibers.

Responses

A sensory receptor is the peripheral component of an afferent axon and the centrally located nerve cell body of that axon.

Sensory receptors convert different types of energy into action potentials; these include sound, light, chemical, thermal, and mechanical energy. Generally, the receptors are specific in that they respond more readily to one form of energy than another. For example, a Krause end-bulb receptor (sensitive to cold) would not generate an action potential if pressure were applied; in such a case, pacinian corpuscles would respond.

Graded Responses

Sensory receptors are subject to graded responses, depending on the intensity of the stimulus. The receptor can be regarded as a generator in which the amount of voltage produced is determined by the stimulus. If the voltage generation reaches threshold for the receptor, a nerve impulse (afferent) is created. As the intensity (amplitude) of the stimulus increases, the frequency of firing increases.

Adaptation

Receptors might not continue to fire at a rate consistent with the intensity of the stimulus, but they are subject to adaptation. The response to a prolonged stimulus might at first show a burst of action potentials at a high frequency, followed by a decrease in rate that quickly returns to zero. Receptors vary as to the degree of their adaptation. The previous response, in which the rate of discharge returns to zero, is characteristic of pacinian corpuscles (sensitive to pressure). This is an example of a phasic receptor organ—that is, one that quickly accommodates to prolonged stimulation. A rapidly adapting receptor is best suited for signaling sudden changes in the environment or vibratory fluctuations. The muscle spindle, which responds to stretch, is an example of a tonic receptor organ with regard to its adaptation. The application of a prolonged stimulus to the muscle spindle elicits a brief volley of action potentials at a high frequency, followed by an action potential rate that slows to a lower level and that is maintained throughout the duration of stimulus. This is known as a tonic receptor organ in the same sense that muscle tone (the result of muscle spindle stimulation) represents a continuous state of low level muscle tension.

PAIN

Pain Reception

Pain is a protective mechanism. Its sensation is aroused by damaging or noxious stimuli from almost all parts of the body, with the exception of the central nervous system (unless there is damage to the pain pathways). The specific receptors for pain are called nociceptors. Pain sensation does not arise from overstimulation of receptors that subserve a different sensation. The receptors are bare nerve endings of sensory neurons (pain neurons) that respond to all intense stimuli. The nerve endings are essentially chemoreceptors, and the pain stimulus (e.g., thermal, chemical, mechanical) produces cell injury, which produces a chemical reaction and causes the nerve to fire. Pain fibers are either myelinated or unmyelinated. The myelinated fibers have a short lag time between stimulus and reaction and the pain has a so-called "bright" quality, whereas unmyelinated fibers have a longer lag time and the pain is more diffuse, with an aching, throbbing quality. Pain fibers, as are the fibers for other sen-

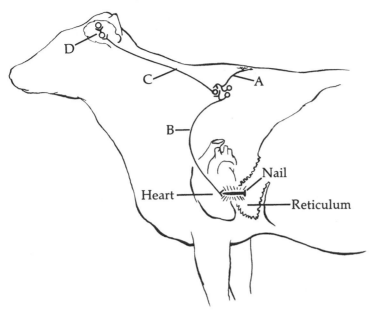

Figure 2.2. The sensory pain pathway. A cutaneous pain afferent fiber (*A*) and a visceral pain afferent fiber (*B*) converge on a common neuron (*C*). Neuron *D* conveys the pain impulse from the thalamus to the cerebral cortex.

sory modalities, are grouped in a specific tract of the spinal cord.

The reaction threshold for pain is highly variable among individuals. What is painful to one person might not be so to another. Furthermore, the diversion of attention from a pained part or painful situation reduces pain perception. This can be demonstrated when a twitch (a handle with a rope loop at one end) is applied to the upper lip of a horse and tightened. The attention to discomfort of the twitch detracts from pain or manipulation of other body parts.

Visceral Pain

Pain does arise from the viscera (the organs within the abdominal, thoracic, and pelvic cavities); the most sensitive parts are the peritoneal and pleural linings of the abdominal and thoracic cavities, respectively. Peritonitis and pleuritis (inflammation of the peritoneum and pleura) evoke severe pain. Some of the thoracic viscera (the heart) might be a source of pain, whereas other viscera (the lungs) might not. Pain from hollow viscera (the intestines) within the abdomen is evoked by severe distention or powerful contractions (spasms). Normal distentions or contractions can be innocuous, but an inflammation can cause these to become painful.

Referred Pain

Referred pain is pain that is felt on the surface of the body. It usually has its source within the thoracic or abdominal viscera. It is caused by a convergence of cutaneous and visceral pain afferent fibers on the same neuron at some point in the sensory pathway (Fig. 2.2). The pain can be identified consciously as cutaneous (referring to the skin) because a previous cutaneous pain was actually seen and perceived as being cutaneous. When the pain source is of visceral origin, however, it is mistakenly perceived as coming from the site of the relevant cutaneous fibers (referred) because their common neuron has the same cerebral projection. Traumatic pericarditis (inflammation of the pericardium caused by perforation from the reticulum) in cattle is a form of referred pain. Pressure applied to the withers causes a painful response in cattle with traumatic pericarditis, whereas a minimal response would be noted in normal cattle. The cutaneous stimulation is additive to that coming from the inflamed heart sac because of the convergence of the nerve fibers.

THE SPECIAL SENSES

Taste

The sense of taste is called gustation. The function of taste in animals appears to be one of discrimination; they appear to be able to discriminate between those substances that are healthful or harmful. Also, foods might be sought that contain nutrients that are lacking in the diet.

Taste Reception

The receptor organ for the sense of taste is the taste bud. Most of the taste buds are located on the tongue in association with the various papillae (Fig. 2.3A), and some are found on the palate, pharynx, and larynx. A collection of taste buds and their locations relative to a circumvallate papilla are shown in Figure 2.3B. A taste bud contains gustatory cells and supporting cells (Fig. 2.3C). The gustatory cells are the receptors for taste sensations. A tiny hair arises from each and extends into the pit of the taste bud. The pit communicates with the oral cavity by way of a pore (Fig. 2.3C). Any substance to be tasted must get into solution and enter the pore of a taste bud. The hair of the gustatory cell that extends into the pit is affected in some way, so that the gustatory cell is stimulated. The generated impulse is transmitted to the brain by branches of cranial nerves VII and IX (anterior two-thirds and posterior third of the tongue, respectively). The afferent ends of these cranial nerve branches originate at the deep ends of taste buds and are in intimate contact with the gustatory cells.

The glands of von Ebner (Fig. 2.3B) are embedded deep within the underlying muscle tissue. Their watery secretion is conveyed to the moatlike furrow that surrounds the papillae by excretory ducts, and the substances to be tasted are dissolved in it.

Taste Sensations

Taste sensations in humans are classified according to verbal reports as being salty, sweet, bitter, or sour. Each taste sensation probably results from some combination of these basic tastes. Much of the current opinion about taste sensations that can be perceived by animals is based on casual observations and folklore.

A common method used to evaluate the sense of taste in animals is the preference test. Accordingly, responses are divided into pleasant, unpleasant, and indifferent. There is considerable individual variation within species. A substance considered to be pleasant by one dog might be regarded as unpleasant or indifferent by others. Similarly, variability of taste exists among pigs in the same litter for the same substances.

Temperature and Taste

In humans, the temperature of a beverage or food markedly affects its taste. The effect of water temperature and its acceptance has been studied in domestic fowl. Acceptability of water decreases as its temperature increases above the ambient temperature. Water for domestic fowl that is placed in sunlight soon becomes warmer than the ambient temperature and is rejected. Chickens will suffer from acute thirst rather than drink water that is 5°C above their body temperature (41°C), but chickens readily accept water down to the level of freezing. Recognition of these preferences is important for maximum productivity and health in poultry production.

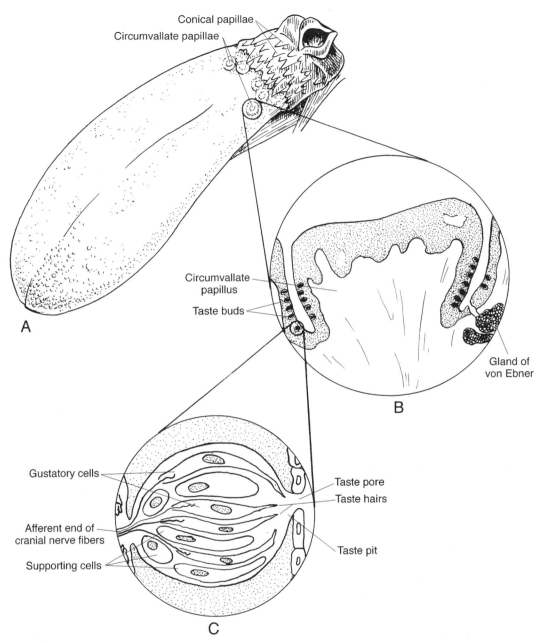

Conical papillae
Circumvallate papillae

Circumvallate
papillus

Taste buds

Gland of
von Ebner

A

B

Gustatory cells

Afferent end of
cranial nerve fibers

Supporting cells

Taste pore
Taste hairs

Taste pit

C

Figure 2.3. Taste buds associated with papillae on the dog tongue. **A**. Fungiform and filiform papillae are represented by the finer dots. Circumvallate and conical papillae are located at the base. **B**. A circumvallate papillus with taste buds lining its moatlike furrow. Glands of von Ebner provide a watery secretion for dissolving substances to be tasted. **C**. A taste bud with its gustatory (taste) cells and supporting cells.

Depraved Appetite

A depraved appetite is recognized in animals when they are seen eating dirt, wood, and other materials not usually considered to be foodstuffs (this is different from similar habits that can develop in some animals). The depraved condition is termed "pica." Its exact cause is difficult to determine, but it could be related to certain dietary deficiencies.

Smell

As development progressed from the simplest animal forms, nerve cell bodies migrated centrally so that only the nerve fibers remained in a peripheral position. Because nerve cell bodies are not regenerated, this central location provided for greater protection from destruction. If the neuron extensions are injured, regeneration can occur to some extent. Central migration did not occur for the nerve cell bodies of cranial nerve I (olfactory), however, and they are found in the mucous membrane of the nasal cavity. They are located in what is known as the olfactory region. The size of the olfactory region is directly related to the degree of development of the sense of smell, and its size varies among species. The individual olfactory receptor of the dog is probably no more sensitive than that of the human, but their larger olfactory region allows dogs to detect odorous substances at concentrations 1:1000 of that detectable by humans.

The sensation of smell is known as olfaction. Animals with a greatly developed sense of smell (most domestic animals) are macrosmatic. A relatively lesser developed sense of smell is known as microsmatic; humans, monkeys, and some aquatic mammals belong to this group. Animals with no sense of smell (e.g., many aquatic mammals) are anosmatic. Macrosmatic animals can become microsmatic or anosmatic and microsmatics can become anosmatic because of disease loss of cells or temporary impair-ment. The peripheral location of the olfactory nerve cell bodies renders them more susceptible to destruction from inflammatory disease. Sensitivity to smell probably decreases with time.

Olfactory Region Structure

A microscopic view of a section taken from the olfactory region is shown in Figure 2.4. Each olfactory receptor cell has a cell body and a nerve fiber extending from each of its ends; one a dendrite and the other an axon (Fig. 2.4). The dendritic process of the olfactory cell extends to the outside of the olfactory region membrane in crevices between the sustentacular cells. The sustentacular cells appear to provide major support to the dendritic processes and allow for the olfactory cell bodies to be shielded from the nasal cavity. At this location there might be several hairlike structures (olfactory cilia) extending into the nasal cavity from the olfactory vesicles (expanded part of a dendrite). Usually they are covered with a thin secretion from the glands of Bowman (subepithelial glands). The ducts of these glands lead through the epithelium to the surface. Their secretion constantly freshens the thin layer of fluid that continuously bathes the olfactory hairs on the surface of the olfactory region. Sniffing allows for the back-and-forth movement of air and provides a greater chance for the substance to be smelled to go into solution. This becomes the stimulus for the impulse to be transmitted to the brain. The axons of the olfactory cells join with others and proceed with them as fibers and branches of the olfactory nerves. Basal cells divide and differentiate into either sustentacular cells or olfactory cells (replacement of a nerve cell). This is a safeguard against loss of smell that might otherwise occur as a result of nasal mucosal disease.

Odor Perception

Considering the great number of smell possibilities, it is unlikely that a specific type

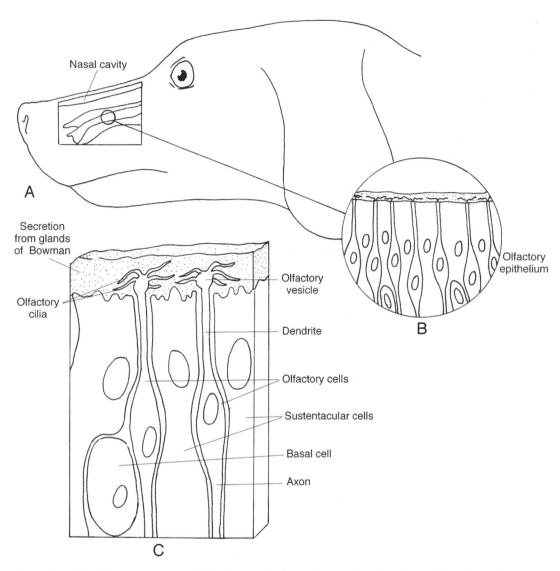

Figure 2.4. The olfactory region of the dog and the cells associated with smell. A. Nasal cavity. B. Olfactory epithelium from nasal cavity mucous membrane. C. Olfactory cells, basal cells, and sustentacular (supporting) cells are associated with olfactory epithelium. Subepithelial glands of Bowman (not shown) provide secretion covering olfactory cilia.

of olfactory cell exists for each smell. It is more probable that basic smells combine to provide the sensation for a particular odor.

Only one odor can be perceived at any one time. Some room deodorants are effective because they can stimulate olfactory cells more than the offensive odor. The offender is not eliminated, it is only "masked." The olfactory cells become adapted to odors so that they do not persist for a particular individual. This is why the smell of fresh baked bread is so apparent when someone enters a bakery, whereas the baker might not even smell it any more.

Pheromones

Animals use odors to communicate with each other. Black-tailed deer and Rocky

Mountain mule deer use the tarsal glands on the insides of their hind legs as transmitters of odors to identify species as friendly or alien to their own kind. The scent is deposited on the skin and hair by the tarsal glands, and communication is established by sniffing other members of their group approximately once each hour. A chemical secreted by one animal that influences the behavior of other animals is known as a pheromone. The first chemical analysis of a mammalian pheromone was accomplished using the deer tarsal gland substance. Some animals have scent glands in the spaces between their hoof pads. Rabbits have a scent gland on their chest and around their anal opening. Cats have glands on their forehead and "mark" people or objects by rubbing their head on them. Pheromones provide for a chemical "language" among animals for certain purposes, such as marking trails or boundaries, recognizing individuals from the same herd or nest, marking the location of food sources, and emitting alarms.

Hearing and Equilibrium

The Ear

EXTERNAL EAR The external ear (Fig. 2.5) consists of the outer visible part (the pinna) and a tube (external acoustic meatus) that extends from the pinna into the substance of the skull to the middle ear (tympanic cavity). The pinna in most animals consists of a funnel-shaped cartilage that is lined on the outside with skin that has a generous amount of hair, and is lined on the inside with relatively hairless skin. Varying degrees of muscle attachment lend mobility to the pinna, which is helpful in localizing and picking up sounds. The funnel-shaped cartilage concentrates sound waves and directs them through the ear canal toward the tympanic membrane, which separates the middle ear from the external ear.

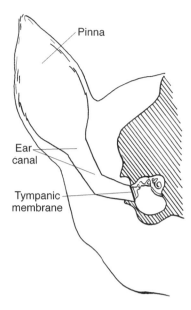

Figure 2.5. Transverse section through the dog head. The external ear (pinna and ear canal) provide for transfer of sound waves to the tympanic membrane. The ear canal in the dog has a vertical and an oblique component.

MIDDLE EAR The middle ear and inner ear are shown in Figure 2.6. The middle ear is separated from the inner ear by membranes that close the vestibular (oval) window and cochlear (round) window. The middle ear communicates with the pharynx by way of the auditory tube (often called the eustachian tube). The auditory tube allows for equalization of pressures between an otherwise closed cavity and the outside. Within the middle ear, a mechanical linkage is provided between the tympanic membrane and the membrane closing the vestibular window by three auditory ossicles (bones). From without inward they are the malleus, incus, and stapes or, more commonly, the hammer, anvil, and stirrup. Amplification of sound waves is provided by leverage of the ossicles and by the greater surface area of the tympanic membrane, which transmits sound waves to the smaller surface area of the vestibular window. Excessively loud

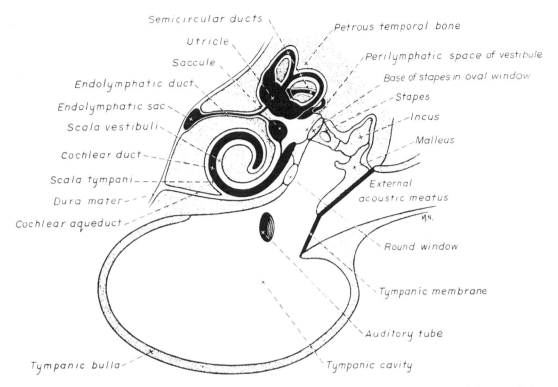

Figure 2.6. The middle ear and inner ear. From Getty R, et al. Macroscopic anatomy of the ear of the dog. Am J Vet Res 1956;17:366.

noises are damped by two skeletal muscles in the middle ear, the tensor tympani and the stapedius (Fig. 2.7). Muscle spindles within these muscles respond to muscle stretch by initiating a reflex that causes the muscles to contract. The degree of stretch is determined by the intensity (loudness) of the sound wave. Loud noises are damped because of excessive muscle stretch and subsequent reflex muscle contraction, which prevents excessive movement of the ossicles.

INNER EAR The inner ear can be divided into two parts according to function: (1) the vestibular portion, which is sensory for position and equilibrium, and (2) the cochlear portion, which is sensory for sound (Fig. 2.8). The cochlear portion receives the cochlear nerve, a branch of the vestibulocochlear nerve (cranial nerve VIII), and the vestibular portion receives the vestibular nerve branch of the same

cranial nerve (VIII). The inner ear is contained within a bony excavation known as the osseous labyrinth (Fig. 2.9). Labyrinth refers to an intricate combination of passages. Because the cochlea is coiled, it can occupy limited space. An uncoiled cochlea would project into the brain.

Vestibular Structure and Function

The vestibular portion is housed in the parts of the osseous labyrinth known as the vestibule and three semicircular canals (anterior, lateral, and posterior). Each semicircular canal leaves and returns to the vestibule (Fig. 2.9). In addition, each semicircular canal is arranged so that it is in a different geometric plane than the others (at right angles to each other). The cochlear portion is housed mostly in the cochlear portion of the osseous labyrinth that departs from the vestibule. Within the

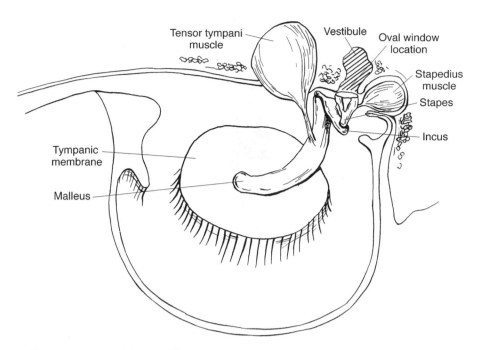

Figure 2.7. Inside view of the middle ear. The malleus is attached to the tympanic membrane, and the stapes is attached to the vestibular window. Muscle spindles in the tensor tympani and stapedius muscles initiate the stretch reflex in response to loud noises and prevent excessive movement of the ossicles.

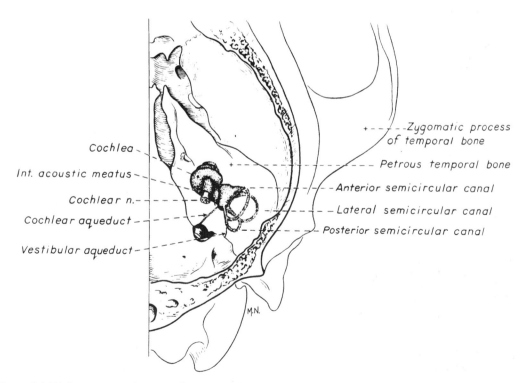

Figure 2.8. Right inner ear (viewed from above). From Getty R, et al. Macroscopic anatomy of the ear of the dog. Am J Vet Res 1956;17:369.

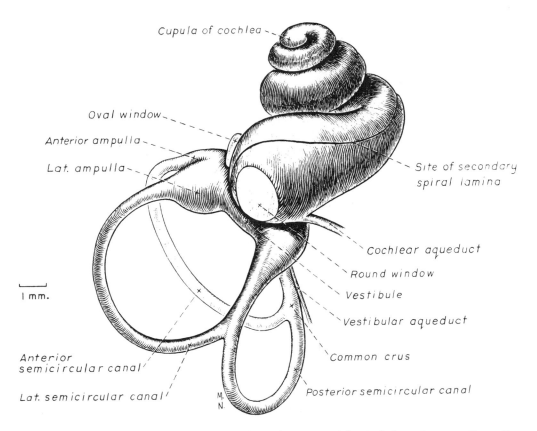

Figure 2.9. Drawing of a latex cast occupying the right osseous labyrinth, lateral aspect. From Getty R, et al. Macroscopic anatomy of the ear of the dog. Am J Vet Res 1956;17:370.

osseous labyrinth is a membranous labyrinth, which is a completely closed connective tissue structure (Fig. 2.10A). It contains a fluid known as endolymph (its composition is similar to that of intracellular fluid). Outside the membranous labyrinth and within the osseous labyrinth is another fluid known as perilymph (its composition is similar to that of cerebrospinal fluid). Within the vestibular portion, the membranous labyrinth also includes three semicircular canals and two sacs within the vestibule, known as the utricle and saccule. Both ends of each semicircular canal open into the utricle, and the utricle communicates with the saccule. The saccule has two other communications: a major one with the membranous labyrinth of the cochlea and another with the endolymphatic duct,

which leads to the endolymphatic sac just outside the dura mater in the skull (see Fig. 2.6). The endolymphatic sac can serve as an absorptive site or can have an expandable potential for endolymph, which is secreted by the epithelial lining of the membranous labyrinth. The perilymph communicates functionally with the subarachnoid space (contains cerebrospinal fluid) through the cochlear aqueduct or perilymphatic aqueduct (Fig. 2.6).

As each membranous labyrinth occupying the semicircular canals leaves the utricle, a dilated portion is noted—the ampulla. Each of the three ampullae contains sensory receptors for equilibrium known as the crista ampullaris (Fig. 2.10B). The utricle and saccule each contains a sensory receptor area known as a macula (Fig. 2.10C).

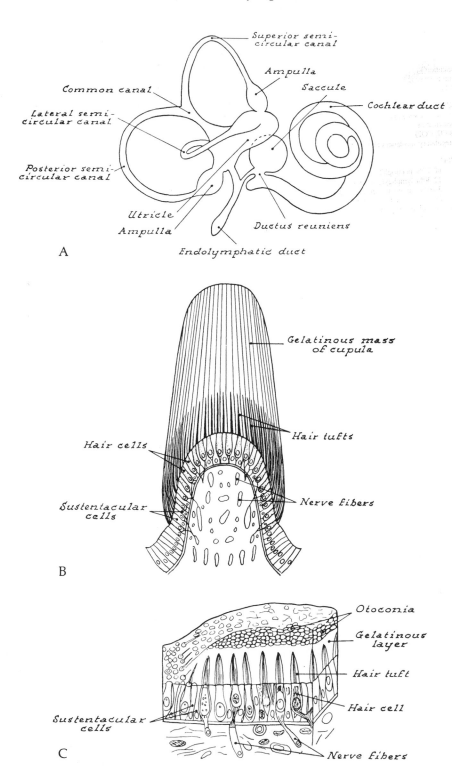

Figure 2.10. Diagrammatic sections of the membranous labyrinth (A), crista ampullaris (B), and macula (C). From Buchanan AR. Functional neuro-anatomy. 3rd ed. Philadelphia: Lea & Febiger, 1957.

The macula receptors are more or less stimulated depending on the position of the head in space (stimulated by the weight of the otoconia on the hair cells). This stimulation and appraisal is provided even when the head is not moving. The cristae, however, are stimulated during head movement so that adjustments can be made to accommodate for the changed equilibrium state. Hair cells of the cristae are stimulated when the head is moved because the hair cells are mechanically moved through the endolymph, which does not move as a result of inertia. When the head stops, the endolymph is finally moved; this stimulates the hair cells in an opposite direction and further accommodation is inhibited. The communication between the endolymphatic sac and other parts of the membranous labyrinth provides a safety valve for keeping the endolymphatic pressure constant.

Cochlear Structure and Function

The extension of the membranous labyrinth into the cochlea is known as the cochlear duct or, more commonly, the scala media. This occupies a central position within the cochlea, extending from one side to the other and dividing the cochlea into a part above the scala media (scala vestibuli) and a part below (scala tympani) (Fig. 2.11). These latter divisions do not communicate with each other except for a small opening at the apex or tip of the cochlea. Along the length of the scala media are a large number of structures, each individually called an organ of Corti (Fig. 2.11). These structures convert sound waves to nerve impulses, which in turn are transmitted to the cerebral cortex to provide the sensation of hearing. The nerve entries for these structures and for the larger basilar cells are arranged so that the thicker base is called the basilar membrane. The location of a particular organ of Corti within the scala media, from the base (near the middle ear)

to the apex of the cochlea, with its individual innervation, determines the frequency of the sound wave perceived (Fig. 2.12).

Sound waves of different frequencies have different transmission patterns from the base to the apex. A weak sound wave (of any frequency) at the base strengthens when it reaches the portion of the basilar membrane that has a natural resonant frequency equal to its own. At this point, the basilar membrane can vibrate easily; the sound wave energy is dissipated and does not travel the remaining distance along the basilar membrane. Therefore, a high-frequency sound wave travels a short distance along the basilar membrane, where it reaches its resonant point and dies out. A low-frequency wave travels a longer distance and a similar phenomenon occurs. All frequencies between high and low are represented at separate points on the basilar membrane between the base and apex of the cochlea.

An organ of Corti is composed of hair cells that have hairs projecting toward the tectorial membrane (Fig. 2.11). Displacement of the hair cell cilia against the tectorial membrane caused by oscillations of the basilar membrane (resulting from dissipation of sound waves) causes the hair cells to depolarize and create a nerve impulse, which is transmitted to the cerebral cortex.

Summary of Sound Reception

The structures traversed and actions initiated for a sound wave to be heard can be summarized as follows (Fig. 2.13):

1. The sound wave is directed into the external auditory meatus by the pinna.
2. The sound wave strikes the tympanic membrane (eardrum) and sets it in motion.
3. The motion of the eardrum is transmitted through the middle ear by the auditory ossicles to the vestibular (oval) window.

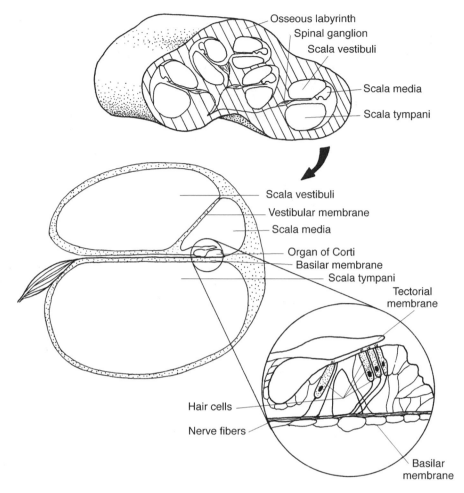

Figure 2.11. The cochlear portion of the inner ear. **A**. Cross section through the cochlea illustrating its coiled nature. **B**. Schematic representation of a section through one of the turns of the cochlea. **C**. Details of an organ of Corti.

4. The vestibular window is set in motion and displaces perilymph in the vestibule of the inner ear.

5. The perilymph (a liquid) is incompressible and thus transmits the sound wave through the scala vestibuli of the cochlea.

6. An organ of Corti at a distance from the base characteristic of the approaching sound wave is stimulated when a sound wave is transmitted to the scala media and from there to the scala tympani.

7. The movement of the liquid in the scala tympani is finally compensated for by an outward movement of the cochlear (round) window into the cavity of the middle ear.

8. The stimulation of hair cells in an organ of Corti initiates a nerve impulse that is transmitted by the cochlear branch of the vestibulocochlear nerve to the brain.

The range of frequencies through which sound can be perceived varies among species. In humans, the limit appears to be

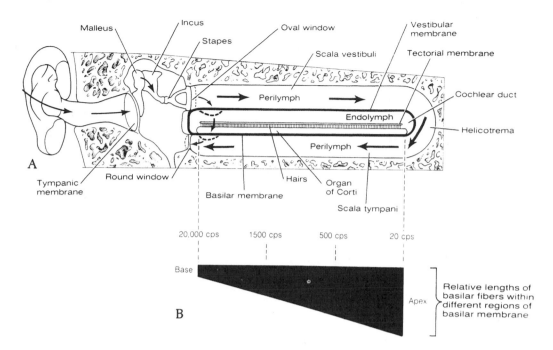

Figure 2.12. **A.** Transmission of pressure waves in the cochlea. When the movement of the stapes is slow, pressure waves are transmitted through the perilymph with no movement of the basilar membrane. With greater movement of the stapes (higher frequency), pressure waves are directed through the endolymph with movement of the basilar membrane and hence sound is perceived. **B.** Graphic representation of regions of the basilar membrane where different sound wave frequencies can cause displacement. From Spence AP, Mason EB. Human anatomy and physiology. 2nd ed. St. Paul, MN: West Publishing, 1983.

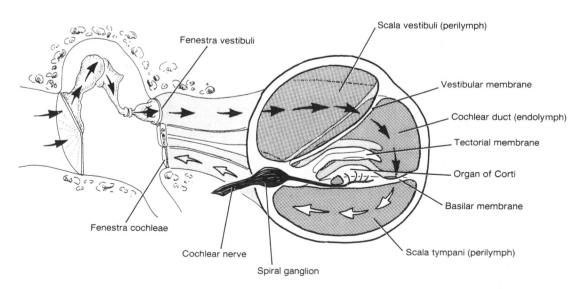

Figure 2.13. Schematic representation of the pathway of sound waves that enter the ear. From Cormack DC. Ham's histology. 9th ed. Philadelphia: JB Lippincott, 1987.

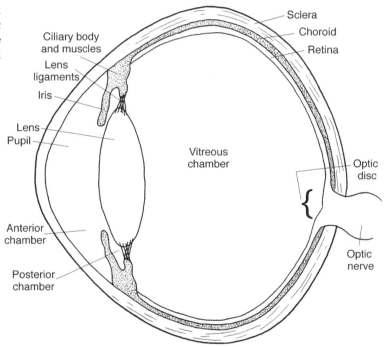

Figure 2.14. The external eye. The medial canthus is on the nasal side. The nasolacrimal duct originates in the medial canthus. The limbus is the junction of the sclera with the iris.

Figure 2.15. Diagram of an eyeball showing its basic structure. The pupil is the opening between the central projection of the iris.

between 20 and 20,000 cycles per second (cps). Dogs can perceive frequencies up to about 50,000 cps, which is the basis for dog whistles. These emit a high-frequency sound that is not perceived by humans, but the dog responds because its organ of Corti is stimulated.

Vision

The receptor organs for vision are the eyes. The receptor stimulus is light and, accordingly, many of the eye structures are adapted for transparency so that light rays can reach the receptors. The parts of the eye as seen from the front (the external eye) are shown in Figure 2.14. The basic structures of the eyeball are shown in Figure 2.15.

Structure and Functions of the Eye

The eye is composed of the eyeball (globe), the optic nerve, and the accessory structures which comprise the eyelids, conjunctivae, lacrimal apparatus, and the muscles of the eyeball.

TUNICS OF THE EYEBALL The eyeball has three distinct layers or coats, known as

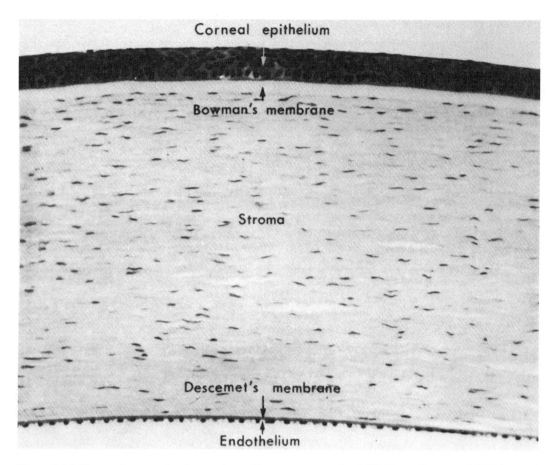

Figure 2.16. Photomicrograph of a section of human cornea (× 160). From Fawcett, DW. Bloom & Fawcett: A textbook of histology. 11th ed. Philadelphia: WB Saunders, 1986.

tunics. The external coat (fibrous tunic) is the supporting layer of the eyeball and is composed of the anterior cornea and posterior sclera. The sclera is the tough, white part of the external tunic. The middle coat is the vascular tunic and is composed of the choroid, ciliary body, and iris. The innermost tunic is the light-sensitive retina (nerve tunic). It consists of several layers; three of its layers are cells. The light-sensitive cell layer consists of the rods (black and white vision) and the cones (color vision). These receptors convert light to a nerve impulse. The retina is black because of the presence of melanin. This black pigmentation not only assists in the absorption

of light, but also prevents uncontrolled reflection to other parts of the eye.

CORNEA The cornea is the transparent, forward continuation of the sclera. It is transparent to allow for the entrance of light. In a cross-sectional view of the cornea, five layers can be identified from the outside to the inside (Fig. 2.16): (1) the corneal epithelium, (2) Bowman's membrane, (3) the stroma, (4) Descemet's membrane, and (5) the endothelium.

There is greater light transmission if the surface area ratio of cornea to sclera is increased. Nocturnal animals have relatively larger corneas than diurnal animals. About 17% of the eyeball in the dog is cornea (a diurnal animal), whereas about 30% of the eyeball in the cat is cornea (a nocturnal animal).

About 90% of the corneal thickness is a result of collagen fibers (called stroma). The collagen fibers have an orderly, laminated arrangement; this is related to the transparent nature of the cornea.

The cornea is avascular (without blood supply) so that blood vessels do not interfere with the inward transmission of light. The cornea is supplied abundantly with nonmyelinated nerve fibers that enter from the limbus and penetrate the outer epithelial layer (Fig. 2.1A). The cornea is one of the most sensitive tissues of the body.

Transparency of the cornea depends further on the degree of its hydration; the normal transparent cornea contains less water than it is able to imbibe. Increased uptake of water with a consequent reduction in transparency can occur as a result of damage to the corneal epithelium or endothelium or a reduction of oxygen. If this occurs, a rearrangement of the collagen fibers results, causing the cornea to become cloudy or white. Other causes of corneal cloudiness or whiteness are thinning from increased intraocular tension, disruption by trauma, or replacement by scar tissue.

THE LENS AND ACCOMMODATION   The lens is positioned between the cornea and retina. It is attached by suspensory ligaments (the zonule) to the ciliary body, which is a thickened forward ridge of the choroid that circumscribes the eyeball. The ciliary body contains three sets of smooth muscle fibers (ciliary muscles), with each set oriented in a different direction. Muscle contractions cause a forward and inward movement of the ciliary body and this decreases the tension on the suspensory ligaments (Fig. 2.17). The reduced tension on the ligaments allows the lens to assume its more normal configuration (because of its elastic lens capsule), that of being more convex (more spherical). A convex lens converges light rays, resulting in a shorter focal distance (a requirement for a short-

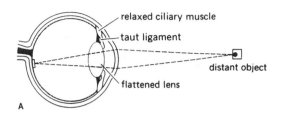

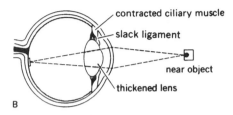

Figure 2.17. Mechanism of accommodation by the lens of the eye. **A.** Relaxation of the ciliary muscles tightens the lens ligaments and causes the lens to become less convex. **B.** Contraction of the ciliary muscles relaxes the lens ligaments and causes the lens to become more convex. From Vander AJ, Sherman JH, Luciano DS. Human physiology: The mechanisms of body function. 4th ed. New York: McGraw-Hill, 1985.

ened eyeball as in hyperopia), thereby changing the point at which the image is formed (Fig. 2.18). When this occurs in response to adjustments needed for near and far objects, it is known as accommodation. Vision is always sharper if the image is formed exactly on the retina.

Accommodation among domestic animals appears limited. This is thought to be true because of the sparsity of ciliary muscles (except in the cat). Lacking adjustments for refraction (ability to bend light rays), some species have substituted an auxiliary feature for accommodation. The shape of the eyeball in the horse is a good example of this. It has been proposed that its shape and accompanying retinal conformation are such that far objects are focused directly behind the lens, the focal distance being just right, and near objects (those on the ground at close range) are focused at a point above the lens (Fig. 2.19). The longer focal distance associated with near objects is not accommodated to the retina by con-

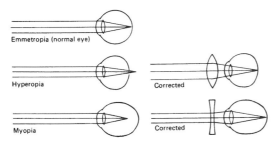

Figure 2.18. Correction of hyperopia with a convex lens and of myopia with a concave (or less convex) lens. In hyperopia (farsightedness) the focal distance is in back of the retina; in myopia (nearsightedness) the focal distance is in front of the retina. From Ganong WF. Review of medical physiology. 17th ed. East Norwalk, CT: Appleton & Lange, 1995.

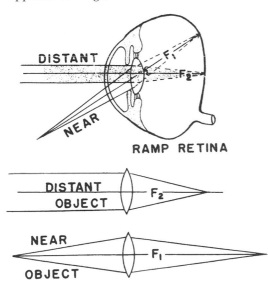

Figure 2.19. Ramp-shaped retina of the horse. This provides a longer focal length for viewing downward (F_1) than for viewing along the axis of the eye (F_2). This means that lower, near objects are in focus without, or with minimal, accommodation. From Prince JH, et al. Anatomy and histology of the eye and orbit in domestic animals. Springfield, IL: Charles C Thomas, 1960.

vergence from a more convex lens, but rather by placing the retina farther from the lens for this image formation. This feature of the horse eyeball is called a ramp retina. Some veterinary ophthalmologists have not been able to verify the differences in

focal distance with the ophthalmoscope, and uncertainty exists about the ramp retina auxiliary feature. Accommodation in the horse is not precise and the tendency to shy (lurch sideways) when approaching near objects is often observed.

IRIS The amount of light allowed to enter the eye is controlled by the iris, which is the colored part of the eye. The allowed opening, of varying size, is called the pupil (Fig. 2.20) The pupil is horizontal in the domestic herbivores and pig, vertical and elliptic in the cat, and circular in the dog. The iris contains two sets of smooth muscles: (1) circularly arranged fibers, innervated by the parasympathetic division of the autonomic nervous system, and (2) radially arranged fibers, innervated by the sympathetic division. Contraction of the circularly arranged fibers decreases the size of the pupil and allows less light to enter the eye, whereas contraction of the radially arranged fibers increases the size of the pupil and allows more light to enter the eye.

Unlike the ventrally located optic disk of most mammals (Fig. 2.15), the cat's disk occupies a central position. Light entering a round, constricted pupil would therefore be projected to the optic disk. The optic disk has no visual receptors and no image is created. In cats, however, constriction of the pupil with a vertical orientation projects light above and below the optic disk to allow for image formation in bright light (which constricts the pupil).

HUMORS OF THE EYE The spaces forward from the lens are divided by the iris into two parts. The space behind the iris and forward from the lens is called the posterior chamber and the space behind the cornea, but in front of the iris, is called the anterior chamber. Projecting from the ciliary body and into the posterior chamber are structures known as ciliary processes (Fig. 2.20). They present a considerable surface area because of their folded arrangement, and they are well vascularized. They actively secrete a liquid into the posterior

Figure 2.20. Schematic representation of the relationship in the dog of the ciliary processes with the ciliary body, the zonular fibers (lens ligaments), and the posterior chamber. The ciliary muscles are a part of the ciliary body and are attached to the zonular fibers. The meshwork represents a collection location for aqueous humor that drains to scleral veins.

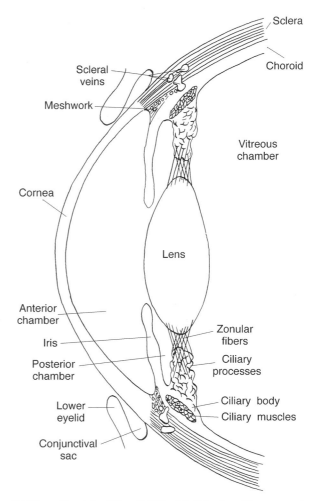

chamber, or the aqueous humor (Fig. 2.21). The aqueous humor has free communication with the anterior chamber and thus occupies all spaces anterior to the lens. The transparent material behind the lens that occupies most of the volume of the eyeball (the vitreous chamber) is called the vitreous body. It does not have the flow characteristics of a liquid; rather, it is more similar to a gelatinous mass—hence, the name vitreous body is more appropriate than vitreous humor.

Aqueous humor can diffuse through the mass of the vitreous body but only slowly. The principal flow of aqueous humor after its formation is through the pupil into the anterior chamber and to where it is reabsorbed at the iridocorneal angle, which is the angle formed where the cornea meets the iris (Fig. 2.22). At this location, a vein, called the canal of Schlemm, encircles the eye. A meshwork of connective tissue separates the canal of Schlemm (venous sinus of sclera) from the anterior chamber. Inasmuch as there is a constant formation of aqueous humor, there must also be a constant removal; this is afforded by reabsorption into the canal of Schlemm. Just like cerebrospinal fluid, it is returned to the blood. Aqueous humor functions to (1) provide nutrition to the avascular lens and cornea, (2) remove waste products of metabolism from these structures, and (3) occupy space and maintain a constant distance for the refractive parts. The pressure maintained by the aqueous humor within the eyeball can be measured; it is about 20 mm Hg in the dog. This pressure maintains the normal shape and firmness of the eyeball. If the reabsorption of aqueous humor is impeded, the pressure increases. This situation is recognized clinically as glaucoma and can lead to blindness if left untreated.

RETINA   The innermost tunic of the eye is the nerve tunic, or retina; it is comprised of ten layers (Fig. 2.23). The photoreceptors, the rods and cones, are located near the outer aspect, immediately inward from the pigmented epithelium. Impulse transmission is directed inwardly toward the vitreous. Considerable convergence of impulses from the photoreceptors occurs on two interposed cell layers. The last cell layer (ganglion cells) has axons that converge at the optic disk to exit the eyeball as the optic nerve.

The retinas of domestic mammals contain mostly rods, and the retinas of domestic birds contain mostly cones. The rods are the photoreceptors associated with black and white vision and the cones are those associated with color vision. The rods are extremely sensitive to light and are used for night vision, whereas cones function best in day vision.

Chemistry of Vision

Light that enters the eye stimulates biochemical reactions in the rods and cones. Chemicals in the rods and cones decompose on exposure to light. The chemical in the rods is called rhodopsin, and the light-sensitive chemicals in the cones are only slightly different from rhodopsin. The reaction scheme shown in Figure 2.24 is characteristic of the visual cycle.

Rhodopsin (also known as visual purple) is a light-sensitive pigment in the outer part of the rod that is located in the pigmented

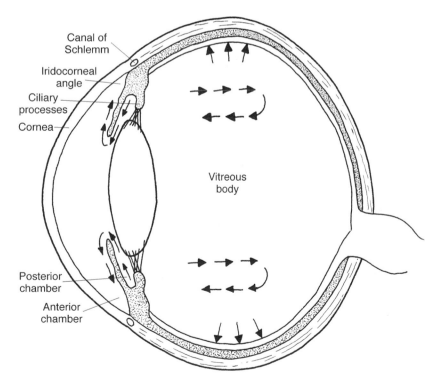

Figure 2.21. Formation of aqueous humor by ciliary processes and its anterior flow. Arrows in vitreous body indicate diffusional flow of aqueous humor through the vitreous body. Some absorption occurs from the vitreous into choroidal vessels.

Figure 2.22. The iridocorneal angle, where the iris meets the cornea. **A.** Section through eyeball. **B.** Detailed section through anterior part of the eye. Here the aqueous humor flows into the veins. From DeCoursey RM. The human organism. 4th ed. New York: McGraw-Hill, 1974.

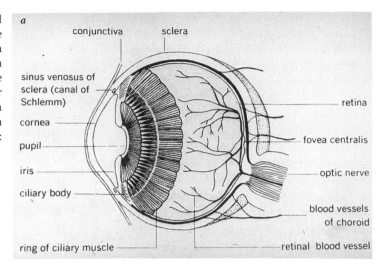

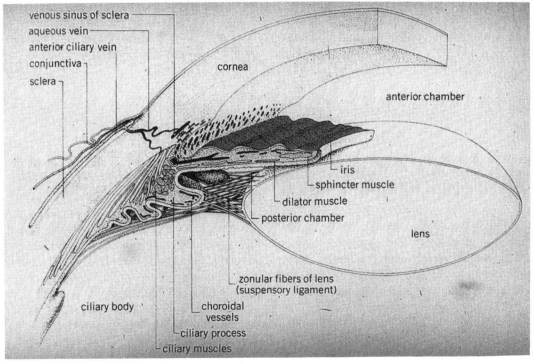

B

epithelium. It is composed of 11-*cis*-retinal (also known as retinene) and scotopsin. Scotopsin is a rod protein, and the similar opsin in cones is photopsin. Exposure of rhodopsin to light energy immediately begins its decomposition, in which a num-

ber of unstable, short-lived (nanoseconds for prelumi-rhodopsin and seconds for metarhodopsin II) intermediates are formed. The final one, metarhodopsin II, triggers highly amplified visual excitation and splits into scotopsin and all-*trans*-retinal. All-*trans*-retinal is chemically the same as 11-*cis*-retinal but has a different physical structure; it is a straight rather than a curved molecule. Its conversion to 11-*cis*-retinal requires the presence of the retinal enzyme isomerase. All-*trans*-retinal is converted to 11-*cis*-retinal, which then recombines with scotopsin to reform rhodopsin.

Rod stimulation is believed to occur at the instant that the rhodopsin molecule becomes excited by light. The stimulation resulting from an instantaneous flash of light can persist for about 0.05 to 0.5 s, depending on the intensity of the light. Rapidly successive flashes with alternating intensity become fused to give the appearance of being continuous. This effect is observed when watching motion pictures or television.

Thus, a relationship exists between vision and vitamin A. A lack of vitamin A results in inadequate formation of rhodopsin. Night vision requires optimum amounts of rhodopsin, and its shortage, because of vitamin A deficiency, is referred to as night blindness.

Adaptation to Varying Light

Dark adaptation refers to an adaptation to relatively dark environments. Because of less light, the concentration of rhodopsin increases, allowing for maximum reaction to the available light. When first entering a

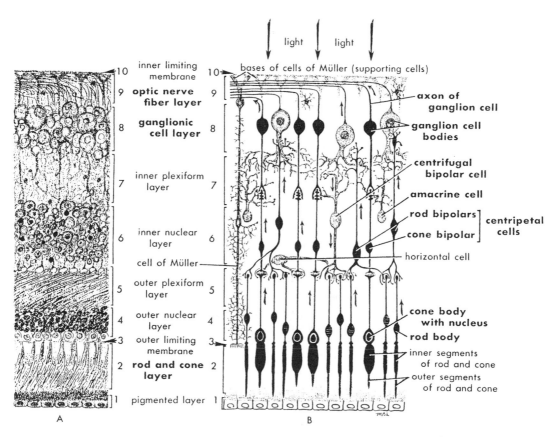

Figure 2.23. The ten layers of the human retina. **A.** Diagram of retinal section (highly magnified). **B.** Schematic representation of the retina. From Crouch JE. Functional human anatomy. 4th ed. Philadelphia: Lea & Febiger, 1985.

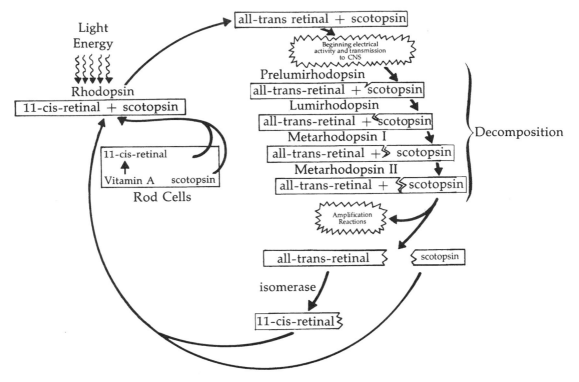

Figure 2.24. Photochemistry of the visual cycle. Metarhodopsin II, called photoexcited rhodopsin, triggers highly amplified visual excitation.

dark room, one might be almost unable to see anything, but after dark adaptation, objects can be perceived more readily.

Light adaptation refers to an adaptation to lighter environments. The higher concentration of rhodopsin decomposes because of the abundance of light. The images perceived seem to be overexposed. Normal vision returns when the rhodopsin concentration is balanced with the available light.

Concurrent with the adaptation processes are the visual reflexes, which increase or decrease the diameter of the pupil (see previous section). Consequently, not only does rhodopsin concentration increase in the dark, but the pupil diameter also increases to allow for maximum light entry. Conversely, rhodopsin concentration decreases in light and pupil size decreases to minimize light entry.

The tapetum is a light-reflecting layer of cells of the inner choroid, located just out-side the retinal-pigmented epithelium (Fig. 2.25). The tapetum is not present throughout the choroid and varies in size among those domestic species in which it is present (e.g., cats, dogs, horses, ruminants). The tapetum allows light that has just stimulated the receptor cells to be reflected back onto them, so that they receive another stimulation. In this way, greater vision is obtained, even with minimal light. The reflected light continues on a forward path through the pupil and out of the eye again. This reflected light is termed "eyeshine," which is when eyes glow at night in the presence of light.

Field of Vision

The field of vision for an animal is the spatial area from which the complete image is formed. The more lateral the placement of

Figure 2.25. Location of the tapetum relative to the retina. The tapetum is shown as a broad band of cell layers between the choroid and the retina. Melanin is absent from the pigmented epithelium of the retina (outer layer of the retina) where tapetum is present. There is a pigmented layer in the choroid to aid light absorption.

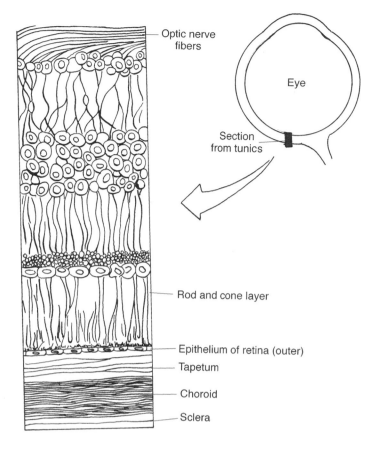

Optic nerve fibers

Eye

Section from tunics

Rod and cone layer

Epithelium of retina (outer)

Tapetum

Choroid

Sclera

the eyes, the larger the field of vision. In fact, some animals might even see everything around them with the exception of objects directly behind their body, which can still be seen with only a slight movement of the head. If the field of vision for each eye overlaps that of the other, a binocular area of vision is formed; conversely, a monocular area is formed if there is no overlap. Binocular vision provides greater depth perception, and this is more pronounced in animals that prey on other animals for food. Greater accuracy of position is necessary before the leap. Such animals characteristically have more forward-placed eyes (Fig. 2.26). In contrast, herbivores (plant eaters) have more laterally placed eyes and have a wider field of vision; this gives greater protection while grazing as far as predator observation is concerned (Fig. 2.27). In all domestic animals, regardless of how far their eyes are situated laterally, there is some central area of overlap providing a zone of binocular vision.

Eyeball Movements

Movements of the eyeball are accomplished by skeletal muscles that are innervated by cranial nerves (Fig. 2.28). Up-and-down, side-to-side, rotational, and inward (retraction) movements are possible. These muscles also hold the eyeball within its orbit against a pad of fat. Side-to-side movements are made by contraction of a laterally placed muscle, up-and-down movements are made by contraction of a dorsally and ventrally placed muscle, and rotational movements are made by contraction of a dorsal or ventral obliquely placed

Figure 2.26. Field of vision of the cat. The large central binocular area results from the forward position of the eyes. From Coulter DB, Schmidt GM. Special senses I: vision. In: Swenson MJ, Reece WO, eds. Dukes' physiology of domestic animals. 11th ed. Ithaca, NY: Cornell University Press, 1993.

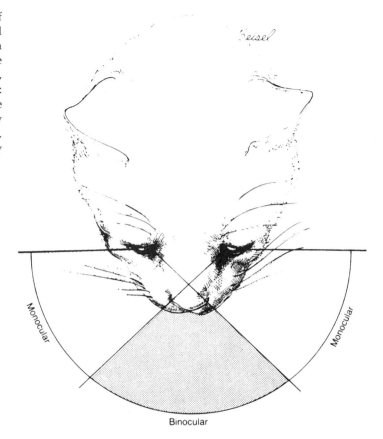

Figure 2.27. Field of vision of the horse. It is relatively large because of the horse's more laterally placed eyes. Note the small binocular area. From Coulter DB, Schmidt GM. Special senses I: vision. In: Swenson MJ, Reece WO, eds. Dukes' physiology of domestic animals. 11th ed. Ithaca, NY: Cornell University Press, 1993.

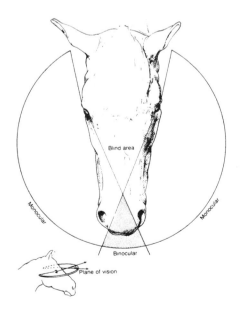

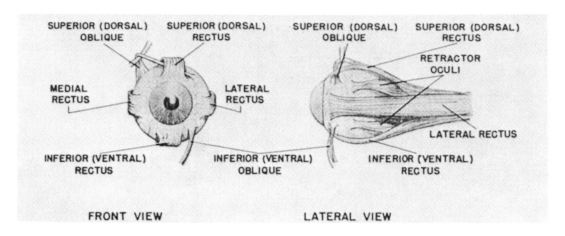

Figure 2.28. Extrinsic muscles of the eye of the dog. From Helper LC. Magrane's canine ophthalmology. 4th ed. Philadelphia: Lea & Febiger, 1989.

muscle. The dorsal oblique muscle rotates the top of the eye medially and the ventral oblique muscle rotates the ventral part of the eye medially. Retractor muscles are absent in humans; they appear to provide protection for animals in situations in which protruding eyeballs would be hazardous. Also, retraction of the eyeball causes the third eyelid (nictitating membrane) to slide over the eyeball and spread the tear film (see below).

Accessory Structures and Their Functions

CONJUNCTIVAE The conjunctivae are the membranes that both line the eyelids and turn back onto the eyeball (Fig. 2.20). The part lining the eyelid is the palpebral conjunctiva and the part turned back onto the eyeball is the bulbar or ocular conjunctiva. The space between the palpebral conjunctiva and the eyeball forms the conjunctival sac. This space is normally minimal and provides a reservoir for the accumulation of tears. It is also used for the application of eye drops and ointments. The conjunctival membrane, because of its superficial location, is useful for examining mucous membrane color. A pink color is considered normal, a blanched appearance indicates lack of blood or anemia, a blue color indicates lack of oxygen, and a yellow color is associated with icterus. The lacrimal apparatus is associated with the formation of lacrimal secretions (tears), transport to the conjunctival sac, and drainage to the nasal cavity (Fig. 2.29). The lacrimal gland is located in the orbit, dorsal to the eyeball. Short ducts carry the secretion into the upper aspect of the dorsal conjunctival sac. The lacrimal secretion keeps the eyeball moist, provides lubrication, and keeps it clean and free of foreign materials. Ducts in the medial aspect of each eye conduct excess secretion to the nasal cavity, where it is dissipated. Glands that secrete a waxy substance, known as meibomian glands, are located along the margin of the eyelids. Their secretion helps to form a dam so that the lacrimal secretion does not ordinarily flow out onto the face.

PRECORNEAL FILM The fluid layer on the cornea is known as the precorneal film (also called the tear film). It consists of an innermost layer of mucin, a middle layer of lacrimal secretions (tears), and an outer oil film.

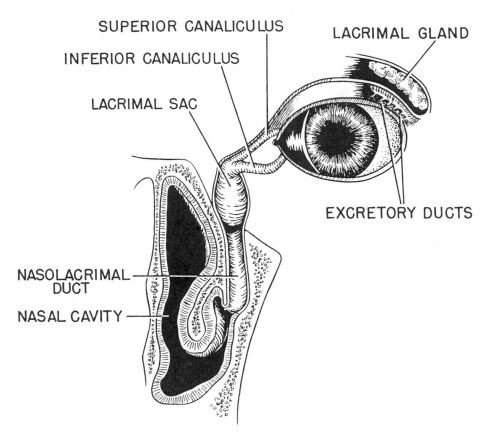

Figure 2.29. The lacrimal production and drainage system of the eye of the dog. The accessory lacrimal glands are not shown. From Helper LC. Magrane's canine ophthalmology. 4th ed. Philadelphia: Lea & Febiger, 1989.

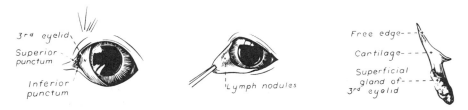

Figure 2.30. Third eyelid in the dog. From Evans HE, deLahunta A. Miller's guide to the dissection of the dog. 4th ed. Philadelphia: WB Saunders, 1996.

The outer oily layer is formed by meibomian glands and accessory sebaceous glands. It reduces the rate of evaporation of the underlying tear layer and also helps to prevent overflow at the lid margin.

The middle layer of fluid is composed of lacrimal secretions, which wet the cornea and reduce evaporation from the eye. It is formed by the lacrimal glands and the accessory lacrimal glands (such as those associated with the third eyelid).

The inner mucinoid layer is formed by the goblet cells of the conjunctiva. In addition to mucin, it contains a high concentration of lysozyme (an enzyme), which can digest bacterial cell walls. Lysozyme is present in most animal tissues and secretions, but it only is found in sufficiently high concentrations to be bactericidal in white blood cells, nasal secretions, and tears. In addition to lysozyme, a gamma globulin protein fraction also contributes to the antibacterial property of tears. Wetability (favorable surface tension between cornea and tears) is provided for by the mucin of the inner layer.

The tear film is reformed each time the eyelids close or when the third eyelid is swept across the eye by eyeball retraction.

THIRD EYELID The third eyelid arises as a fold from the ventromedial aspect of the conjunctiva (visible part shown as membrane nictitans in Fig. 2.14). It is well developed in the dog, is highly mobile, and is large enough to cover the entire anterior face of the cornea. The third eyelid is reinforced by a T-shaped cartilage surrounded at its base by a gland that contributes to the tear film (Fig. 2.30). Pigs and cattle also have a second, deeper gland. The third eyelid becomes prominent when all the muscles of the eyeball are caused to contract, as in some clinical situations such as strychnine poisoning. The contraction retracts the eyeball and puts pressure on the cartilaginous plate, pushing it forward. Lymph nodules are also present on the underside of the third eyelid. When they become inflamed in the dog they often protrude; the condition is referred to as "cherry eye."

STUDY AIDS—THE SENSORY ORGANS

Sensory Receptors and Their Functions

1. What are the special senses?
2. Are pain, cold, heat, touch and pressure sensations known as special senses?
3. To what group of sensory receptors do muscle spindles and Golgi tendon organs belong?

4. Differentiate between a phasic and a tonic receptor. Are muscle spindles tonic or phasic receptors?
5. What is the name for receptors specific for pain?
6. Can a receptor for cold or heat send an afferent impulse to the cerebral cortex to be recognized as pain?
7. How is pain that arises from the intestines produced?
8. What are the most sensitive visceral structures that produce pain?
9. What is a good example of referred pain in cattle?

Taste

1. What is the physiologic name for taste?
2. What is a function of taste in animals?
3. Where are most of the taste buds located?
4. Study the location of taste buds relative to papillae and the glands of von Ebner.
5. To stimulate taste hairs, what part of a taste bud must *dissolved* substances enter?
6. How are taste substances classified in animals?
7. At what temperature does water rejection occur for poultry?
8. What is meant by depraved appetite in animals?

Smell

1. What is the physiologic name for smell?
2. Where are the nerve cell bodies for smell located?
3. Why do dogs have a better sense of smell than humans?
4. Differentiate between anosmatic, microsmatic and macrosmatic.
5. What is the function of the glands of Bowman secretion?
6. What is the function of olfactory epithelial basal cells?
7. Can more than one odor be perceived at one time?

8. What is meant by adaptation to smell?
9. What are pheromones?
10. What are some functions of animal pheromones?

Hearing and Equilibrium

1. Be able to follow the motion initiated by a sound wave from the tympanic membrane through the cochlear window (round window).
2. What is the function of the two striated muscles located in the middle ear?
3. What reflex is inherent to the function of the middle ear muscles?
4. What are the respective functions of the vestibular and cochlear portions of the inner ear?
5. Why is the cochlea coiled?
6. Differentiate between membranous labyrinth and osseous labyrinth and their respective fluids.
7. How are the cristae (located in the semicircular canals) stimulated?
8. How are the macula receptors stimulated?
9. What are the divisions of the cochlea brought about by extension of the membranous labyrinth into the cochlea?
10. Which cochlear division contains the organ of Corti?
11. What function is served by the organs of Corti?
12. Summarize sound reception (which relates to item 1 in this list).

Vision

1. Identify the parts of the external eye.
2. Identify the basic structures of the eyeball.
3. What is the normal arrangement of the corneal stroma?
4. Does the cornea have a blood supply?
5. Are there nerve fibers in the cornea?
6. How is accommodation accomplished by the lens of the eye?
7. What is the extent of accommodation among domestic animals?
8. How is the size of the pupil changed?

9. Are pupil shapes the same among all animals?
10. What would be the impact of a centrally located optic disk and a constricted circular pupil?
11. Review the production, location, circulation, function, and drainage of aqueous humor.
12. What visual chemical begins to decompose when excited by light and stimulates retinal rod cells?
13. What is the tapetum and how does it provide for better vision in reduced light?
14. What is meant by field of vision? Binocular vision? Monocular vision?
15. Describe the conjunctiva.
16. If the nasolacrimal duct were plugged, explain the reason for a horse's wet face.
17. What is "cherry eye" in the dog?

SELF-EVALUATION— THE SENSORY ORGANS

1. A green dye placed into the conjunctival sac of a horse should later appear in the nasal cavity (near the nostrils) if the nasolacrimal apparatus is functioning properly.
   a. true
   b. false
2. A chemical odorous signal secreted by one animal to influence the behavior of another animal is known as a:
   a. pheromone
   b. scent
   c. perfume
   d. pheroscent
3. The fluid that provides nutrition to the avascular (without blood supply) cornea and lens is:
   a. vitreous humor
   b. good humor
   c. aqueous humor
   d. endolymph
4. The radially arranged muscles of the iris that dilate the pupil are innervated by the:

a. sympathetic division of the autonomics
b. parasympathetic division of the autonomics

5. Which one of the following cells from the olfactory region might provide for return of the smell sensation after olfactory receptor cell destruction?
   a. sustentacular cells
   b. olfactory receptor cells
   c. basal cells

6. The tear film:
   a. has little function
   ⌐b. provides optical, mechanical, lubricating, and bactericidal functions (WOW!)
   c. is a good movie
   d. is secreted by glands in the nasal cavity

7. High frequency sounds are dissipated (and thus stimulate appropriate cells for the sense of hearing):
   a. near the base of the cochlea (closest to the vestibule)
   b. near the tip of the cochlea (farthest from the vestibule)
   c. near the base of the semicircular canals
   d. in the curved portion of the semicircular canals

8. The taste bud is a receptor organ for olfaction.
   a. true
   b. false

9. The greatest number of taste buds are associated with the:
   a. nasal cavity
   b. tongue papillae
   c. cheek
   d. pharynx

10. Pheromones are associated with which one of the following special senses?
    a. taste
    b. smell
    c. hearing
    d. vision

11. Water that is colder (even down to freezing) than environmental temperature is readily accepted by chickens and turkeys, whereas they may refuse water (water that has been sitting in the sun) that is higher than their body temperature.
    a. true
    b. false

12. Which one of the following statements best explains why most domestic animals are macrosmatic?
    a. their individual receptors are more sensitive
    b. they are better able to sniff
    c. they have a more extensive epithelium containing the receptors

13. Muscles in the middle ear that are attached to the auditory ossicles:
    a. amplify sound waves
    b. protect the ear from excessive amplification
    c. help direct sound waves into the ear canal

14. Animals with eyes that are placed well forward on the head (such as the cat) have a more extensive field of vision than animals with eyes placed laterally, but they have a more restricted binocular vision.
    a. true
    b. false

15. Which one of the following statements about the ciliary body is FALSE?
    a. it is a part of the vascular tunic
    b. contains ciliary muscles which when contracted *decrease* tension on lens ligaments, causing the lens to become more convex
    c. has secretory processes known as choroid plexus
    d. ciliary muscles within are *poorly* developed in most domestic animals

16. The function of the tapetum is:
    a. to convert light to a nerve impulse
    b. focus light upon the retina
    c. reflect light back to rod cells in the retina
    d. secrete aqueous humor

17. Which one of the following statements about the cornea is FALSE?
    a. the ratio of corneal area to eyeball area varies among animal species
    b. it is devoid of blood vessels
    c. it is well supplied with bare nerve endings for pain reception
    d. it is normally clear because of random arrangement of collagen fibers
18. Which one of the following statements about the retina is FALSE?
    a. the light sensitive cells (rods and cones) are on the inside (nearest vitreous)
    b. it has highest metabolic rate per unit of weight of any tissue in body
    c. it may be damaged by deficiency or excess of oxygen
    d. it appears black because of outer pigment layer (in choroid if have tapetum)
19. Dark adaptation (greater vision in the dark) implies a depletion of rhodopsin
    a. true
    b. false
20. The movement of fluid in the membranous semi-circular canals moves hair cells of the ampullae therein. This apprises the brain about:
    a. equilibrium
    b. hearing
    c. smell
    d. pain
21. Which component of the ear relies upon fluid conduction of sound waves for its function?
    a. external ear
    b. middle ear
    c. vestibular apparatus
    d. cochlea
22. Muscle spindles and Golgi tendon organs belong to the class of sensory receptors known as:
    a. interoceptors
    b. nociceptors
    c. exteroceptors
    d. proprioceptors

23. Stimulation of a Krause end-bulb (cold receptor) can result in the pain sensation.
    a. true
    b. false
24. Pain arising from the viscera that is felt on the surface of the body is known as:
    a. heart pain
    b. window pain
    c. referred pain
    d. pleuritis or peritonitis
25. Which one of the following is NOT associated with gustation in animals?
    a. papillae, taste buds, tongue
    b. taste pore, pit, taste hairs
    c. pleasant, unpleasant, indifferent
    d. pheromone
26. Which one of the following is NOT associated with olfaction in animals?
    a. pica
    b. sniffing
    c. adaptation
    d. macrosmatic, microsmatic, anosmatic
27. Equalization of pressure between the middle ear and the body exterior is accomplished by way of the:
    a. pinna
    b. ear canal
    c. auditory tube (eustachian tube)
    d. cochlear duct
28. What proprioceptive sensory organ is present in the middle ear skeletal muscles that responds to stretch and dampen loud sounds?
    a. bare nerve endings
    b. muscle spindle
    c. Golgi tendon organ
    d. Vater-Pacinian corpuscle
29. The observation of a pig with its head tilted and an awkward sense of body balance (equilibrium) would indicate malfunction within the
    a. vestibular structure of the inner ear
    b. cochlear structure of the inner ear
    c. vestibular structure of the middle ear
    d. cochlear structure of the middle ear

30. The first fluid displaced by the inward movement of the stapes is:
    a. endolymph in the scala media (cochlear duct)
    b. endolymph in the vestibule
    c. perilymph in the vestibule
    d. perilymph in the scala media

31. The sensory receptor of the inner ear that converts sound energy to a nerve impulse is known as the:
    a. organ of Corti
    b. crista ampullaris
    c. macula
    d. harmonica

32. The cornea is normally clear and transparent because the collagen fibers (stroma):
    a. have a lamellar (parallel) arrangement
    b. are randomly arranged
    c. have a good blood supply
    d. have a poor oxygen supply

33. For the lens to become more convex and increase convergence of incoming light, the ciliary muscles must:
    a. relax
    b. contract

34. It appears that accommodation in domestic animals (as judged by ciliary muscle development) is:
    a. limited and some may have auxiliary features
    b. well developed in all species

35. What are the two avascular structures of the eye that receive nutrition and have waste products removed by the aqueous humor?
    a. retina and choroid
    b. iris and ciliary muscles
    c. lens and cornea
    d. canal of Schlemm and sclera

36. An expanded field of vision with more limited binocular vision would be noted in animals that have:
    a. more laterally-placed eyes
    b. more forward-placed eyes
    c. a centrally-placed eye

37. When someone asks you what causes "eyeshine" in animals, you are now able to say that it is caused by reflective cells in the inner choroid known as the:
    a. cone
    b. vitreous body
    c. ramp retina
    d. tapetum

SUGGESTED READINGS

Buchanan AR. Functional neuro-anatomy. 3rd ed. Philadelphia: Lea & Febiger, 1957.

Chibuzo GA. The tongue. In: Evans HE, ed. Miller's anatomy of the dog. 3rd ed. Philadelphia: WB Saunders, 1993:396–414.

Cormack DH. Ham's histology. 9th ed. Philadelphia: JB Lippincott, 1987.

Coulter DB, Schmidt GM. Special senses I: vision. In Swenson MJ, Reece WO, eds. Dukes' physiology of domestic animals. 11th ed. Ithaca: Cornell University Press, 1993:803–815.

Crouch JE. Functional human anatomy. 4th ed. Philadelphia: Lea & Febiger, 1985.

De Coursey RM. The human organism. 4th ed. New York: McGraw-Hill, 1974.

Dellman HD. Textbook of veterinary histology. 4th ed. Philadelphia: Lea & Febiger, 1993.

Evans HE, deLahunta A. Miller's guide to the dissection of the dog. 4th ed. Philadelphia: WB Saunders, 1996.

Fawcett DW. Bloom & Fawcett: A textbook of histology. 12th ed. New York: Chapman & Hall, 1994.

Ganong WF. Review of medical physiology. 17th ed. East Norwalk, CT: Appleton & Lange, 1995.

Getty R, Foust HL, Presley ET, Miller ME. Macroscopic anatomy of the ear of the dog. Am J Vet Res 1956;17:364.

Helper LC. Magrane's canine ophthalmology. 4th ed. Philadelphia: Lea & Febiger, 1989.

Kare MR, Beauchamp GK, Marsh RR. Special senses II: taste, smell, and hearing. In: Swenson MJ, Reece WO, eds. Dukes' physiology of domestic animals. 11th ed. Ithaca: Cornell University Press, 1993:816–835.

Prince JH, Diesem CD, Eglitis I, Ruskell GL. Anatomy and histology of the eye and orbit in domestic animals. Springfield, IL: Charles C. Thomas, 1960.

Spence AP, Mason EB. Human anatomy and physiology. 4th ed. St. Paul, MN: West Publishing Co., 1992.

Stryer L. Biochemistry. 4th ed. New York: WH Freeman, 1995.

Vander AJ, Sherman JH, Luciano DS. Human physiology: The mechanisms of body function. 6th ed. New York: McGraw-Hill, 1994.

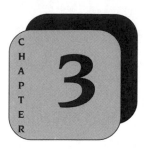
Muscle

Movements of the skeleton, changes in the amount of blood supplied to body parts, transport of ingesta through the intestinal tract, generation of body heat, and circulation of blood are examples of muscle function. Because of these diverse functions throughout the body, and because considerable work is required to perform them, it is not surprising that 45 to 50% of the body weight is represented by components of the muscular system.

CLASSIFICATION

There are three types of muscle cells of the animal body: smooth, cardiac, and skeletal.

Smooth Muscle

Smooth muscle is so named because it has no visible striations. The individual cells are spindle-shaped and have a centrally located nucleus (Fig. 3.1). Smooth muscles are regulated by the autonomic nervous system and are located in visceral structures that require movements of an automatic nature. Aggregates of myofilaments in smooth muscle are composed of the contractile proteins actin and myosin. The filaments are not arranged in order (as in skeletal muscle), which accounts for the lack of visible striations.

Cardiac Muscle

Cardiac muscle is found only in the heart. It is regulated by the autonomic nervous system, like smooth muscle. In contrast to smooth muscle, however, on microscopic examination cardiac muscle shows striations characterized by alternating light and dark bands. Cardiac muscle is composed of elongated, branching cells with irregular contours at their junction with other cells (Fig. 3.2). The boundary area where the end of a cell anastomoses (joins) with the next cell is known as an intercalated disk. This highly specialized cell membrane structure facilitates the transmission of nerve impulses from one cell to the next. Each cell has one nucleus (sometimes two) that is centrally located.

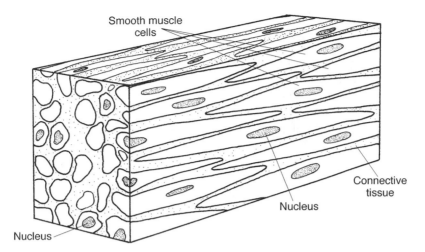

Figure 3.1. Smooth muscle cells exposed in their longitudinal and cross-sectional planes. The cells are characteristically spindle-shaped and have a centrally located nucleus.

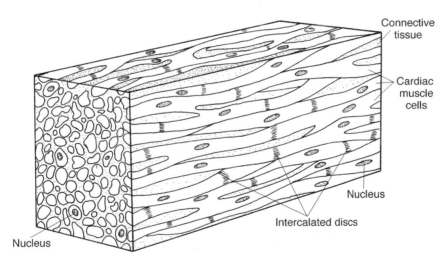

Figure 3.2. Cardiac muscle cells exposed in their longitudinal and cross-sectional planes. Note elongated, branching cells with irregular contours at their junction with other cells.

Skeletal Muscle

Skeletal muscle cells (fibers) of many animals can be one of three types: (1) red or dark, (2) white or pale, or (3) intermediate, with characteristics between those of red and white fibers (Fig. 3.3). Red muscle fibers are characterized by having more myoglobin and more mitochondria than white fibers. All muscles are probably a mixture of these three types, but in some animals the red and in others the white predominate. A striking example of this is the crimson red pectoralis muscle (breast muscle) of pigeons, which contrasts sharply with the stark white color of the chicken pectoralis muscle. Red muscle fibers usually contract more slowly and fatigue less readily than white muscle fibers. In birds, the amount of red pigmentation in the pectoralis muscle can be correlated directly with the ability for sustained flight. Geese and ducks, as well as pigeons, are known for their sustained flight, and they have a predominance of red pectoralis muscle fibers.

Skeletal muscle comprises the major portion of the muscle mass of the animal body. An individual skeletal muscle fiber can extend the length of the muscle of which it is a part. As is characteristic of cardiac muscles, skeletal muscles are also striated when viewed microscopically. They are not branched and do not anastomose (thus, no intercalated disk), and a nerve impulse to each muscle fiber is required for its stimulation. Multiple, peripherally arranged nuclei are present in each cell (Fig. 3.4), in contrast to both smooth and cardiac muscle cells.

Skeletal muscles are often described according to the type of movement performed. They are flexors if they are located on the side of the limb toward which the joint bends when decreasing the joint angle. They are extensors if they are located on the side of the limb toward which the joint bends when increasing the joint angle. Adductors are muscles that pull a limb toward the median plane and abductors

pull a limb away from the median plane. Sphincters are arranged circularly to constrict body openings. Muscles are strategically located to best serve the structure they

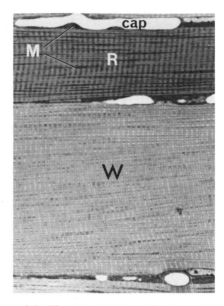

Figure 3.3. Photomicrograph of skeletal muscle showing red fibers (R) and white fibers (W). Red fibers have more mitochondria (*M*) packed between their myofibrils, especially in association with capillaries (*cap*). From Cormack DC. Ham's histology. 9th ed. Philadelphia: JB Lippincott, 1987.

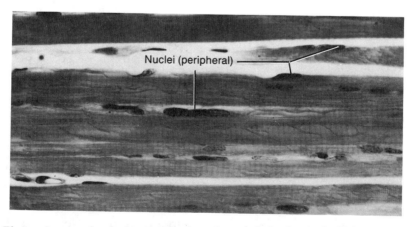

Figure 3.4. Photomicrograph of a longitudinal section of skeletal muscle fibers. Note the striations and the multiple, peripherally located nuclei. From Cormack DC. Ham's histology. 9th ed. Philadelphia: JB Lippincott, 1987.

affect. Lack of adduction occasionally occurs in the hind limbs of cows after parturition or calving. The adductor muscles are supplied by the obturator nerves (one to each leg), each of which passes through an opening (obturator foramen) in the birth canal. Its injury during the calving process can be followed by the inability to adduct one or both of the hind legs (obturator paralysis).

ARRANGEMENT

The function of muscles is to contract or shorten. In doing this, they move a body part or body contents, or they provide resistance to some movement. A primary consideration for muscles to accomplish a desired result is their arrangement. Accordingly, the muscle cells might be arranged in sheets, sheets rolled into tubes, bundles, rings (sphincters), or cones, or they might remain as discrete cells or clusters for more precise or less forceful action. The emptying of visceral structures (e.g., urinary bladder, stomach, heart) or the conveyance of intestinal contents or organ secretions, as provided by smooth and cardiac muscle, is accomplished because of their intimate association with the affected part. Apart from the skeletal

muscle sphincters, the effects of skeletal muscle can be noted at a point some distance from their location. This means that their contraction must be transmitted somehow to the affected part. For this to happen, one end of the muscle must be relatively fixed or anchored and the other end must be attached directly or by a tendon to the movable part. Accordingly, the anatomic description of a skeletal muscle sometimes refers to its origin and insertion, the origin being the least movable end and the insertion the most movable end. Contraction of skeletal muscle brings the origin and insertion closer together and, when attachments involve two bones, one or both of the bones will move.

SKELETAL MUSCLE HARNESSING

The harness for skeletal muscle fibers is composed of connective tissue elements (epimysium, perimysium, endomysium) that are continuous from the individual muscle fibers to the connective tissue of the structure to which the muscle attaches and on which it exerts its pull when it contracts. Often the connective tissue of the structure to which it is attached is a tendon (Fig. 3.5).

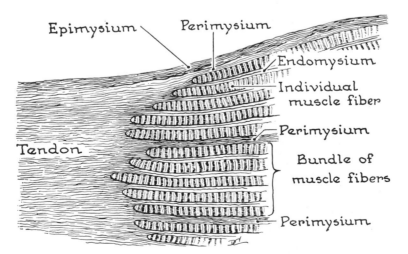

Figure 3.5. Longitudinal section of a muscle. The connective tissue elements of muscle are continuous with a tendon. From Ham AW. Histology. 7th ed. Philadelphia: JB Lippincott, 1974.

Figure 3.6. The division of muscles into smaller parts, down to myofibrils. From Feduccia A, McCrady E. Torrey's morphogenesis of the vertebrates. 5th ed. New York: John Wiley & Sons, 1991.

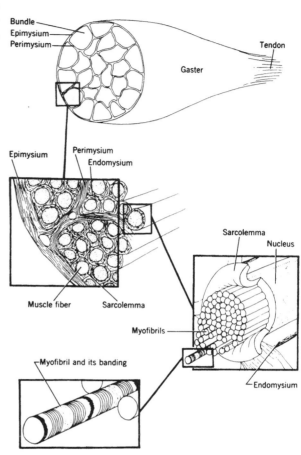

A broad connective tissue sheet that fulfills a similar function is an aponeurosis. The connective tissue elements of skeletal muscle are as follows:

1. Muscle fibers that comprise a muscle bundle are attached by their cell covering (sarcolemma) to a connective tissue division, the endomysium.
2. The endomysium is continuous with connective tissue that envelops muscle bundles, the perimysium.
3. The perimysium is continuous with connective tissue that envelops the muscle (collection of muscle bundles), the epimysium.
4. The epimysium is continuous with the tendon or aponeurosis, which can travel some distance for its attachment.

Some muscles seem to arise directly from a bone, and their attachment could be considered a fleshy attachment. These muscle cells, however, do have a short tendinous attachment to the periosteum of the bone.

MICROSTRUCTURE OF SKELETAL MUSCLES

To understand how muscles contract, the microstructure of skeletal muscle fibers must be understood. A muscle fiber varies considerably in length, and often it is as long as the muscle of which it is a part.

Muscle Fiber Division

The division of muscles into smaller parts, down to myofibrils, is shown in Figure 3.6.

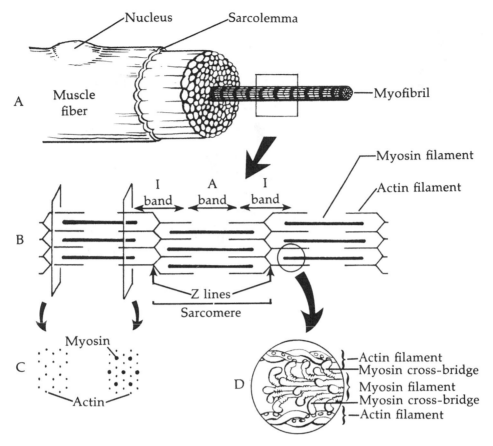

Figure 3.7. The division of myofibrils into sarcomeres. **A.** Cross section of a muscle fiber. **B.** Longitudinal arrangement of myofilaments within sarcomeres. **C.** Spatial arrangement of the myofilaments within a sarcomere. **D.** Further details of the relationship between actin and myosin molecules.

Depending on the diameter of the muscle fiber, there might be several hundred to several thousand myofibrils within one muscle fiber. Each myofibril has striations or banding. The further division of myofibrils into repetitive units (sarcomeres) and their components is shown in Figure 3.7. Sarcomeres contain the protein myofilaments, actin and myosin, which, by their arrangement, give rise to striations (Fig. 3.7A). Inasmuch as the striations are characteristic of the muscle fiber, it is apparent that the sarcomeres of a myofibril are in alignment with the sarcomeres of all the other myofibrils of the muscle fiber. The Z line is located at each end of a sarcomere and is common to both sarcomeres that it separates. Actin filaments project from the Z line into the sarcomeres that it separates (Fig. 3.7B). Thus, each sarcomere has actin filaments projected toward its center from each end. The actin of two sarcomeres common to the same Z line comprise an I band. The myosin filaments are centrally located within a sarcomere and, coupled with the overlap of actin filaments, provide for the dark banding (A band) of the characteristic striations (Fig. 3.8). The actin and myosin filaments have a regular, spatial arrangement to each other, as shown in the cross section of a myofibril (Fig. 3.7C),

Figure 3.8. Photomicrograph of a longitudinal section of a skeletal muscle fiber. Shown is the characteristic banding. From Cormack DC. Ham's histology. 9th ed. Philadelphia: JB Lippincott, 1987.

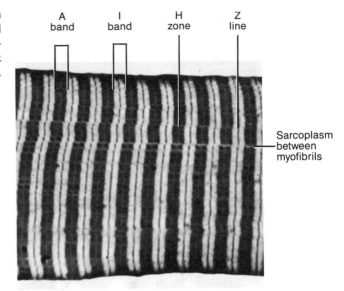

which has a 2:1 ratio of actin to myosin. A longitudinal section of the spatially arranged myofilaments shows cross linkages extending from the myosin filaments toward the actin filaments (Fig. 3.7D). During muscle fiber shortening, the actin filaments appear to slide deeper into the myosin filaments.

Sarcotubular System

Skeletal muscle fibers contain a network of tubules known as the sarcotubular system. These tubules are located within the muscle fiber but are outside the myofibrils. The sarcotubular system is composed of two separate tubule sets, with each set having a different arrangement among the myofibrils (Figs. 3.9 and 3.10). The tubules that are arranged parallel to the myofibrils and encircle them are known as the sarcoplasmic reticulum. The tubules that are arranged transversely (right angles) to the myofibrils are known as the T tubules. T tubules extend transversely from one side of the fiber to the other. They open to the outside of the fiber, and therefore their lumens contain extracellular fluid. The T-tubule openings are regularly spaced throughout the length of the muscle fiber

because of their orientation to each sarcomere. Similarly, their openings are regularly spaced around the circumference of the fiber so that all myofibrils are intimately served by the sarcotubular system.

In reference to a sarcomere, the T-tubules are located near the junction of the actin filaments with the myosin filaments. Therefore, each sarcomere is in close proximity to two T tubules (Fig. 3.10). The individual tubules of the sarcoplasmic reticulum are located regularly throughout the length of the muscle fiber between the T tubules, and they in turn contain intracellular fluid. The T tubules do not open into the sarcoplasmic reticulum; instead, the bulbous ends of the sarcoplasmic reticulum are associated closely with the T tubules. The point of closeness of a T tubule with the bulbous ends of two adjoining sarcoplasmic reticula is known as a triad. The principal function of the sarcotubular system is to provide a means for conduction of an impulse from the surface of the muscle fiber to its innermost aspects.

Neuromuscular Junction

Each skeletal muscle fiber is provided with one specialized area, the neuromuscu-

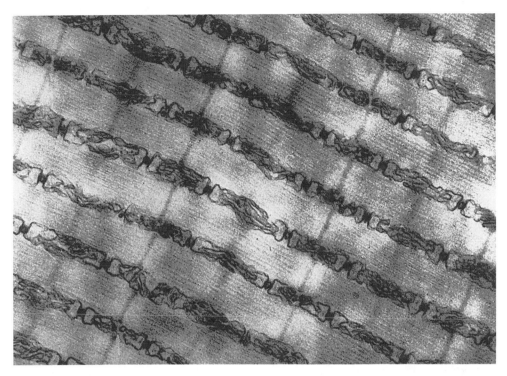

Figure 3.9. Longitudinal section of sarcoplasmic reticulum that surrounds myofibrils. The cross section of T tubules, which are at right angles to the sarcoplasmic reticulum, appear as circular structures between the bulbous ends of each sarcoplasmic reticulum. From Fawcett DW. The cell. 2nd ed. Philadelphia: WB Saunders, 1981.

lar junction. This junction is the intimate association of the terminal branch of a nerve fiber with the muscle fiber (Fig. 3.11). The nerve fiber ending is not continuous with the muscle fiber—there is a space between the neuromuscular junction and the muscle fiber. This space is centrally located on the surface of the muscle fiber. A nerve fiber can have a number of terminal branches, with each one going to a separate muscle fiber (Fig. 3.12). A motor unit consists of a nerve fiber and the muscle fibers that it innervates. A motor unit ratio of 1:150 means that one nerve fiber is innervating 150 muscle fibers, whereas a ratio of 1:4 means that one nerve fiber is innervating four muscle fibers. Hypothetically, a smaller ratio is helpful if greater precision is required for muscle contraction.

SKELETAL MUSCLE CONTRACTION

Depolarization of Muscle Fibers

The neuromuscular junction functions as an amplifier for a nerve impulse. The arrival of a spinal or cranial nerve impulse at the neuromuscular junction results in the release of acetylcholine (ACh) into the space between the nerve fiber terminal branch and the muscle fiber. The release of ACh is accelerated because calcium ions from the extracellular fluid enter the prejunctional membrane when the nerve impulse arrives. ACh is the stimulus that increases the permeability of the muscle fiber membrane for sodium ions, after which membrane depolarization begins. Depolarization proceeds in all directions

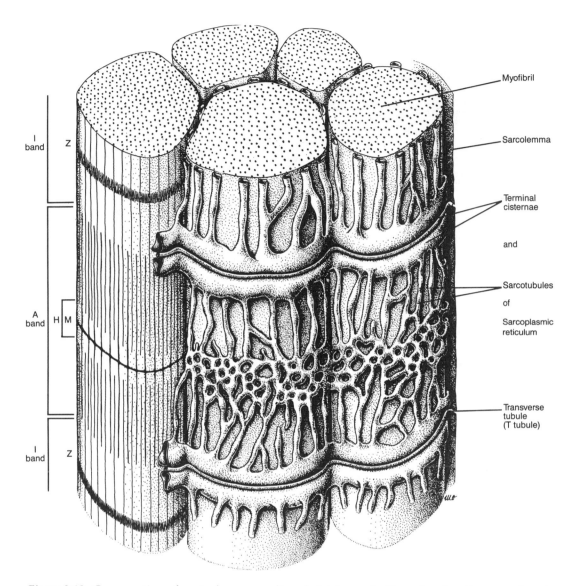

I band — Z

A band — H M

I band — Z

Myofibril

Sarcolemma

Terminal cisternae

and

Sarcotubules of Sarcoplasmic reticulum

Transverse tubule (T tubule)

Figure 3.10. Cross section of part of a mammalian skeletal muscle fiber, showing the sarcoplasmic reticulum that surrounds myofibrils. Two transverse (T) tubules supply a sarcomere and are in close association with the sarcoplasmic reticulum. The T tubules open to the surface of the myofibril. From Cormack DC. Ham's histology. 9th ed. Philadelphia: JB Lippincott, 1987.

from the neuromuscular junction, and an impulse is generated. The impulse is conducted into all parts of the muscle fiber by the sarcotubular system (see previous text). Because the impulse initiates muscle contraction, a more synchronized contraction results when all parts of the fiber are depo-larized nearly simultaneously as a result of sarcotubular transmission.

A low concentration of calcium in the extracellular fluid is recognized clinically in dairy cows after calving (parturient paresis, or milk fever) as a state of semi-paralysis caused by partial neuromuscular

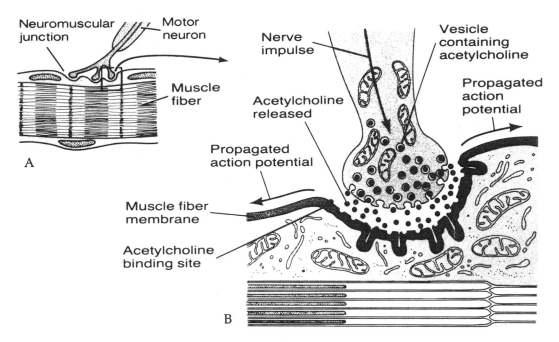

Figure 3.11. A neuromuscular junction. **A.** General structure. **B.** Magnification of junctional area showing the events that occur following nerve impulse transmission. From Spence A, Mason EB. Human anatomy and physiology. 2nd ed. Redwood City, CA: Benjamin-Cummings, 1983.

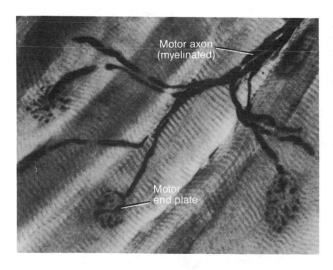

Figure 3.12. Photomicrograph showing the distribution of terminal branches from a nerve fiber to individual muscle fibers to comprise a motor unit. A motor end-plate is a small, flattened mound on the muscle fiber surface formed by the axon terminal branch and its myelin covering. From Cormack DC. Ham's histology. 9th ed. Philadelphia: JB Lippincott, 1987.

block. When the calcium ion concentration is low, the amount of ACh released is lowered; this might not be sufficient to cause neuromuscular transmission and thus neuromuscular block results.

Almost immediately after its release, ACh is hydrolyzed by the enzyme acetyl-cholinesterase into acetic acid and choline. Therefore, the next depolarization must await the arrival of the next nerve impulse.

The tubules of the sarcoplasmic reticulum have a relatively high concentration of calcium ions. Depolarization of these tubules results in a simultaneous release of

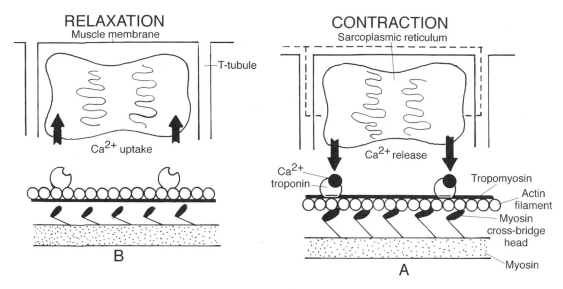

Figure 3.13. A cycle of contraction followed by relaxation. **A.** The dashed line indicates transfer of depolarization to the sarcoplasmic reticulum. Depolarization is followed by Ca^{2+} release with diffusion to the myofibrils. Ca^{2+} binds to troponin, removing blocking action of tropomyosin. Myosin cross-bridge heads attach to active sites on actin and bend toward center of myosin molecule. **B.** ATP binds to cross-bridge heads causing their detachment from actin. Ca^{2+} is returned to the sarcoplasmic reticulum using energy supplied by ATP. Removal of CA^{2+} from troponin restores blocking action of tropomyosin.

calcium ions into the sarcoplasm, which in turn diffuse rapidly into the myofibrils (Fig. 3.13). The presence of calcium ions within the myofibrils initiates the contraction process. The calcium ions are returned rapidly by active transport to the sarcoplasmic reticulum after contraction is initiated and are released again when the next nerve impulse arrives.

Contraction Process

The shortening, or contraction, process involves an interaction between the actin and myosin filaments. There is a natural attraction for actin and myosin molecules involving active sites on the actin molecule. Attraction is inhibited during relaxation because the active sites are covered, but when calcium ions enter the myofibril, the active sites are uncovered. The projecting portions of the myosin molecules (cross bridges) attach to the active sites and bend toward the

center, causing the actin to slide toward the myosin molecule center (Fig. 3.14).

The actin filament has three major components (all protein)—actin, tropomyosin, and troponin (Fig. 3.15). Actin and tropomyosin are arranged in helical strands interwoven with each other. Troponin is located at regular intervals along the strands and contains three proteins, two of which bind actin and tropomyosin together and the third of which has an affinity for calcium ions. Active sites (places where myosin cross bridges attach) are located on the actin strands and are normally covered by the tropomyosin strands. When calcium ions bind to the troponin complex, however, it is believed that a conformational change occurs between the actin and tropomyosin strands and causes the active sites to be uncovered. The uncovered sites favor activation of the natural attraction that exists

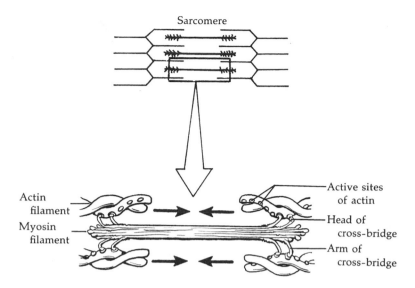

Figure 3.14. The components of the actin and myosin myofilaments associated with contraction of the sarcomere. Arrows indicate the direction of actin movement during contraction (shortening of myofibrils).

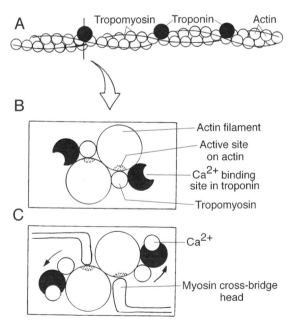

Figure 3.15. Conformational changes of the actin filament after calcium binding. **A.** The actin filament with its three proteins, actin, troponin, and tropomyosin. The vertical line indicates the cross-section location for **B** and **C. B.** The active sites on actin are covered by tropomyosin. **C.** Ca^{2+} binds to troponin resulting in a conformational change that exposes the active sites on actin. Myosin cross-bridge heads attach to actin active sites, and myofibril contraction begins.

between actin and myosin. A number of changes occur in the heads of the myosin cross-bridges that cause muscle contraction and these are summarized as follows (Fig. 3.16) (assume that cross-bridge heads have just bound with adenosine triphosphate (ATP) and have detached from the active sites of the actin filaments):

1. Adenosine triphosphatase (ATPase) of the myosin cross-bridge heads hydro-

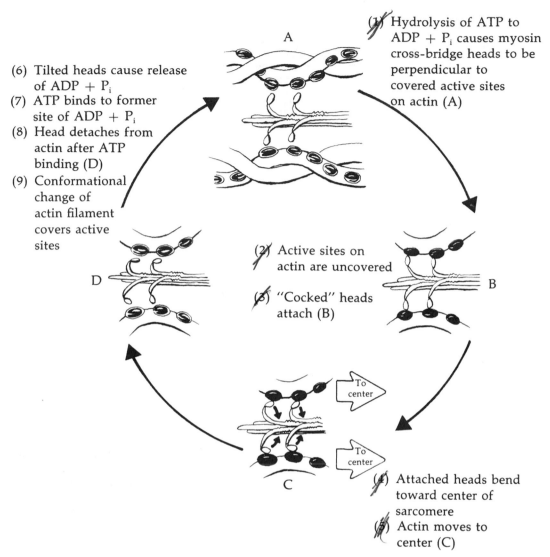

(6) Tilted heads cause release of ADP + P$_i$
(7) ATP binds to former site of ADP + P$_i$
(8) Head detaches from actin after ATP binding (D)
(9) Conformational change of actin filament covers active sites

(1) Hydrolysis of ATP to ADP + P$_i$ causes myosin cross-bridge heads to be perpendicular to covered active sites on actin (A)

(2) Active sites on actin are uncovered

(3) "Cocked" heads attach (B)

(4) Attached heads bend toward center of sarcomere
(5) Actin moves to center (C)

To center

To center

Figure 3.16. The sequence of actin and myosin interaction. This results in muscle shortening.

lyze ATP to adenosine diphosphate (ADP) + inorganic phosphorus (P$_i$), leaving the ADP + P$_i$ bound to the heads.

2. Energy from the hydrolysis of ATP "cocks" the heads so that they increase their angle of attachment to the cross-bridge arm and become perpendicular to the active sites of the actin filaments.

3. After depolarization of the sarco-tubular system, calcium ions diffuse from sarcoplasmic reticulum into myofibrils and bind to the troponin complexes, whereby actin filament active sites are uncovered; calcium ions are returned rapidly to sarcoplasmic reticulum once the short-ening process begins (ATP required for return).

4. Natural attraction of myosin to actin is now permitted, and the "cocked" heads bind with active sites.

5. Bonds with actin cause conformational change in heads ("uncocking"), causing them to bend (tilt) toward cross-bridge arms (toward center of sarcomere), pulling actin with it (energy derived from previous ATP hydrolysis).

6. Tilted heads cause release of ADP + P_i and expose sites on heads for binding of new ATP.

7. Binding of new ATP causes detachment of myosin cross-bridge heads from actin filaments.

8. ATPase of heads hydrolyzes ATP as before, cocking the heads; process is repeated when the next neuromuscular transmission causes depolarization of the sarcotubular system.

9. Repetition of the process causes the actin filaments to be pulled further into the center, thus shortening the sarcomere.

The immediate energy for muscle contraction is thus derived from ATP, forming ADP + P_i. The amount of ATP in muscle fibers is limited, and rephosphorylation of ADP must occur so that contraction can continue. This is accomplished by transfer from creatine phosphate (CP), which is about five times more plentiful than ATP, according to the following reaction:

$$CP + ADP \xrightarrow{kinase} C + ATP$$

Because the amount of CP is also limited, the necessary rephosphorylation of creatine (C) and ADP is ultimately derived from intermediary metabolism within the muscle cell and from the associated reoxidation of reduced cofactors that occurs in the electron transport chain of the mitochondria. The presence of ATP is required for relaxation, or detachment of the myosin from the actin, and also for the return of calcium ions to the sarcoplasmic reticulum.

Muscle contraction is only about 25% efficient in regard to the accomplishment of work. The nonwork portion is dissipated as heat. This heat source is important to the body for the maintenance of body heat. Body cooling results in shivering, which is an attempt by the body to generate heat by muscle contraction.

Contraction Versus Contracture

Muscle shortening can occur in the absence of action potentials. This type of shortening is referred to as rigor or physiologic contracture, as opposed to contraction. The actin and myosin filaments remain in a continuous contracted state because sufficient ATP is not available to bring about relaxation (see previous section). Contracture that occurs after death is referred to as rigor mortis. Lack of ATP for relaxation in this case endures, however, and relaxation only occurs as a result of postmortem autolysis caused by enzymes released from the lysosomes 12 to 24 hours after death. Those muscles that were most active just before death are those that develop rigor mortis first (i.e., greater exhaustion of ATP and CP associated with greater activity).

Contraction Strength

Contraction strength varies and is achieved by multiple motor unit summation or by wave summation. The stimulation of one motor unit causes a weak contraction, whereas the stimulation of a large number of motor units develops a strong contraction. This is known as motor unit summation. All gradations of contraction strength are possible, depending on the number of motor units stimulated. Increasing the strength of contraction by wave summation occurs when the frequency of contraction is increased. When a muscle is stimulated to contract before the muscle has relaxed, the strength of the subsequent contraction, as measured by the height of a lifted load, is

Figure 3.17. Increasing muscle strength by increasing the frequency of contraction. This is known as wave summation. Tetany occurs when individual contractions are fused and cannot be distinguished from each other. From Carlson AJ, Johnson V. The machinery of the body. 4th ed. Chicago: University of Chicago Press, 1953.

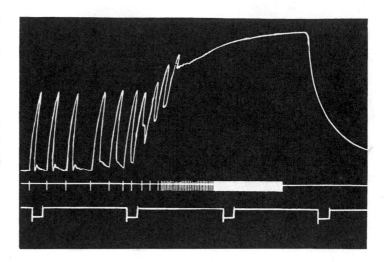

increased. When the frequency is sufficient such that the individual muscle twitches become fused into a single prolonged contraction, the strength is at a maximum; this condition is known as tetany (Fig. 3.17).

TETANUS Tetanus is a bacterial disease caused by a potent neurotoxin elaborated by the organism *Clostridium tetani*. The neurotoxin reaches the central nervous system and prevents release of an inhibitory transmitter (glycine). The resulting sensitivity to excitatory impulses, unchecked by inhibitory impulses, produces generalized muscular spasms (tetany). Tetanus has been called lockjaw because the masseter muscles that close the mouth are stronger than the muscles that open the mouth and the jaws remain in a closed (locked) position.

TREPPE Muscles appear to "warm up" to a maximum contraction state. This can be demonstrated by applying stimuli of equal intensity a few seconds apart to muscle. Each successive muscle twitch has slightly more strength than the previous one, until optimal contraction strength is reached (Fig. 3.18). This phenomenon is referred to as treppe, or the staircase phenomenon. Successive stimulations are believed to provide for an increasing concentration of calcium ions in the sar-coplasm during the beginning contractions of rested muscles.

Comparison of Contraction Among the Three Muscle Types

Brief structural differences among the three muscle classifications were noted earlier. The contraction process for all three is generally similar in that actin filaments slide between myosin filaments and cause a shortening of the cell. There is a greater similarity in arrangement of these filaments between cardiac and skeletal muscle (hence, their common description as striated muscle). The myofibrils of cardiac muscle constitute most of the muscle fiber, but instead of being discrete and cylindric, as in skeletal muscle, they join together and are of variable diameter. This might be related to the more circular contraction of the heart (cardiac muscle) as compared to the more linear contraction of skeletal muscle.

Whereas the work of skeletal muscle fibers is harnessed to connective tissue elements, cardiac muscle fibers anastomose with each other. Thus, the contraction of each joins with others to decrease the diameter of their respective heart chamber. Also, each skeletal muscle fiber receives separate stimulation through a spinal or cranial

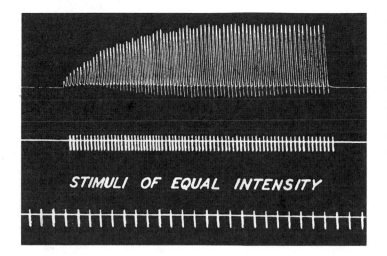

Figure 3.18. The staircase phenomenon of skeletal muscle. This is also known as treppe. Successive stimuli of the same intensity produce contractions of increasing strength. From Carlson AJ, Johnson V. The machinery of the body. 4th ed. Chicago: University of Chicago Press, 1953.

STIMULI OF EQUAL INTENSITY

nerve and neuromuscular junction, but cardiac muscle receives its stimulus from rhythmic, contractile, and specialized cardiac muscle cells known as pacemakers. The autonomic nervous system regulates the pacemakers. Conduction of stimulation is from cell to cell (through the intercalated disk) and from special conduction fibers (Purkinje fibers in the ventricular walls). The sarcotubular system of cardiac muscle is not as well developed as that of skeletal muscle.

Smooth muscle myofilaments are not aligned into myofibrils, as in cardiac and skeletal muscles. Furthermore, a higher ratio of actin to myosin exists (15:1 instead of 2:1). The actin filaments are attached to dense bodies, which are dispersed inside the cell, and some are also attached to the cell membrane. The dense bodies correspond to the Z lines of skeletal muscle and are held in place by a framework of structural proteins that link one dense body to another. The actin filaments from two separate dense bodies extend toward each other and surround a myosin filament, thereby providing a contractile unit that is similar to a contractile unit of skeletal muscle (Fig. 3.19).

There also are differences between the contraction of smooth muscle and striated muscle. The cycle of attachment and detachment of cross-bridge heads that extend from myosin to actin is much slower in smooth muscle. This provides for prolonged tonic contraction in contrast to rapid contractions of skeletal muscle. The slower cycles are a result of the much lower ATPase activity on the myosin cross-bridge heads than in skeletal muscle, and the heads remain in an "uncocked" position for a longer time. Coupled with the slower frequency of attachment-detachment cycling is the lower energy requirement for sustaining the same tension of contraction in smooth muscle as in skeletal muscle. This is important from the standpoint of energy conservation wherein smooth muscle organs (e.g., urinary bladder, intestines) must maintain tone throughout the day and night.

Smooth muscle cells are able to shorten a much greater percentage of their total length than skeletal muscle. This feature enables a smooth muscle organ, such as the urinary bladder, to reduce its lumen diameter from its expanded state to virtually zero.

The neuromuscular junctions associated with smooth muscle are diffuse junctions. The autonomic nerve fibers that innervate smooth muscle do not make direct contact with the muscle fibers but form diffuse junctions that secrete their transmitter substance into the interstitial fluid whereupon

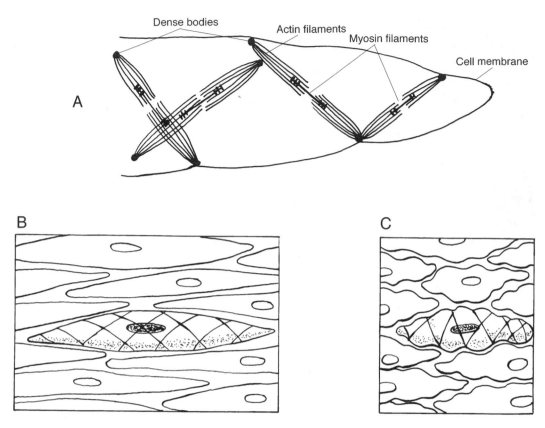

Figure 3.19. Contraction of smooth muscle. **A**. Physical structure of smooth muscle. Dense bodies attach either to the cell membrane or to an intracellular structural protein that links several dense bodies together. The dense bodies are functionally similar to Z lines. **B**. A translucent view of a relaxed smooth muscle cell. **C**. A translucent view of a contracted smooth muscle cell.

it diffuses to the smooth muscle cells. The vesicles of the terminal axons contain either ACh or norepinephrine, depending on whether the postganglionic terminal fiber is parasympathetic or sympathetic, respectively. The vesicle secretion may be excitatory or inhibitory depending on the receptors that are located on the smooth muscle membrane. The receptors determine whether the smooth muscle will be excited or inhibited and also which one of the two transmitters will be effective in causing the excitatory or inhibitory response. The sarcotubular system of smooth muscle fibers is poorly developed. Counterparts to the T tubules are vesicles just under the cell membrane that open onto the surface of the fiber.

CHANGES IN MUSCLE SIZE

Hypertrophy and Hyperplasia

An increase in individual muscle fiber size is referred to as hypertrophy. It is common in skeletal, cardiac, and smooth muscle cells. Postnatal growth of skeletal muscle fibers is not accomplished by an increase in the number of muscle fibers but rather by the addition of myofibrils to the periphery and of sarcomeres to the tendinous ends. An increase in the number of muscle fibers is called hyperplasia. Regeneration of skeletal muscle fibers is possible from so-called satellite cells, but this requires an intact endomysium for successful repair. An increase in cardiac muscle size is similar to that of skeletal muscles in that it involves hypertrophy and not hyperplasia. Regeneration of cardiac muscle fibers does not occur. Smooth muscle organs can increase their size by hypertrophy and by hyperplasia, so smooth muscle has considerable regenerative ability.

Atrophy

A decrease in the size of a muscle is referred to as atrophy. When a body part has been immobilized for a period of time, the muscles become smaller (referred to as disuse atrophy). Loss of the nerve supply to a muscle results in denervation atrophy. This was formerly a common condition in harnessed draft horses. The presence of the collar presses on the suprascapular nerve that supplies the two major muscle masses of the shoulder blade. The resulting denervation causes the muscles of the shoulder to atrophy, resulting in a condition known as sweeny (also called shoulder slip).

STUDY AIDS—MUSCLE

Classification, Arrangement, Harnessing

1. What kinds of nerves are associated with the activity of smooth, cardiac, and skeletal muscle?
2. What is the principal distinguishing characteristic between smooth muscle and cardiac and skeletal muscle?
3. What is the function of an intercalated disc in cardiac muscle?
4. What is the functional difference between red and white skeletal muscle fibers?
5. What is the difference between an adductor and an abductor skeletal muscle?
6. What is the difference between the origin and insertion of a skeletal muscle?
7. Differentiate between epimysium, perimysium, and endomysium. Which of these is associated most intimately with individual muscle fibers?

Microstructure of Skeletal Muscles

1. Is a muscle fiber the same as a muscle cell?
2. Understand the division of a muscle fiber into myofibrils; myofibrils into sarcomeres; sarcomeres into myofilaments; and myofilaments into actin and myosin.
3. Be able to sketch a sarcomere and the spatial arrangement of the myofilaments.
4. Relate the striations (banding) of skeletal muscle to the myofilaments.
5. Which tubule set of the sarcotubular system opens to the outside of the muscle fiber and contains extracellular fluid?
6. What is the location of the sarcoplasmic reticulum relative to T tubules and myofibrils?
7. What is the function of the sarcotubular system?
8. What is a neuromuscular junction and how many are there for each muscle fiber?
9. What is a motor unit?

Skeletal Muscle Contraction

1. Describe the chain of events that initiate muscle fiber membrane depolarization.
2. What is the association of Ca^{2+} to ACH release? How is this related to milk fever in dairy cows?
3. What is the trigger for release of Ca^{2+} from the sarcoplasmic reticulum? Where do the Ca^{2+} go following their release?
4. Study the molecular basis of muscle contraction with emphasis on sequence and relate to shortening and relaxation of muscle fibers.
5. What molecule appears to be necessary for relaxation?
6. What causes rigor mortis?
7. What is muscle tetany? Is this a reflection of motor unit or wave summation?
8. How is the bacterial disease tetanus related to CNS neurotransmitters?

9. What characteristic of muscle contraction is generally similar among smooth, cardiac, and skeletal muscle fibers?
10. Differentiate harnessing, innervation, and stimulus conduction between cardiac and skeletal muscle.
11. Do smooth muscle fibers have actin and myosin, a neuromuscular junction, a harnessing system, and a sarcotubular system?
12. What is the difference between hyperplasia and hypertrophy?
13. How do skeletal muscle fibers hypertrophy (grow in size) after birth?
14. Is regeneration of skeletal, cardiac, and smooth muscle fibers possible?
15. What is muscle atrophy?

SELF-EVALUATION—MUSCLE

1. Muscle fibers that contract more slowly and fatigue less readily are:
   a. red fibers
   b. white fibers
2. In skeletal muscle fibers, the sarcomeres of a myofibril are in alignment with the sarcomeres of all the other myofibrils.
   a. true
   b. false
3. Which tubule set of the sarcotubular system releases Ca^{2+}, when depolarized, for their diffusion to the myofibrils?
   a. transverse tubules
   b. sarcoplasmic reticulum
4. What chemical substance is released from vesicles at the neuromuscular junction upon the arrival of a nerve impulse?
   a. succinylcholine
   b. epinephrine
   c. acetylcholine
   d. curare
5. Which one of the following is the smallest component of a skeletal muscle?
   a. sarcomere
   b. myosin
   c. myofibril
   d. muscle fiber

6. Rigor mortis most probably occurs when:
   a. actin and myosin are detached
   b. Ca^{2+} is depleted
   c. insufficient ATP is available for relaxation
   d. contraction frequency is rapid and sustained
7. The sarcotubular system:
   a. is located within muscle fibers but outside of the myofibrils
   b. is a system within each of the myofibrils
   c. has no direct communication (openings) with extracellular fluid (ECF)
   d. consists of a nerve fiber and the muscle fibers that it innervates
8. The function of Ca^{2+} at the level of myofilaments is to:
   a. uncover active sites on actin so that the "cocked" projections of myosin may make an attachment
   b. depolarize the muscle fiber membrane
   c. initiate acetylcholine release
   d. block pores to prevent Na^+ inrush
9. The refractory period for a nerve or muscle fiber refers to:
   a. the time period of depolarization
   b. the time period when they may again be stimulated
   c. the total time period of the action potential
   d. the time period when they can not be stimulated no matter how strong the stimulus
10. Muscles showing an increase in size of their individual muscle fibers are said to have undergone:
    a. atrophy
    b. treppe
    c. hypertrophy
    d. gangrene
11. Conduction of depolarization from the surface of a muscle fiber to its inner aspects is accomplished by the:
    a. neuromuscular junction
    b. actin filaments
    c. endomysium
  — d. sarcotubular system

12. The skeletal muscle harness component most intimately associated with the sarcolemma is the:
    a. endomysium
    b. perimysium
    c. epimysium

13. A pelvic delivery of an unusually large calf has caused a cow to be down and unable to bring her hind legs together. Obturator nerve paralysis is suspected and the affected muscles are classified as:
    a. abductors
    b. adductors
    c. extensors
    d. flexors

14. What chemical begins the depolarization of skeletal muscle fibers after a nerve impulse initiates its release?
    a. Ca^{2+}
    b. acetylcholine
    c. succinylcholine
    d. acetylcholinesterase

15. After depolarization of the sarcoplasmic reticulum, what chemical is released that initiates the contraction process?
    a. ATP
    b. tropomyosin
    c. Ca^{2+}
    d. ACh

16. Increased muscle strength associated with tetany is an example of:
    a. wave summation
    b. motor unit summation
    c. *Clostridium tetani* neurotoxin activity

17. Myosin cross-bridge heads detach from actin active sites when the cross-bridge heads bind:
    a. Ca^{2+}
    b. ATP
    c. creatine phosphate
    d. $ADP + P_i$

18. Rigor mortis is an example of _____ that results from a depletion of _____ and a failure of cross-bridge heads to _____ to/from actin. (Select choice below that has respective words for blanks above.)
    a. contraction; Ca^{2+}; attach
    b. relaxation, Ca^{2+}; attach
    c. contracture; ATP; detach
    d. contraction; ATP; detach

19. Muscle tone:
    a. is a state of complete muscle relaxation
    b. is a state of muscle tension (contraction) that enables an animal to assume and remain in an erect position
    c. refers to the sound made by contracting muscle
    d. is an autonomic nervous system function

20. Cardiac muscle cells have separations between adjacent cells known as intercalated discs. Their function is to:
    a. regenerate new cells
    b. provide a location for neuromuscular junctions
    c. provide for low electrical resistance and thus facilitate depolarization from one cell to the next
    d. release Ca^{2+} for initiation of muscle contraction

21. The Ca^{2+} that is released begins the contraction process by:
    a. "cocking" the myosin filament crossbridge heads
    b. rephosphorylating ADP
    c. exposing actin filament crossbridge binding sites
    d. facilitating ACH release from the neuromuscular junction

22. Dense bodies (correspond to Z lines) and intermediate filament bundles are associated with shortening of the longitudinal axis of:
    a. smooth muscle cells
    b. skeletal muscle cells
    c. cardiac muscle cells

SUGGESTED READINGS

Carlson AJ, Johnson V. The machinery of the body. 4th ed. Chicago: University of Chicago Press, 1953.

Cormack DC. Ham's histology. 9th ed. Philadelphia: JB Lippincott, 1987.

Fawcett DW. The cell. 2nd ed. Philadelphia: WB Saunders, 1981.

Feduccia A, McCrady E. Torrey's morphogenesis of the vertebrates. 5th ed. New York: John Wiley & Sons, 1991.

Guyton AC. Textbook of medical physiology. 8th ed. Philadelphia: WB Saunders, 1991.

Kelley DE, Wood RL, Enders AC. Bailey's textbook of microscopic anatomy. 18th ed. Baltimore: Williams & Wilkins, 1984.

Spence AP, Mason EB. Human anatomy and physiology. 4th ed. St. Paul, MN: West Publishing, 1992.

Vander AJ, Sherman JH, Luciano DS. Human physiology: the mechanisms of body function, 6th ed. New York: McGraw-Hill, 1994.

Bones, Joints, and Synovial Fluid

Bones are cellular structures whereby the extracellular fluid environment of the cell is surrounded by a rigid, calcified frame. The framework of one bone, when combined with all the other bones of the body, comprises what is commonly known as the skeleton. The skeleton gives an identifiable form to the body of an animal and provides protection to the cranial, thoracic, abdominal, and pelvic viscera. Also, the medullary cavity of the bones is the principal location of blood formation, and the calcified regions act as a "sink" and a "source" for many of the needed minerals (cations and anions). Because of the attachment of muscles to bones, movement of the body parts is enabled. Bones are dynamic structures that are capable of accommodating to different loads and stresses by remodeling their shape. Also, function can be restored to broken bones (fractures) by the process of bone repair after appropriate fixation (alignment) of the bone parts.

An important aspect of bone study is the movable union between two bones, known as a joint. This union is enclosed by a joint capsule. The inner aspect of the joint capsule is lined with a synovial membrane, which produces synovial fluid that provides for lubrication and nutrition of the joint surface.

The physiology of bones, joints, and synovial fluid is important, not only because of the association of bones with other body systems, but also because bone and joint diseases are frequently encountered in animals.

Structure and Function

The bones of the body are generally similar among the animals but vary according to size, shape, and number. The skeleton of the horse (Fig. 4.1) is shown as an example that features the general arrangement of the bones with each other. The bones of the

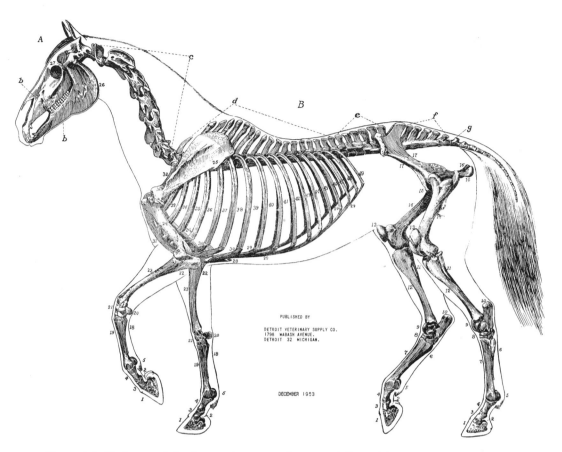

Figure 4.1. Skeleton of the horse. Anatomical names followed by common names in parenthesis (where present) are referenced to the numbers and letters on the illustration. 1. Distal phalanx (coffin bone). 2. Distal sesamoid (navicular bone). 3. Middle phalanx (short pastern bone). 4. Proximal phalanx (long pastern bone). 5. Proximal sesamoid. 6. Metatarsal II (medial small metatarsal or splint bone). 7. Metatarsal III (large metatarsal or cannon bone). 8. Central and third tarsal bones. 9. Talus. 10. Calcaneal tuber. 11. Fibula. 12. Tibia. 13. Patella. 14. Femur. 15. Pubis. 16. Ischial tuber. 17. Ilium. 18. Metacarpal II (medial small metacarpal or splint bone). 19. Metacarpal IV (lateral small metacarpal or splint bone). 20 and 21. Carpal bones (carpus). 22. Ulna. 23. Radius. 24. Humerus. 25. Scapula. 26. Mandible (ramus). 27. Skull. 28. Xiphoid cartilage. 29. Costal arch. 30. Costal cartilages of true ribs. 31. Sternum. 32-39. Ribs (true ribs). 40-49. Ribs (false ribs). A. Head. B. Trunk. b. Maxilla (upper jaw) and mandible (lower jaw). c. Cervical vertebrae. d. Thoracic vertebrae. e. Lumbar vertebrae. f. Sacrum (sacral vertebrae). g. Caudal vertebrae.

skeleton are classified as belonging to either the axial skeleton or appendicular skeleton. Those of the axial skeleton lie on the long axis (midline) of the body and include the skull, vertebrae, and those bones attached to the vertebrae (the ribs) and the ventral connection of the ribs (the sternum). The appendicular skeleton is made up of the bones of the front (pectoral) and hind (pelvic) limbs and their respective pectoral girdle (shoulder) and pelvic girdle (pelvis). The pectoral girdle is composed of the scapula, clavicle, and coracoid, and the pelvic girdle is composed of the ilium, ischium, and pubis.

The structure of a long bone (e.g., the femur) is shown in Figure 4.2. A longitudi-

nal section is shown to reveal its inner structure. Compact and spongy characteristics are noted. Compact bone appears to be solid, whereas spongy bone (also called cancellous bone) has the appearance of a sponge. In spongy bone, there are trabeculae (spicules) of mineralized tissue, and the empty spaces between the trabeculae occupy a considerable volume. In living animals, the regions between the trabeculae are filled with bone marrow. The rigidity and strength of long bones is caused not only by the hardness of its compact bone but also by the scaffolding arrangement of the trabeculae, which are generally parallel to lines of maximum stress and therefore act as pillars for stress points (Fig. 4.2). The epiphysis refers to either extremity of a long bone, and the diaphysis is the cylindrical shaft situated between the two epiphyses. The metaphysis is the expanded or flared part of the bone at the ends of the diaphysis. The diaphysis contains the marrow (medullary) cavity that is surrounded by a thick-walled tube of compact bone. The medullary cavity, or bone marrow, is the site of blood cell production. A small amount of spongy bone may line the inner surface of the compact bone. The epiphyses consist chiefly of spongy bone with a thin outer shell of compact bone. The epiphyseal plate (also called physis) is composed of hyaline cartilage and represents the point of growth in a longitudinal direction. Hyaline cartilage is the ordinary type and is so-named because its matrix is a glassy-bluish-white (*hyalos* is the Greek word for glass) and is somewhat translucent. In mature bones, the cartilage has been replaced by bone, and epiphyseal lines remain where the plate last existed. The contact area of the bone that articulates with its neighboring bone at a movable joint is covered with articular cartilage (described later in this chapter).

With the exception of the joint surfaces, all other outer surfaces of the bone are covered with periosteum. The periosteum is

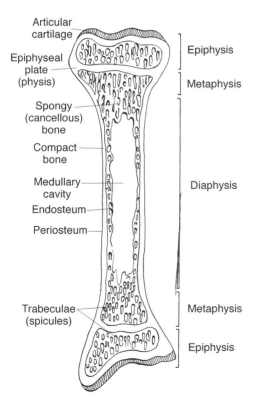

Figure 4.2. The structure of a long bone. The endosteum and periosteum designations refer only to their locations. Note the parallel arrangement of the trabeculae to form scaffolding for maximum strength in response to its assumed load.

composed of an outer fibrous layer and an inner cell-rich layer containing osteoblasts (if bone formation is in progress) or other cells that can become osteoblasts in response to an appropriate stimulus. Osteoblasts synthesize and secrete the organic substance of bone and participate in the mineralization of the organic matrix. The periosteum is responsible for the increase in diameter of bones and also functions in the healing of fractures. The endosteum is the lining tissue of all surfaces of the bone that face the medullary cavity and also of the trabeculae of the spongy bone. It is only one cell thick and the cells can become osteoblasts when stimulated.

Figure 4.3 is a three-dimensional illustration showing the appearance of both a cross section and a longitudinal section of the shaft of a mature long bone. The channels that run parallel to the long axis of the bone are the haversian canals, which contain blood vessels that communicate with blood

vessels serving the external surfaces and marrow cavity. The latter blood vessels are perpendicular to the long-axis of the bone and are contained within Volkmann's canals. The unit of structure of compact bone is the haversian system (also known as an osteon), which consists of a central haversian canal surrounded by concentric layers of bone, the lamellae. Bone cells, the osteocytes, are contained within small cavities known as lacunae (little lakes). The osteocytes communicate with each other and with the haversian canal through a branching network of canals, the canaliculi. The interstitial fluid for the osteocytes is contained within the lacunae and canaliculi. It diffuses through the canalicular network from the blood vessels in the canals for maintenance of the osteocytes. Facilitation of fluid transport may be caused by periodic contraction of the osteocytes. Haversian systems are absent in spongy bone, but concentric lamellae with enclosed lacunae and

Figure 4.3. Three-dimensional view of the shaft of a long bone. From Ham AW. Histology. 1st ed. Philadelphia: JB Lippincott, 1950.

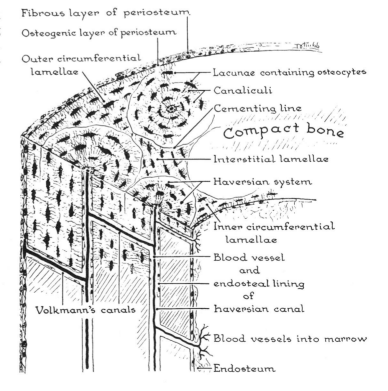

A

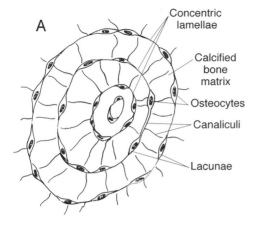

Concentric lamellae

Calcified bone matrix

Osteocytes

Canaliculi

Lacunae

B

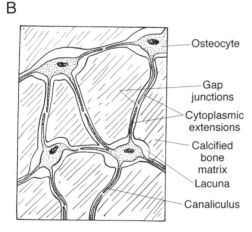

Osteocyte

Gap junctions

Cytoplasmic extensions

Calcified bone matrix

Lacuna

Canaliculus

Figure 4.4. An osteon (haversian system). **A**. Concentric lamellae showing osteocytes within their lacunae and their communicating canaliculi. **B**. Cytoplasmic extensions of osteocytes into canaliculi for communication with other osteocytes

osteocytes with intercommunicating canaliculi are present. In addition to the concentric lamellae that make up the haversian system, other lamellar patterns occur in the form of interstitial lamellae and outer and inner circumferential lamellae. The outer and inner circumferential lamellae are produced by the osteoblasts that cover the outer and inner surfaces of the bone while it is in the process of attaining its full width. During this time, haversian systems develop, and this gives the inner aspect of the outer circumferential lamellae and the outer aspect of the inner circumferential lamellae an interrupted appearance. Their uninter-

rupted aspects, however, gives the outer and inner lamellar surfaces a smooth look. The interstitial lamellae are remnants of older haversian systems or of circumferential lamellae.

Four different types of cells are associated with bone: osteoprogenitor cells, osteoblasts, osteocytes, and osteoclasts. The first of these, osteoprogenitor cells, comprise the population of cells in the innermost layer of the periosteum, the endosteal lining cells of the marrow cavities, and the lining cells of the haversian canals and Volkmann's canals. Their stimulation leads to the more active secretory cell, the osteoblast. Where active bone formation is not occurring, the surfaces are covered by bone lining cells which are analogous to osteoprogenitor cells except that they represent a more quiescent state.

The osteoblast is the differentiated bone-forming cell responsible for the production of bone matrix. Its secretion of collagen and ground substance makes up the initial unmineralized bone or osteoid. The osteoblast is also associated with calcification of the matrix.

The osteocyte is the mature bone cell and represents a transformed osteoblast. It is enclosed by the bone matrix that it had previously laid down as osteoid when it was an osteoblast. Osteocytes maintain the bone matrix and are able to synthesize and resorb matrix to a limited extent. They extend their cytoplasmic processes through the canaliculi to contact, by means of gap junctions, similar processes of neighboring cells. The gap junctions have a low electrical resistance that permit ionic and small molecule flow between cells. Communication among the osteocytes is thus possible, such that the outermost cells, as well as those closest to blood vessels, can respond to stimuli (e.g., hormones). The osteocyte is smaller than its previous state as an osteoblast because of reduced perinuclear cytoplasm. The appearance of osteocytes within their calcified bone matrix lacunae and their cytoplasmic extensions into the canaliculi is shown in Figure 4.4.

Osteoclasts are large, motile, often multinucleated bone-resorbing cells. Their precursors are stem cells in blood-producing tissue of bone marrow and spleen. These stem cells differentiate into bone-resorbing monocytes and then fuse with others to form the large multinucleated osteoclasts. Osteoclasts are considered to be members of the diffuse mononuclear phagocyte system (MPS).

Although osteoprogenitor cells, osteoblasts, and osteocytes are featured as distinct cell types, they should be regarded as different functional states of the same cell type.

Composition of Bone

On a wet-weight basis, adult bone is approximately 25% water, 45% mineral, and 30% organic matter. Calcium constitutes about 37% of the mineral content and phosphorus constitutes about 18.5%. On a dry-weight basis, the mineral content is between 65% and 70%, whereas the organic fraction is 30% to 35%. The organic fraction is about 90% collagen which is converted to gelatin when heated in aqueous solution. Several different elements are incorporated in the mineral phase of bone, but the major constituents are calcium and phosphorus.

Bone Formation

Bone formation (ossification) is identified according to the environment in which it is formed as either heteroplastic, endochondral, or intramembranous. Ossification is heteroplastic if it is formed in tissue other than the skeleton. This type occurs with the os penis of some animals and the os cordis of the bovine heart but mostly it is pathologic. Endochondral ossification is that which develops from cartilage. It is preformed mostly in the fetus but continues after birth from cartilage plates located between the metaphysis and epiphysis, and from the periosteum that surrounds the cortex. Most long bones are developed by this method. Intramembranous bone formation is that which is formed without the intervention of cartilage. These bones are preformed in a fibroid membrane which is then infiltrated with osteoid tissue that later becomes calcified. Bones formed by this method are the flat bones of the skull and face, the mandible, and the clavicle. The previously mentioned mechanisms refer only to the manner in which existing bone was originally formed. Remodeling of bone is established on the preexisting bone, and the mechanism of remodeling is identical whether the original bone was formed by endochondral or intramembranous ossification. The sequence of actual bone formation during remodeling consists of osteoblasts laying down osteoid tissue, which is subsequently calcified.

Growth of Long Bones After Birth

Increase in length of a bone depends on the presence of a cartilage plate (epiphyseal plate), wherein four zones are recognized which extend from the epiphysis to the diaphysis (Fig. 4.5). These are termed zones of reserve cartilage (the youngest), proliferation, hypertrophy, and calcified matrix (the oldest). Beyond the zone of calcified matrix are the developing trabeculae that comprise the spongy bone of the metaphyses.

Cartilage does not have a blood supply, and nutrition of the cartilage cells (chondrocytes) depends on diffusion of extracellular fluid from its source to the chondrocytes that lie within their lacunae. Also, unlike osteocytes, chondrocytes are still able to divide after they have become embedded in cartilage matrix. When the chondrocytes from the zone of reserve cartilage undergo division, the chondrocytes become organized into distinct columns, and a zone of proliferation is recognized that is directed towards the

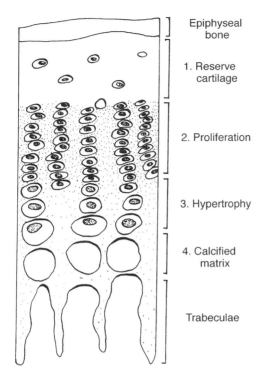

Figure 4.5. The four zones of a cartilage (epiphyseal) plate.

1. Reserve cartilage
2. Proliferation
3. Hypertrophy
4. Calcified matrix

Epiphyseal bone

Trabeculae

hypertrophied cells previously occupied the space between the linear bands of compressed cartilage matrix (now calcified). What are seen as trabeculae (columns) in longitudinal sections, in reality constitute a honeycombed structure in cross-sections, and the spaces seen between the trabeculae in longitudinal sections are seen as tunnels in cross sections.

The tunnels are now invaded from the diaphysis by capillaries, and osteoblasts line up along the sides of the tunnels and deposit bone on their inner surfaces (Fig. 4.6B). The osteoblasts continue to divide whereby each division of osteoblasts pushes the original osteoblast layer closer to the capillary in the center. Concentric lamellae of bone substance are thus established with osteocytes occupying lacunae and canaliculi. After several layers of bone (concentric lamellae) have been deposited, the tunnel is reduced to a narrow canal, which contains a blood vessel, some osteoblasts or osteogenic cells, and perhaps a lymphatic (Fig. 4.6C). This arrangement is known as a haversian system, the unit of structure of compact bone.

While a long bone is growing in length, it is also growing in width. New layers of bone are being added to the outside of the shaft at the same time bone is dissolved away from the inside of the shaft. Although the shaft of the bone becomes wider, its walls do not become unduly thick and the width of the marrow cavity gradually increases. The shaft of a bone grows in width by the appositional mechanism (Fig. 4.7). The periosteum provides the osteogenic layer and by repeated proliferation, new bone is formed to fill in the grooves between the longitudinal ridges of haversian systems that were formed while the bone was elongating. The same process of appositional growth occurs on the inner aspect of the bone shaft from endosteum. The bone formed from the periosteum and endosteum accounts for the outer and inner circumferential lamellae, respectively (Fig. 4.3).

diaphysis. The columns are formed because of chondrocyte capture within lacunae. Each daughter cell within a lacunae produces matrix and this causes the cartilage matrix to expand from within. This has the effect of pushing the epiphysis away from the diaphysis, thus, elongation of the bone.

Each division of chondrocytes brings about larger cells; hence the zone of hypertrophy. This has the effect of compressing the matrix into linear bands between the columns of hypertrophied cells. After several divisions, the hypertrophied cells become further removed from the epiphyseal plate and become active in bringing about calcification of the cartilage matrix. Calcification, coupled with increasing distance from the nutritional source, causes the chondrocytes to die, and the matrix becomes the zone of calcified matrix. A cross-section at this level (Fig. 4.6A) would show that tunnels now exist where nests of

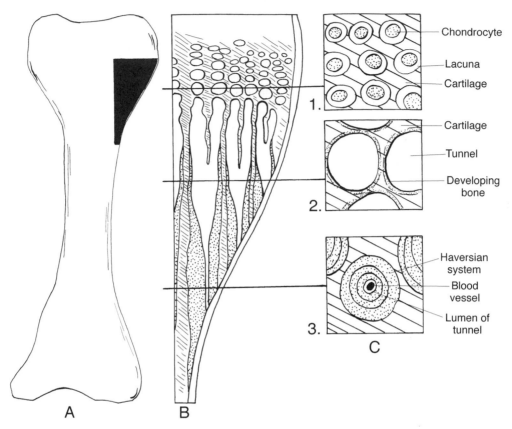

Figure 4.6. Illustrations to show the appearance presented both by longitudinal and by cross-sections of different areas of the epiphyseal plate and metaphysis at the periphery of a growing shaft. **A**. The blackened area is the location on the long bone for illustrations **B** and **C**. **B**. Horizontal lines extend to their respective cross-sections. White areas are tunnels or openings to tunnels. The oblique lines represent cartilage and the stippled structures represent calcified matrix. **C1**. Chondrocytes in their lacunae in the zone of hypertrophy. **C2**. Tunnels formed in the zone of calcified matrix. Trabeculae are composed of both cartilage and bone. **C3**. Haversian system transforming tunnels into compact bone.

Bone Remodeling

As described previously, the growth of bones does not simply involve an increase in their thickness. Rather, there is a coordinated formation of new bone at the outer surfaces and resorption of bone at the inner surfaces (Fig. 4.8). This occurs as well to the bones of the calvarium to accommodate the growing brain during its maturation. In each instance, the two processes of appositional growth and bone resorption are the only ways the shape and size of a bone can change during prenatal and postnatal life.

As this applies to long bones of the body, the shape of the bone does not grossly change during growth, and its marrow cavity is enlarged to assure a sufficient amount for blood cell requirements. During growth, haversian systems are being formed, resorbed, and remodeled. The general process for new haversian systems is initiated generally by osteoclasts concurrent with the invasion of blood vessels (Fig. 4.9). The osteoclasts are on the leading edge of the invading blood vessels. New tunnels are thus formed by erosion through the endosteal surface that are oriented with the

How a layer of bone is formed on a surface. (Appositional growth).

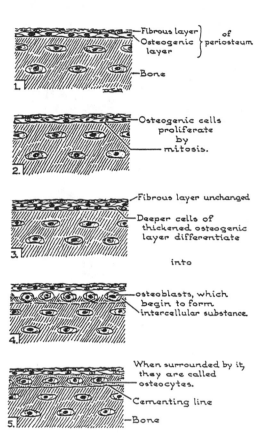

Figure 4.7. Bone growth by apposition. From Ham AW. Histology. 1st ed. Philadelphia: JB Lippincott, 1950.

long axis of the shaft. A layer of osteoblasts forms on the surface of the eroded tunnel (that has a central blood vessel) and concentric lamellae are formed as previously described for haversian systems. The blood vessels grow and branch, with accompanying osteoclast and osteoblast activity, whereby new channels are made and new haversian systems form to fill them.

In addition to the remodeling that occurs to accommodate growth, remodeling also occurs in response to stress placed upon bones. Reduction in bone mass accompanies loss of muscle mass and decreased mobility, whereas an increase in muscle mass and exercise is accompanied by an increase in bone mass. Therefore, the organization of bone changes to meet mechanical and other stresses placed on the skeleton, and it represents a balance between bone formation and bone resorption.

Bone Repair

Bone fractures are the most common consequences of bone injury. Fractures can result in separation of bone parts with loss of alignment, separation of periosteum and endosteum, and severe bleeding that is followed by clot formation. The torn blood vessels can be those that supply Volkmann's canals, haversian systems, and the periosteum and endosteum at the fracture site. In the vicinity of the disrupted blood supply, the osteocytes begin to die and the periosteum and bone marrow become necrotic. The acute inflammatory condition that follows brings phagocytic cells into the area for clearance of blood clot components and necrotic tissue. New blood vessels enter the damaged area and new bone formation begins. Bone formation does not occur until a blood supply has been established.

The most common type of bone repair involves the formation of a callus. This type takes place when the broken ends are not perfectly realigned and stabilized. A collar of repair tissue forms around the external surface of each broken end, and when a bridge is formed across the break, it is known as the external callus. The healthy intact periosteum is the source of the osteogenic cells for the external callus, whereas endosteum is the source for the internal callus. Depending on the richness of the periosteal capillaries, the callus will be composed either of spongy bone or cartilage. Inadequate blood supply predisposes to cartilage formation. When cartilage is formed, it is subsequently replaced by bone. The transformation from cartilage to bone is similar to that previously described for growth of long bones from the epiphyseal plate. The chondrocytes

Figure 4.8. Remodeling of bone. From Cormack DC. Ham's histology. 9th ed. Philadelphia: JB Lippincott, 1987.

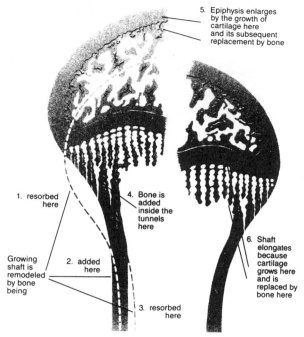

5. Epiphysis enlarges by the growth of cartilage here and its subsequent replacement by bone

1. resorbed here

4. Bone is added inside the tunnels here

6. Shaft elongates because cartilage grows here and is replaced by bone here

Growing shaft is remodeled by bone being

2. added here

3. resorbed here

Figure 4.9. Osteoclastic activity that precedes bone remodeling. Osteoclasts advance a resorption cavity into the bone and are immediately followed by a vascular loop accompanied by precursor cells that multiply and differentiate into osteoblasts. Osteoblasts lay down new layers of osteoid. Canaliculi are formed and osteoblasts become osteocytes. Successive layers of new bone are deposited to give the concentric lamellar rings of haversian bone. From Whittick WG. Canine orthopedics. 2nd ed. Philadelphia: Lea & Febiger, 1990.

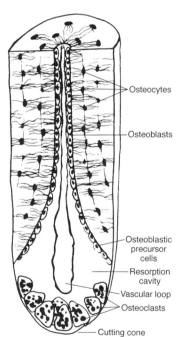

Osteocytes

Osteoblasts

Osteoblastic precursor cells

Resorption cavity

Vascular loop

Osteoclasts

Cutting cone

hypertrophy and the cartilage matrix becomes calcified. The calcified cartilage is removed and replaced with spongy bone after the entrance of blood vessels. Any dead bone that was incorporated into the callus is removed by the action of osteoclasts and is replaced by bone formed by osteoblasts that move into the spaces created by osteoclastic activity. As compact bone is formed at the fracture site, the spongy bone in the periphery of the callus is no longer needed to provide strength, and therefore it is resorbed. Final remodeling occurs when stresses associated with normal use return. A summary of fracture healing is shown in Figure 4.10.

Joints and Synovial Fluid

The connection between any of the skeleton's rigid component parts is known as a joint. These connections are also described as articulations. The study of

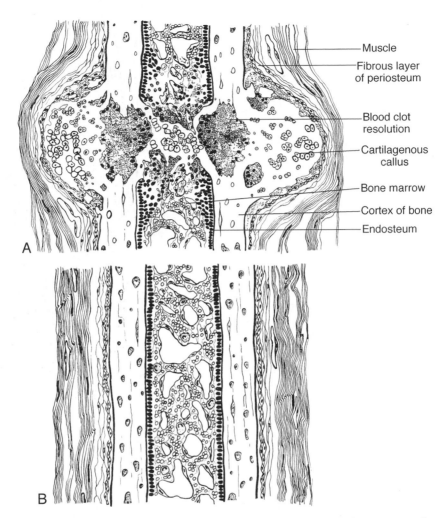

Figure 4.10. Bone fracture repair. **A.** Fracture has been reduced and immobilized. Repair involves the appearance of a palpable callus. A cartilaginous callus precedes the mineralized callus. **B.** Fracture completely healed. The bone has been remodeled to conform to lines of stress. Original fracture site is obliterated. From Whittick WG. Canine orthopedics. 2nd ed. Philadelphia: Lea & Febiger, 1990.

joints is termed arthrology and inflammation of joints is termed arthritis. Arthritis is a common malady among domestic animals; therefore, this brief study of the anatomy and physiology of joints is intended to assist students' understanding of joint diseases.

Synovial joints are those that allow one surface to glide over another (Fig. 4.11). This motion is facilitated by the presence of articular cartilage on each bone surface of the articulation and also by the presence of synovial fluid. The synovial joint is enclosed by a joint capsule. Synovial fluid is contained within the joint capsule and is secreted by its inner membrane, the synovial membrane. The outer layer of the joint capsule is a fibrous layer that extends from the periosteum of each bone and contributes to the stability of the joint. A meniscus within the joint capsule serves a cushioning function.

Synovial Membrane

The synovial membrane is a vascular connective tissue that lines the inner surface of the joint capsule but does not cover the bearing surfaces (the articular cartilage). Synoviocytes within the synovial membrane synthesize synovial fluid by an active, energy-requiring process.

The chief functions of synovial fluid are joint lubrication and nourishment of the articular cartilage. It is a sticky, viscous fluid, often like egg-white in consistency. It is usually slightly alkaline and ranges from colorless to deep yellow. The color and viscosity vary with species and type of joint. Fluid from large joints is usually less viscous than that from small joints. The viscosity of synovial fluid is due almost entirely to hyaluronic acid. Other chemical constituents of synovial fluid are those that are normally present in blood plasma. Synovial fluid normally contains a few cells that are mostly mononuclear. Examination of the cellular and chemical content and physical characteristics can be a valuable diagnostic aid when evaluating joint disease.

Articular Cartilage

Adult articular cartilage is usually hyaline in nature, avascular, aneural, and has an acellular matrix that surrounds a relatively small number of cells called chondrocytes. It is a highly specialized connective tissue with biochemical and biophysical characteristics that enable it to play a dual role as a shock absorber and as a bearing surface. During the growth period, articular cartilage provides the growth zone for endochondral ossification in the epiphysis. During growth, articular cartilage is capable of regeneration and thus repairs defects that may arise. However, when growth ceases, it loses much of its power of repair. Cartilage is a resilient and elastic tissue that becomes thinner when compressed and slowly regains its original thickness when the pressure is released. Intermittent pres-

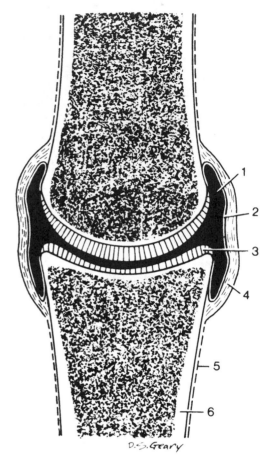

Figure 4.11. Synovial joint in section. 1, Joint cavity; 2, synovial membrane; 3, articular cartilage; 4, fibrous layer of joint capsule; 5, periosteum; 6, compact bone. From Dyce KM, Sack WO, Wensing CJG. Textbook of veterinary anatomy. Philadelphia: WB Saunders, 1987.

sure associated with compression and release of compression causes cartilage to thicken by taking up fluid. Synovial fluid is absorbed by this spongelike property and diffuses through the cartilage matrix to provide for its nutrition. Other possible sources of nourishment for articular cartilage include diffusion from epiphyseal vessels that loop through subchondral bone, and diffusion of fluid from capillaries associated with the arterial circle around the joint at the line of capsular attachment.

Lubrication of the Joints

The fluids that lubricate a synovial joint are the synovial fluid and fluid pressed from articular cartilage during compression. Substances within synovial fluid that contribute to its lubricating properties are hyaluronic acid and a glycoprotein known as lubricin. Both of these substances are secreted by the synovial membrane and lubricate the articular surface during light loads associated with minimal articular cartilage compression. During heavy loads, the synovial membrane fluids are displaced from the articular cartilages, and the compression causes fluid from the cartilage to be expressed and form a layer between the opposing surfaces. The lubrication provided by the cartilage fluid is known as weeping lubrication. Articular cartilage has been compared to a stiff sponge; it resists tensile stresses, exhibits elastic deformation under load, contains a high proportion of extracellular fluid (hyperhydrated), and exudes fluid under pressure (which is of major importance in lubrication).

Blood, Lymph, and Nerve Supply of Joints

The blood and nerve supply of a synovial joint is shown in Figure 4.12. The arteries that supply a joint and adjacent bone generally have a common origin. These arteries usually enter the bone near the line of capsule attachment and form a network around the joint. Capillaries from this network are one of the sources of nutrition to articular cartilage that was noted in the previous section. Lymph vessels are present with blood vessels, and the lymph vessels that leave a joint drain into regional lymph nodes. Diffusion between the joint cavity and the blood and lymph capillaries takes place readily.

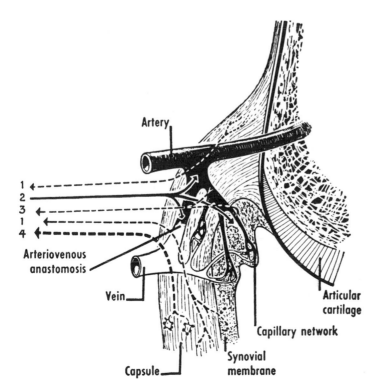

Figure 4.12. Blood and nerve supply of a synovial joint. An artery is shown supplying the epiphysis, joint capsule, and synovial membrane. Note the arteriovenous anastomosis. The articular nerve contains (1) sensory fibers (mostly pain) from the capsule and synovial membrane, (2) autonomic fibers (postganglionic, sympathetic to blood vessels), (3) sensory fibers (pain, and others with unknown functions) from the adventitia of blood vessels, and (4) proprioceptive fibers from Ruffini endings and from small lamellated corpuscles (not shown). Arrows indicate direction of conduction. From Gardner E, Gray DJ, O'Rahilley R. Anatomy. 4th ed. Philadelphia: WB Saunders, 1975.

Nerve supply to a joint has two principal functions. A first function has to do with pain and reflex responses that may accompany joint disease. A second function is associated with their role in posture, locomotion, and kinesthesia, which is a sense mediated by stimulation of end organs in muscles, tendons, and joints in response to body movements and tension (see proprioceptors, Chapter 2). The pain fibers are distributed within the fibrous layer and synovial membrane of the joint capsule.

STUDY AIDS—BONES, JOINTS AND SYNOVIAL FLUID

Structure and Function

1. Differentiate between the axial and appendicular skeleton.
2. What is another name for spongy bone?
3. Are the trabeculae (spicules) associated with compact or spongy bone?
4. How do trabeculae contribute to the strength of long bones?
5. Differentiate between epiphysis, metaphysis, and diaphysis.
6. How are bones associated with blood cell formation?
7. What is the epiphyseal plate? What parts of the bone does it separate?
8. What is periosteum and endosteum?
9. What is the unit of structure of compact bone? Describe it.
10. What are lacunae and canaliculi? Where is bone interstitial fluid located?
11. What are interstitial and circumferential lamellae?
12. How are osteoprogenitor cells, osteoblasts, and osteocytes related?
13. Is the osteocyte more mature than the osteoblast?
14. How do osteocytes maintain communication with each other?
15. What is the name of the bone-resorbing cells? What is their origin?

Composition of Bone

1. What percent of adult bone is water?
2. On a dry weight basis, what percent of adult bone is mineral content?
3. What part of bone is converted to gelatin when it is heated in aqueous solution?
4. What two elements are the major constituents of the mineral phase of bone?

Bone Formation

1. What method of bone formation is represented by the os penis of some animals and the os cordis of the bovine heart?
2. What is endochondral ossification?
3. What method of bone formation forms the flat bones of the skull and face?

Growth of Long Bones After Birth

1. What is the name of the oldest zone within the epiphyseal plate?
2. Visualize the elongation of a bone by virtue of cells dividing, secreting matrix, and thus pushing the zone of reserve cartilage away from the diaphysis.
3. Does cartilage have a blood supply?
4. Are cartilage lacunae connected by canaliculi?
5. What causes chondrocytes to die?
6. What previously occupied the tunnels that exist in the zone of calcified matrix?
7. Note the invasion of the tunnels by capillaries as a prerequisite for new bone formation.
8. Visualize the development of lamellae (layers) around the capillary such that the tunnel is reduced to a narrow canal (a haversian system).

9. As a bone grows in width, why don't the walls become unduly thick? What is the appositional mechanism of bone growth?
10. What osteogenic layer accounts for the outer circumferential lamellae? The inner circumferential lamellae?

Bone Remodeling

1. What cell provides for the erosion needed to form new channels during the process of bone remodeling?
2. After the erosion, what sequence of events forms new haversian systems?
3. How is bone mass correlated with increased muscle mass and exercise?

Bone Repair

1. What happens to osteocytes, the periosteum, and bone marrow when the blood supply is disrupted after bone fracture?
2. Will bone repair occur if a blood supply is not restored to a fracture site?
3. As related to bone repair, what is a callus?
4. What is the source of the osteogenic cells for the external and internal callus?
5. What determines whether or not a callus will be composed of spongy bone or cartilage?
6. What eventually happens to a cartilage callus?
7. Will spongy bone be replaced by compact bone at the fracture site?
8. What determines when remodeling of initial bone repair will occur?

Joints and Synovial Fluid

1. What is another name for the connection between component parts of the skeleton that is otherwise known as a joint?
2. What is the term used to describe inflammation of a joint?
3. What facilitates the two surfaces of a synovial joint to glide over each other?

4. What is a joint capsule?
5. What part of the joint capsule secretes synovial fluid?

Synovial Membrane

1. Does the synovial membrane cover the articular cartilage?
2. What are synoviocytes?
3. What are the chief functions of synovial fluid?
4. What component of synovial fluid provides for its viscosity?
5. What is the difference in viscosity of synovial fluid among joints of different sizes?
6. Are normal plasma constituents common to synovial fluid?

Articular Cartilage

1. Describe adult articular cartilage. Does it have cells, blood vessels, and a nerve supply?
2. What provides the growth zone for endochondral ossification of the epiphysis?
3. How does intermittent pressure on articular cartilage relate to its nutrition?

Lubrication of the Joints

1. What substances in synovial fluid contribute to its lubricating properties?
2. How does compression on articular cartilages contribute to lubrication?
3. What is weeping lubrication?

Blood, Lymph, and Nerve Supply of Joints

1. Does an artery that supplies a bone also supply its joints?
2. Does the capillary network of a joint provide nutrition to an articular cartilage?
3. Do joints have a lymph drainage?
4. What functions are served by nerves that supply joints?

5. Are there pain nerve fibers in articular cartilage? What is the distribution of pain nerve fibers that are associated with a joint?

SELF-EVALUATION—BONES, JOINTS, AND SYNOVIAL FLUID

1. The front and hind limbs and their respective shoulder and pelvic girdle are parts of the:
   a. axial skeleton
   b. appendicular skeleton
2. The cylindrical shaft of a long bone is known as the:
   a. epiphysis
   b. metaphysis
   c. diaphysis
3. The principal location of hematopoiesis (blood cell production) occurs in the:
   a. joint capsule
   b. medullary cavity of the diaphysis
   c. epiphyseal plate
   d. lacunae
4. The outer surface of bones (with the exception of joint surfaces) is covered by:
   a. the endosteum
   b. hyaline cartilage
   c. periosteum
   d. osteoblasts
5. Osteoblasts:
   a. are the hematopoietic cells of bone
   b. synthesize and secrete the organic substance of bone
   c. are bone-dissolving cells
   d. are the mature cells of bone
6. The interstitial fluid of osteocytes:
   a. is contained within lacunae and canaliculae
   b. diffuses from blood vessels with in haversian canals
   c. serves osteocytes in all concentric lamellae, even the outermost
   d. is described in a, b, and c, above

7. Stimulation of osteoprogenitor cells leads directly to:
   a. osteoclasts
   b. osteocytes
   c. osteoblasts
   d. chondrocytes
8. Production of osteoid and its subsequent calcification is accomplished by:
   a. osteoclasts
   b. osteocytes
   c. osteoblasts
   d. chondrocytes
9. Bone cells that represent transformed osteoblasts, communicate with each other by gap junctions in canaliculae, and maintain bone matrix are:
   a. osteoprogenitor cells
   b. osteoblasts
   c. osteoclasts
   d. osteocytes
10. Osteoclasts:
    a. are transformed osteocytes
    b. are large bone-resorbing cells considered to be members of the diffuse mononuclear phagocytic system
    c. are active in producing bone matrix
11. Calcium and phosphorus:
    a. are the major constituents of the mineral phase of bone and exist in a ratio of 2:1 (calcium:phosphorus)
    b. represent the organic matter of bone
    c. are never recovered from bone once they are deposited in the mineral phase
12. The os penis, os cordis, and pathologic bone deposits represent:
    a. endochondral bone formation
    b. intramembranous bone formation
    c. heteroplastic bone formation
13. Most long bones are developed:
    a. without the intervention of cartilage
    b. by endochondral ossification
    c. by heteroplastic ossification
14. The epiphyseal plate:
    a. is a cartilage plate between the epiphysis and diaphysis
    b. has a profuse blood supply
    c. has no distinguishable zones
    d. is located on only one end of a long bone

15. Bone forms:
    a. in both directions from the epiphyseal plate
    b. towards the diaphysis with a lifting effect on the epiphyseal plate
    c. because the chondrocytes never die
    d. because the zone of reserve cartilage dies
16. Haversian systems:
    a. are the units of structure of compact bone
    b. develop within tunnels formed in the zone of calcified matrix
    c. develop when capillaries invade the tunnels formed by nests of dead chondrocytes
    d. are represented by a, b, and c
17. Remodeling of bone:
    a. occurs during growth and in response to stress placed upon bone
    b. does not occur (once formed, not removed)
    c. does not involve osteoclastic activity
18. A prerequisite for fracture repair is:
    a. the alleviation of pain
    b. perfect realignment
    c. reestablishment of a blood supply
    d. splinting
19. Callus formation after bone fracture:
    a. is the most common type of bone repair
    b. is located on the external surface only
    c. whether on the internal or external surface, the osteoblasts originate from the periosteum
    d. does not revert to compact bone and subsequent remodeling
20. The synovial membrane:
    a. covers the bearing surface (articular cartilage) of a joint
    b. is the outer fibrous layer of a joint capsule that contributes to the stability of the joint
    c. is the lining inner surface of a joint capsule that contains synoviocytes which secrete synovial fluid

21. The chief function(s) of synovial fluid is (are):
    a. to serve as an adhesive to hold bones together at a joint
    b. to provide for a popping noise when bones are pulled apart
    c. to provide for joint lubrication and nourishment of the articular cartilage
22. Synovial fluid:
    a. viscosity is due almost entirely to hyaluronic acid
    b. color is always yellow
    c. viscosity is the same in all joints
    d. contains numerous cells
23. Adult articular cartilage is:
    a. supplied with nerves and blood vessels
    b. smooth but very rigid
    c. a resilient and elastic tissue that becomes thinner when compressed and regains original thickness when pressure is released
24. Nutrition of adult articular cartilage:
    a. is not needed
    b. is provided by synovial fluid and fluid that diffuses from capillaries in the joint capsule
    c. is provided from capillaries that infiltrate its substance
25. Which one of the following items best describes lubrication of synovial joints?
    a. they don't need it because they are smooth
    b. aqueous humor
    c. hyaluronic acid and lubricin that are secreted by the synovial membrane
    d. secretions of the choroid plexus
26. Nerve fibers for pain:
    a. are located in articular cartilage
    b. are located in the joint capsule
    c. do not exist in association with synovial joints

SUGGESTED READINGS

Cormack DH. Ham's histology. 9th ed. Philadelphia: JB Lippincott, 1987.

Fawcett DW. Bloom and Fawcett: A textbook of histology. 12th ed. New York: Chapman and Hall, 1994.

Ham AW. Histology. 1st ed. Philadelphia: JB Lippincott, 1950.

Ross MH, Romrell LJ, Kaye GI. Histology: a text and atlas. 3rd ed. Baltimore: Williams & Wilkins, 1995.

Wasserman RH, Kallfelz FA, Lust G. Bones, joints, and synovial fluid. In: Swenson MJ, Reece WO, eds. Dukes' physiology of domestic animals. 11th ed. Ithaca: Cornell University Press, 1993:536–572.

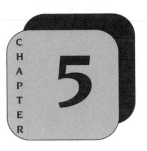

Body Water

Water is the most abundant constituent of the body fluids, comprising about 60% of the total body weight. It is the solvent for the many chemicals of the body, and the solutions thus formed provide the diffusion media for the body cells. Cells receive and expel materials through diffusion.

The physical properties of water make it ideal for this transport function. It has a relatively high specific heat whereby heat from the cells is absorbed with a minimum of temperature increase. Water also provides the lubrication necessary for minimizing friction associated with fluid flow, cell movement, and movement of body parts.

PHYSICOCHEMICAL PROPERTIES OF SOLUTIONS

Diffusion

Simple diffusion refers to the random movement of molecules, ions, and suspended colloid particles under the influence of brownian (thermal) motion. If a concentration gradient (differential) exists, molecules, ions, and colloidal particles tend to move from the area of their higher concentration to the area of their lower concentration. The movement is specific to each substance—that is, Na^+ will diffuse from the area of its higher concentration to the area of its lower concentration, regardless of the presence and concentrations of other substances. If the molecules and ions are dispersed equally, the random motion continues but does not accomplish net movement or flow; this represents a state of equilibrium.

Barriers to diffusion are generally the membranes of cells. These consist of a lipid bilayer, which is a thin film of lipid only two molecules thick through which fat-soluble substances (especially carbon dioxide and oxygen) can readily diffuse (Fig. 5.1). There might be facilitated diffusion for other substances in which a carrier is required (Fig. 5.2). Facilitated diffusion for any substance, however, still occurs from the area of its higher concentration to that of its lower concentration. Because cell membranes are predominantly lipid, they are relatively hydrophobic (water repelling), and the diffusion of water through the lipid bilayer proceeds with difficulty, but water

111

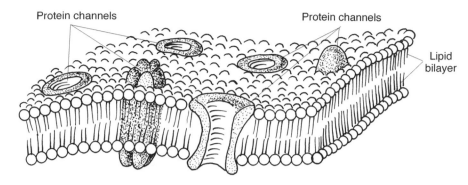

Figure 5.1. Structure of a cell membrane. The lipid bilayer is represented by a thin film of lipid that is two molecules thick. The protein channels (pores) may be comprised of a single protein or a cluster of more than one protein. The channels may have specificity for certain substances or they may be restrictive because of size. Virtually all water diffuses through the protein channels.

Figure 5.2. A postulated mechanism for facilitated diffusion. **A.** The transported molecule enters the carrier protein channel and binds with the receptor. **B.** Subsequent to binding, the carrier protein undergoes a conformational change to open the channel on the opposite side, and transported molecule is released, causing return of the carrier protein to its original conformation. From Vander AJ, Sherman JH, Luciano DS. Human physiology: the mechanisms of body function. 6th ed. New York: McGraw-Hill, 1993.

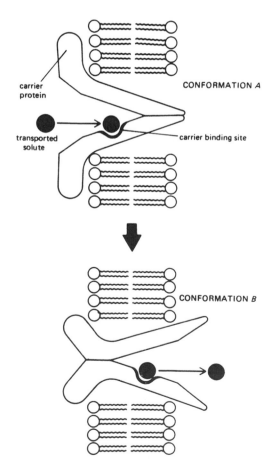

can diffuse through protein channels. Protein channels consist of large protein molecules interspersed in the lipid film; they provide structural pathways ("pores") not only for water, but also for water-soluble substances. Some substances might be excluded from diffusion through the pores because of their large size; conversely, diffusion might be facilitated because of other factors, such as a substance's relatively smaller size, its electrical charge (e.g., negative pore charge assists Na$^+$ diffusion), or the protein channel's specificity (e.g., specific ion channels). Other protein channels act as carrier proteins for transport or substances in a direction opposite to their natural diffusion direction. This is known as active transport.

Osmosis and Osmotic Pressure

The most abundant substance in the body that diffuses is water. Diffusion of water occurs throughout the body relatively easily. The amount diffusing into cells is usually balanced by an equal amount diffusing out. Osmosis is the process by which two aqueous solutions that differ in their concentration of water and are separated by a membrane that is permeable (permits passage) to water, but not to its solutes, allow a net diffusion of water from the side having the highest water concentration to the side having the lowest water concentration. When comparing water concentrations of solutions, it is implied that the solution with the highest water concentration has the lowest solute concentration. A situation in which osmosis could occur is illustrated in Figure 5.3. Net diffusion has occurred from the compartment with the highest water concentration to the one with the lowest water concentration.

The quantitative measure of the tendency for water to osmose is the osmotic pressure. This is the pressure that would have to be applied to the compartment with the lowest water concentration to prevent net diffusion of water from the compartment with the highest water concentration. The number of particles in a solution (i.e., ions, molecules) determines its osmotic pressure. The greater the number of particles, the higher the osmotic pressure. For two aqueous solutions of NaCl separated by a membrane that permits diffusion of

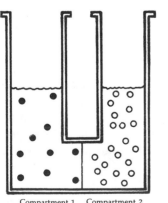 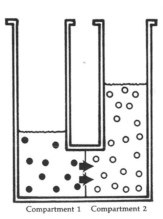

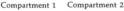

Figure 5.3. Osmosis. **A.** Before osmosis. **B.** During osmosis. Equal volumes of aqueous solutions (solutes represented by black circles and open circles) are placed in compartments that are separated by membranes permeable to water but not to the solutes. The aqueous solution in compartment 1 has the highest concentration of water (lowest concentration of solute). Osmosis (diffusion of water) occurs from compartment 1 to compartment 2 (highest water concentration to lowest water concentration) and the water level rises in compartment 2.

water, but not NaCl, the highest osmotic pressure is measured for the solution with the highest concentration of NaCl (lowest concentration of water). Water diffuses to the area of greatest osmotic pressure. This is really a potential pressure because it is the pressure that would have to be applied to prevent osmosis (i.e., in the body, osmosis is not prevented when water imbalances exist).

One mole of an undissociated (not ionized) substance is equal to 1 osmole (osm). If a substance dissociates into two ions (NaCl → Na^+ and Cl^-), 0.5 mole of the substance equals 1 osmole. The number of particles, not the mass of the solute, determines osmotic pressure.

Accordingly, osmolar concentrations are used to prepare solutions that exert specific osmotic pressures or to express the osmotic strength of solutions (e.g., urine, plasma, NaCl). One liter of a solution that contains 300 milliosmoles (mOsm) (0.3 osm) of glucose (undissociated) exerts the same osmotic pressure as one that contains 300 mOsm of NaCl. Similarly, the osmolarity of a urine sample that is measured as 300 mOsm exerts the same osmotic pressure as the previous solutions of glucose and NaCl.

Tone of Solutions

The membranes of the body vary in their permeabilities and allow certain solutes (as well as water) to diffuse through them. They are selectively permeable membranes. The measured osmotic pressure for a solution containing solutes that could diffuse through membranes would then not be an index for its tendency to cause osmosis. Instead, the tone of a solution is defined, which is the effective osmotic pressure. Only those particles (molecules, ions) for which the membrane is not permeable contribute to the tone. The principles of osmosis continue to prevail, except that now water diffuses to the greatest effective osmotic pressure. Figure 5.4 illustrates the tone of solutions. Two solutions of equal volumes and particle numbers are shown to be separated by a membrane that permits the passage of water and the particles in compartment 2. Each solution has the same measured osmotic pressure (same concentration of particles). Because compartment 1 has particles that cannot diffuse through the membrane, these particles are the ones that contribute to an effective osmotic pressure and, because the solution in compartment 2 has no effective osmotic pressure (because particles are diffusible), water diffuses to the greatest effective osmotic pressure, or from compartment 2 to compartment 1. In this example, the net diffusion of water stops when the pressure resulting from the weight of the solution in compartment 2 opposes the diffusion resulting from the effective osmotic pressure in compartment 1.

From a practical standpoint, the tone of solutions that can be infused into the blood of animals is usually compared to the solution inside red blood cells (erythrocytes). The solution of erythrocytes is in osmotic equilibrium with plasma (the fluid part of blood). An infused solution is hypotonic if it has a lower effective osmotic pressure than the solution of erythrocytes, and it is hypertonic if it has a higher effective osmotic pressure than the solution of erythrocytes.

The effect of solutions with different tones on erythrocytes is illustrated in Figure 5.5. An erythrocyte placed into solution A enlarges. This solution must have a lower effective osmotic pressure than the erythrocyte solution (water diffuses to the higher effective osmotic pressure) and is classified as hypotonic to plasma. In solution B there is no change in the size of the erythrocytes. The solution in the beaker and in the erythrocyte must have the same effective osmotic pressure, and the beaker solution is classified as isotonic to plasma. The erythrocyte in solution C decreases in size, indicating a loss of erythrocyte water to the beaker solution. In this case, the higher effective

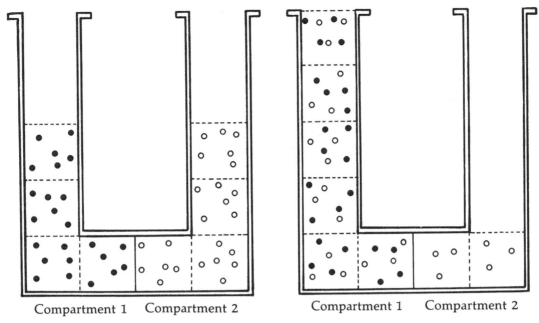

Figure 5.4. Hypothetical example of tone of solutions. **A.** Before osmosis. **B.** After osmosis. Two aqueous solutions (solutes represented by black circles and open circles) of equal osmotic pressure are separated by a membrane permeable to water and open circle solutes. Effective osmotic pressure is exerted only by black circle solute, and water diffuses to compartment 1. At equilibrium, open circle solute has a new, lower concentration that is equal throughout compartments 1 and 2. (Dashed lines represent divisions of equal volume.)

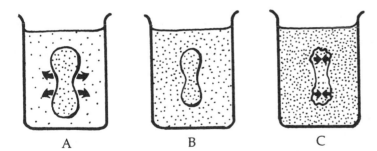

Figure 5.5. Effect of the tone of solution on erythrocytes (red blood cells). **A.** The solution is hypotonic and the erythrocyte expands. **B.** The solution is isotonic and no change occurs in erythrocyte size. **C.** The solution is hypertonic and the erythrocyte decreases in size.

osmotic pressure is found in solution C (water diffuses to the higher effective osmotic pressure). The loss of water from erythrocytes caused by hypertonic solutions makes the cells wrinkled in appearance, and they are said to be crenated.

Solutions that cause erythrocytes to enlarge can be sufficiently hypotonic to cause hemolysis (rupture) of the erythrocytes. Hemoglobin (red in color) in the erythrocyte imparts its color to the solu-tion. Plasma from an animal in which hemolysis has occurred has some degree of redness, depending on the extent of the hemolysis (plasma is usually light yellow to colorless). When this occurs it is known as hemoglobinemia. Sometimes hemoly-sis occurs to such an extent that hemoglo-bin enters the kidney tubules and appears in the urine. In this condition, called hemoglobinuria, a red color is imparted to the urine.

DISTRIBUTION OF BODY WATER

Total Body Water and Fluid Compartments

The total body water (TBW) is the sum of the water that is contained in arbitrary divisions of its distribution between the intracellular and extracellular compartments. The extracellular compartment can be divided further into interstitial, intravascular (the plasma volume), and transcellular compartments. The divisions of TBW among the compartments are shown in Figure 5.6.

The terms water and fluid are nearly the same but do differ inasmuch as a fluid, as found in the body, contains not only water but also solutes. The measurement of a compartment's volume usually includes the entire space occupied by the water and solutes. For example, blood plasma is a fluid, and the measurement of its volume is larger than the space occupied by the water it contains. For practical purposes, the compartments are referred to as fluid compartments because the fluid volume rather than water volume is that which is usually measured.

TBW is variable and depends mostly on the amount of fat in the body. A lean animal might have water equivalent to 70% of its body weight, whereas an obese animal might only have 45% of its body weight as water because of the nature of fat cells (the cytoplasm is almost filled with fat). The fat and water are immiscible and most of the cell mass is fat, rather than water. The average animal (neither fat nor lean) probably has water equivalent to 60% of its body weight.

Intracellular and Extracellular Fluid

About two-thirds of the body water is found within the cells; this comprises the intracellular fluid (ICF). The amounts given for percentage of body weight are average values and can vary. All the water that is not in cells is considered to be extracellular, or outside the cells. This includes the interstitial fluid (ISF), intravascular fluid (IVF), and transcellular fluid (TCF).

The ISF is that which immediately surrounds the cells (Fig. 5.7). It is outside the cells and the capillaries. In addition to the elastic and collagen fibers of the intercellular substance, an amorphous ground substance is present; its principal component is hyaluronic acid. Hyaluronic acid is a highly hydrated gel that holds tissue fluid in its interstices. Because of the gel form, fluid is not observed to flow and accumulate in lower body parts, nor does fluid flow from a cut surface.

The IVF is the liquid part of blood known as plasma. About 92% of the plasma volume (PV) is water; the remaining 8% of PV is mostly protein.

TCF is the fluid found in body cavities and is usually minimal. It includes

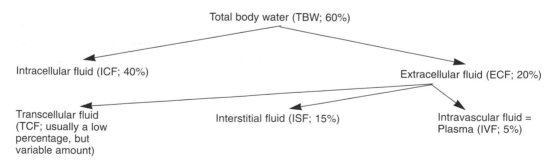

Figure 5.6. Total body water and its distribution among the fluid compartments.

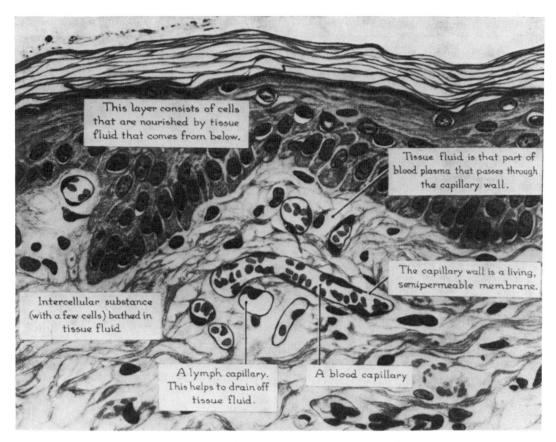

This layer consists of cells that are nourished by tissue fluid that comes from below.

Tissue fluid is that part of blood plasma that passes through the capillary wall.

The capillary wall is a living, semipermeable membrane.

Intercellular substance (with a few cells) bathed in tissue fluid

A lymph capillary. This helps to drain off tissue fluid.

A blood capillary

Figure 5.7. Skin and its subcutaneous composition as an example of the environment for cells. Elastic and collagen fibers are present but the main substance is hyaluronic acid. Most interstitial water is in combination with hyaluronic acid, giving it the characteristics of a gel. From Ham AW. Histology. 7th ed. Philadelphia: JB Lippicott, 1974.

intraocular fluid and cerebrospinal fluid. The most plentiful TCF is in the digestive tract. Its amount is greatest in ruminants, in which stomach compartments for fermentation are found.

WATER BALANCE

From day to day in any one animal the water content of the body remains relatively constant, with a balance between gains and losses. An example of daily water balance is shown in Table 5.1. The water turnover for the nonlactating cow is 29 L/day and is 56 L/day for the lactating cow. The water intake in both cases is equal to the output—there is water balance. The "pool" size is constant, but the water in the pool changes (water turnover). The output of the lactating cow has increased, not only because of the obvious milk production, but also because of the greater fecal output associated with eating nearly twice as much and because of greater urine and vapor losses associated with increased metabolism.

Water Gain

Water gains occur by ingestion of water in food and drink and from metabolic water. The food eaten by animals contains a variable amount of water; the usual drink

TABLE 5.1. Daily Water Balance of Holstein Cows Eating Legume Hay (values in liters)

Balance	Nonlactating	Lactating
Intake		
Drinking water	26	51
Food water	1	2
Metabolic water	<u>2</u>	<u>3</u>
Total	29	56
Output		
Feces	12	19
Urine	7	11
Vaporized	10	14
Milk	<u>0</u>	<u>12</u>
Total	**29**	**56**

From Houpt TR. Water and electrolytes. In: Swenson MJ, Reece WO, eds. Dukes' physiology of domestic animals. 11th ed. Ithaca, NY: Cornell University Press, 1993.

is water or, in the very young, milk. Metabolic water is derived from the chemical reactions of metabolism in the cell mitochondria. At the end of the electron transport chain, hydrogen is combined with oxygen to form water; this is metabolic water. This is also the point at which oxygen is taken up by the body. The electron transport chain is the chemical site for the oxidation of reduced cofactors involved in the transformations of the citric acid (Krebs) cycle. An example of this is the oxidation of the reduced cofactor, NADH (reduced nicotinamide-adenine dinucleotide), by oxygen through the cytochrome electron transport system in the mitochondria:

$$2\ NADH + \tfrac{1}{2}O_2 \rightarrow 2\ NAD^+ + H_2O$$

The metabolism of proteins, carbohydrates, or fats requires different amounts of cofactors, with the greatest amounts required for fats. Accordingly, the yield of metabolic water is greater for a certain amount of fat than for an equal amount of protein or carbohydrate. For example, the water yield from each of 100 g of protein, carbohydrate, and fat is 40, 60, and 110 mL, respectively. Energy in the form of adenosine triphosphate (ATP) is formed during the transfer of electrons. The amount of metabolic water formed varies but could be substantial under certain conditions. In the domestic animals, it is said to average about 5 to 10% of daily water gain and it can approach 100% of the water gain for some small desert rodents.

Water Loss

Water loss from the body is classified as either an insensible loss or a sensible loss. Insensible losses are associated with vapor losses and occur constantly by evaporation from the skin and by loss of water vapor in exhaled air. Inhaled air becomes saturated with water vapor in the respiratory passages and lungs, but there is no body mechanism to remove moisture from the respiratory gases before exhalation. Sensible losses are the visible losses; they are part of the urine, feces, and body secretions that leave the body and are not subject to evaporation. Sensible losses can become excessive in certain conditions, such as diarrhea, and threaten body stores of water.

Water Requirements

No linear relationship exists between basal water needs and body weight.

Accordingly, a 500-kg cow does not require ten times more water than a 50-kg calf. The basal daily needs for water (that needed to maintain water balance), however, are related to caloric expenditure. Under basal metabolism conditions (e.g., resting animal, thermally neutral environment, fasting state), caloric expenditure is related linearly to body surface area. The cow might require only three to four times more water than the calf because her body surface area is three to four times greater. If the ECF (20% of body weight) is considered to be that from which emergency water is drawn, the 500-kg cow has 100 kg of fluid and the 50-kg calf has only 10 kg. Therefore, the cow has considerably more reserve on which to draw to supply basal needs for water than does the calf. In other words, the cow has ten times more reserve water to supply her needs, and her needs are only three to four times greater than the calf's. It is because of the more limited reserves associated with their relatively higher needs that calves become distressed more quickly in conditions of uncontrolled water loss (such as diarrhea).

DEHYDRATION, THIRST, AND WATER INTAKE

Dehydration

In dehydration, the immediate source of water lost from the body is the extracellular fluid, and this is followed by a shift from the intracellular to the extracellular fluid. A loss of water equal to 10% of the body weight is considered to be severe for most animals. The concentrations of electrolytes (ions) in the body fluids do not continue to increase during dehydration, but are excreted by the kidney in proportion to the water loss. With continuing dehydration, water and electrolytes are depleted. Therefore, rehydration requires not only water, but also appropriate electrolytes.

Stimulus for Thirst

When water losses exceed water gain, there is an effort on the part of the kidneys to conserve water. Also, animals are provided with a thirst mechanism to recognize the need for water intake greater than that provided by food and metabolic water. Thirst is the conscious desire for water. Central to the thirst mechanism is a thirst center located in the hypothalamus of the brain and represented by thirst cells. The thirst cells are stimulated by an increase in their osmoconcentration (loss of water and increased salt concentration). Osmoconcentration of the thirst cells is a consequence of dehydration (see previous section).

Another stimulus of thirst is the hormone angiotensin II. This is formed in response to low blood pressure to bring about changes to increase blood pressure (e.g., salt retention, peripheral vasoconstriction, water ingestion). A loss of blood volume, as in hemorrhage (an isotonic fluid loss), results in lowered blood pressure, and angiotensin II is formed. The thirst stimulation previously described causes an animal to drink water, which is subsequently absorbed, and blood volume and blood pressure are restored toward normal.

Relief of Thirst

An experiment can be performed with a dog to demonstrate the effect of dehydration on thirst stimulation. A hypertonic NaCl solution is injected intravenously, which increases the osmoconcentration of plasma and subsequently that of the thirst cells in the hypothalamus. Water that was previously offered to the dog and ignored is now consumed. The amount consumed is approximately equal to the amount that would have been needed to make the hypertonic solution isotonic. Even though the water ingested was not absorbed, the dog's thirst was relieved.

Thirst can be temporarily relieved by wetting the mouth and pharynx and by distention of the stomach that accompanies water ingestion. The former method is used by many people seeking relief from thirst. The latter can be demonstrated by distending a balloon placed into the stomach. Both these temporary relief methods help prevent overingestion. A brief time is required after either method for water to be absorbed and to lower the osmoconcentration of thirst cells or to increase blood pressure, depending on what stimulus produced the thirst. Thirst is an important mechanism for maintaining water balance. Water must be adequately provided for animals, or ill health, discomfort, and loss of production can ensue.

Adaptation to Water Lack

Throughout history, certain animals have had to adapt to conditions of water lack because of their habitat (little adaptation has been necessary, however, for cattle, swine, dogs, and cats). The problem is compounded by exposure to high temperatures. Indian cattle breeds (Zebu and Brahman) are more tolerant of heat than European breeds because of greater sweating (and hence cooling) and not because of any special water conservation mechanism. Adequate water must be provided. Camels, donkeys, and sheep, however, have adapted for coping with periods when water is not available.

Camels

The means whereby the dromedary (one-humped camel) has adapted to water lack has received the most interest. Many legends have been associated with this camel and its ability to survive for long periods in the desert without water. It was thought that the metabolism of hump fat, and the greater metabolic water yield from it, provided the extra water needed, but this notion has generally been discredited. The amount of fat in the hump is not great and, even though more metabolic water is derived from fat

metabolism, more energy (ATP) is also produced. Consequently, only half as much fat is metabolized as would be the case for protein and carbohydrate, resulting in about the same water production.

The most important finding is the camel's ability to endure a degree of dehydration equal to about 30% of its body weight, compared to 10 to 12% for most other animals. This permits it to survive longer when water is not available. Another adaptive mechanism is the camel's ability to store body heat (resulting in a body temperature increase) during the day rather than dissipate it. In one day, the camel's body temperature might range from 34.2 to 40.7° C (as compared to 38 to 39.3° C for the dairy cow). Water is thus conserved because heat dissipation requires the evaporation of water. The camel awaits the cool desert night to dissipate the stored heat. The camel also has summer fur, which is most prominent on its back; this is effective in reducing solar heat gain. Finally, the camel can ingest water up to 25% of its body weight in just a few minutes, which permits rehydration at the infrequently found watering spots. The lowering of plasma osmotic pressure that occurs when such a large volume of water is absorbed after ingestion does not appear to bother the camel, whereas hemolysis might occur in other species. The oval, biconcave erythrocytes of the camel are more resistant to osmotic hemolysis. Although the camel can concentrate its urine and dehydrate its feces, these are not significant factors in regard to the camel's ability to withstand water deprivation.

Sheep and Donkeys

Sheep and donkeys are also notable in their ability to withstand water lack. They are similar to the camel in that they can endure dehydration up to about 30% of their body weight. Also, the sheep and donkey are similar to the camel in being able to drink almost 25% of their body weight in water at one time without harmful effects. The sheep is protected from solar heat gain by its wool covering and excretes dry feces and relatively concentrated urine. The donkey dissipates heat by sweating more than the camel and sheep; its survival time is correspondingly less. Because sheep do not sweat as much as camels and donkeys, evaporative heat loss by way of the respiratory passages is a more important factor in sheep.

STUDY AIDS—BODY WATER

Physicochemical Properties of Solutions

1. What parts of a cell membrane (proteins or lipids) account for the diffusion of water soluble substances? What parts are considered to be the pores?
2. How does facilitated diffusion differ from simple diffusion?
3. A membrane separates two NaCl solutions that permits diffusion of water but not NaCl. The NaCl concentration on Side A and Side B is 0.15M and 0.3M, respectively. This means that:
   a) osmosis occurs from Side A to Side B
   b) osmosis occurs from Side B to Side A
   c) there will be no osmosis
4. Solution 1 has an effective osmotic pressure greater than solution 2. Which solution (1 or 2) has the greater tone?
5. What is the fate of erythrocytes placed into a hypotonic solution?

Distribution of Body Water

1. What percent of the body weight is composed of water?
2. What are the two major body water compartments and what percent of the body weight is represented by each?
3. What substance gives interstitial water the characteristics of a gel?

Water Balance

1. What is the derivation of metabolic water? Why does 5g of fat yield more metabolic water than 5g of protein or carbohydrate?
2. What are examples of insensible water loss?
3. Why are excess water losses (e.g., diarrhea) more critical in young animals than in adults of the same species?

Dehydration, Thirst, and Water Intake

1. What is the immediate source (compartment) of water lost from the body?
2. Define thirst.
3. What are two stimuli to thirst?
4. How can thirst be temporarily relieved?

Adaptation to Water Lack

1. Why are Indian cattle breeds more tolerant of heat than European breeds?
2. How has the camel adapted to limited water availability?
3. How much water loss (percent of body weight) can most animals withstand?

SELF-EVALUATION—BODY WATER

1. Which one of the following body fluid compartments would represent about 40% of the body weight?
   a. transcellular
   b. intravascular
   c. intracellular
   d. extracellular
2. A selectively permeable membrane allows the passage of water and substance X but not substance Y. Equal volumes of aqueous solution X and aqueous solution Y are placed on opposite sides of the membrane. After equilibrium, which side will contain the greater volume?
   a. the side that originally contained solution X
   b. the side that originally contained solution Y

3. Erythrocytes are placed in a solution that causes them to hemolyze. The solution must be:
   a. isotonic
   b. hypertonic
   c. hypotonic

4. A different solution is placed on either side of a selectively permeable membrane. Water diffuses from side A to side B. Which side has the greater effective osmotic pressure for this to occur?
   a. side A
   b. side B

5. Water lost from the body when air is exhaled is considered a vapor loss or insensible loss. Compared to water lost in feces or urine, it is insignificant.
   a. true
   b. false

6. The water requirement of a 1000 lb cow is about 30 liters each day. If a calf weighs 100 lbs. and has about 1/5 of the body surface area of the cow, what would be its approximate water requirement each day?
   a. 30 liters
   b. 3 liters
   c. 6 liters

7. Which one of the following statements is correct as it relates to tolerance to dehydration?
   a. cattle (may lose up to 30% of body weight in H_2O) have better tolerance than sheep
   b. sheep (may lose up to 25 to 30% of body weight as H_2O) have better tolerance than cattle and pigs
   c. sheep, cattle and pigs have same tolerance
   d. sheep (may lose up to 12% of body weight in H_2O) have better tolerance than pigs (may lose up to 5% of body weight as H_2O)

8. If the effective osmotic pressure in the plasma becomes greater than the effective osmotic pressure within the thirst cells in the hypothalamus, which of the following would be predicted?
   a. animal would seek water
   b. animal would not seek water

9. Solution 1 has a greater effective osmotic pressure than solution 2. Which one of these solutions has the greater tone?
   a. solution 1
   b. solution 2

10. What is the fate of erythrocytes that are placed into a hypotonic solution?
    a. they increase in volume
    b. they decrease in volume
    c. there is no change in volume

11. A membrane separates aqueous solution A from aqueous solution B. It is determined that solution A has the greater effective osmotic pressure. Therefore, water will diffuse from:
    a. solution B to solution A
    b. solution A to solution B
    c. there would be no net diffusion of water

12. Interstitial fluid is a component of:
    a. the intracellular fluid compartment
    b. the extracellular fluid compartment
    c. the transcellular fluid compartment

13. Metabolic water is derived from the reoxidation of cofactors (such as NAD) that are reduced during the metabolism of carbohydrates, proteins, and fat. Which one of the following has the most cofactors/100g reduced during their metabolism?
    a. carbohydrate
    b. protein
    c. fat

14. The basal daily needs for water are directly related to:
    a. body weight
    b. caloric expenditure and body surface area
    c. animal color

15. Thirst can be stimulated by:
    a. osmoconcentration of the extracellular fluid
    b. low blood pressure associated with blood loss
    c. both a and b

SUGGESTED READINGS

Ham AW. Histology. 7th ed. Philadelphia: JB Lippincott, 1974.

Houpt TR. Water and electrolytes. In: Swenson MJ, Reece WO, eds. Dukes' physiology of domestic animals. 11th ed. Ithaca, NY: Cornell University Press, 1993:9–21.

Reece WO. Physicochemical properties of solutions. In: Swenson MJ, Reece WO, eds. Dukes' physiology of domestic animals. 11th ed. Ithaca, NY: Cornell University Press, 1993:1—8.

Vander AJ, Sherman JH, Luciano DS. Human physiology: the mechanisms of body function. 6th ed. New York: McGraw-Hill, 1993.

Wilson RT. The camel. New York: Longman Group, 1984.

6

Blood and its Functions

The blood vascular system evolved to provide for the transport of nutrients to the cells after they had become so numerous and distant from the surface that diffusion was no longer adequate. The circulating medium came to be known as blood. The functions of blood are generally related to transport (e.g., nutrients, oxygen, carbon dioxide, waste products, hormones, heat, and immune bodies). There are additional functions of blood relating to its role of maintaining fluid balance and pH equilibrium in the body. Because blood must be maintained in a closed system for transport efficiency, it is provided with a mechanism for preventing blood loss if the normally closed system is opened.

COMPOSITION OF BLOOD

Blood is composed of cells and plasma. The cells of blood are the (1) erythrocytes (red blood cells, RBCs), (2) leukocytes (white blood cells, WBCs), and (3) platelets, also known as thrombocytes. Plasma is the liquid component of blood within which the cells and colloids are suspended and other transported substances are dissolved.

General Characteristics and Their Determination

Hematocrit

The relative proportion of cells to plasma is a clinically useful measure that can be determined by the hematocrit. Hematocrit means to centrifuge; by centrifugation, a column of blood can be divided into its component parts according to their relative specific gravity (Fig. 6.1). Accordingly, the erythrocyte mass occupies the lower portion and is known as the packed cell volume (PCV), the leukocytes and platelets occupy the middle portion, known as the "buffy coat," and the plasma occupies the top portion. The PCV is the most useful for helping to distinguish abnormal conditions.

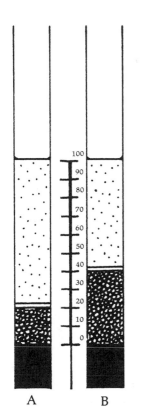

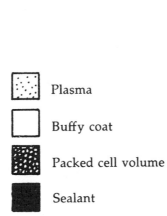

Plasma

Buffy coat

Packed cell volume

Sealant

Figure 6.1. The microhematocrit as it might appear for an anemic (A) and a normal (B) animal. The buffy coat occupies an insignificant volume and is not accounted for. Accordingly, in the normal hematocrit, the plasma volume would be noted as 60%.

For greater precision of measurement and for uniformity, a standard procedure (microhematocrit method) is used in the determination of the hematocrit. A thin column of blood is allowed to fill about three-fourths the length of the capillary tube. One end of the tube is sealed with putty and it is then centrifuged for 5 minutes at 11,000 rpm. The centrifuge used is a microhematocrit centrifuge. The proportion of the blood column length occupied by the RBCs can be obtained by measurement. PCV values are reported as percentages.

Blood Color

The red color of blood is imparted by the hemoglobin contained within the erythrocytes. Gradations of color from bright red to bluish-purple are seen, depending on the degree of saturation of hemoglobin with oxygen. The greater the saturation, the brighter the red color. Plasma is yellow to colorless, depending on the quantity and species examined. Plasma that is ordinarily light yellow when observed in a test tube might be almost colorless in a capillary tube. The color of plasma results principally from the presence of bilirubin, a degradation product of hemoglobin. It is a darker yellow in the cow and even darker in the horse, which has a relatively high bilirubin concentration.

Blood Volume

Blood volume is a function of the lean body weight and is generally 8 to 10% of the body weight. Blood volume cannot be measured directly because exsanguination (removal of blood) results in the loss of only about 50% of the blood; the remainder is trapped in capillaries, venous sinuses, and other vessels. The erythrocyte or plasma volume can be measured by various techniques. If one or the other is measured, and the PCV is known, the blood volume can be calculated according to the hematocrit relationship. An equality exists stating that the ratio of the plasma volume (PV) to the blood volume (BV) is the same as the hematocrit ratio; i.e., the ratio of the plasma portion of the hematocrit (1 – PCV, its decimal equivalent) to the whole of the hematocrit (1, which represents all components of blood). Accordingly,

$$PV/BV = \frac{1-PCV}{1}$$

Solving for BV, the equation becomes BV = (PV × 1)/(1 – PCV). Assuming that a 12.5 kg dog has a PCV of 40% and a measured PV of 600 ml, its BV is derived as follows: BV = (600 × 1)/(1 - 0.4) = 600/0.6 = 1000 ml. Translated to ml/kg of body weight (1000 ml/12.5 kg), the value becomes 80 ml/kg. Further calculation shows that this is the same as 8% of the body weight if correction for specific gravity is not made and if 1 ml of blood is considered to weigh 1 g.

Blood pH

Blood has a pH of about 7.4. Venous blood is slightly more acidic than arterial blood. Thus, if the arterial blood pH is 7.4, one would expect the venous blood pH to be about 7.36. The higher acidity of venous blood is related to the transport of carbon dioxide; higher concentrations of CO_2 exist in venous blood. The hydration of carbon dioxide in venous blood ($CO_2 + H_2O \leftrightarrow H_2CO_3 \leftrightarrow H^+ + HCO_3^-$) forms hydrogen ions, thus resulting in its higher acidity.

The pH symbol is the chemical notation for the logarithm of the reciprocal of the hydrogen ion concentration [H^+] in gram-atoms per liter of solution. For monovalent substances, equivalent measurements are the same as gram-atom measurements; when the pH is 7.4, the [H^+] is 0.00000040

g-atoms of H^+ in 1 L of solution, or 40 nEq (nanoequivalents). When the [H^+] doubles or halves, the pH changes by 0.3 units as follows:

pH	[H^+]
7.4	Normal
7.1	Double normal
7.7	Half-normal
6.8	Four times normal

Even though the pH might seem to change very little, the [H^+] changes considerably. Therefore, the pH of the body fluids must be regulated precisely.

Leukocytes

Classification and Appearance

Leukocytes are classified either as granulocytes, containing granules in the cytoplasm, or as agranulocytes, containing few, if any, granules in the cytoplasm. There are three types of granulocytes, named according to which component of the H&E stain (hematoxylin, basic and colored blue; eosin, acidic and colored red) stains their granules. Neutrophils are neither markedly acidophilic nor basophilic and incorporate both basic and acidic components into their granules. Basophils only accept the basic (hematoxylin) component and eosinophils only accept the acidic (eosin) component. There are two types of agranulocytes: monocytes and lymphocytes. Granulocytes and monocytes are produced in the bone marrow from a myeloid stem cell known as a myeloblast. Lymphocytes originate from a lymphoid stem cell in lymph tissue, such as lymph nodes, spleen, tonsils, and various lymphoid clusters in the intestine and elsewhere. The different types of leukocytes are shown in Figure 6.2.

The nuclei of the granulocytes assume various shapes as they proceed to maturity (Fig. 6.3). The nuclei of the mature forms are generally divided into lobes or segments connected by filaments; these are sometimes called segmented cells. The younger forms have a nucleus that appears

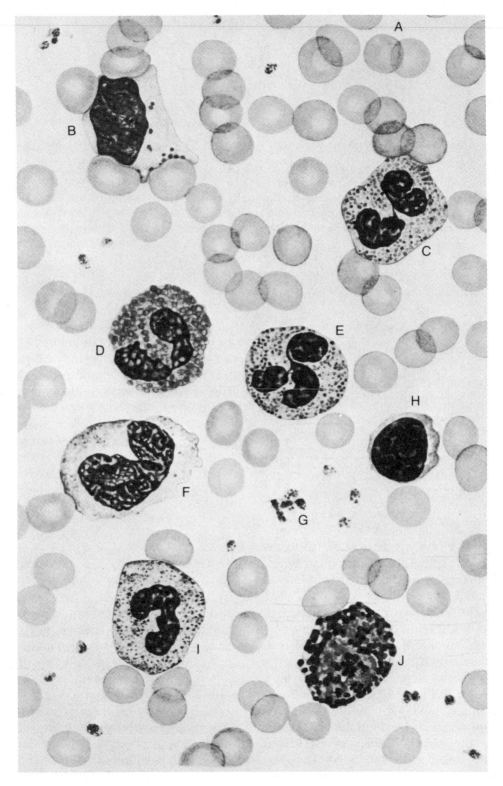

Figure 6.2. Cell types found in smears of normal peripheral blood. **A.** Erythrocytes. **B.** Large lymphocyte. **C** and **E.** Segmented neutrophils (granules stain light pink to bluish-black). **D.** Eosinophil (granules stain reddish-orange). **F.** Monocyte. **G.** Platelets (thrombocytes). **H.** Lymphocyte. **I.** Band neutrophil (granules stain various shades of pink and blue). **J.** Basophil (granules stain dark blue). From Diggs LW, Sturm D, Bell A. Morphology of human blood cells. Abott Park, IL: Abbott Laboratories, 1985. Reproduction of morphology of human blood cells has been granted with approval of Abbott Laboratories, all rights rserved by Abbott Laboratories.

Granulocyte

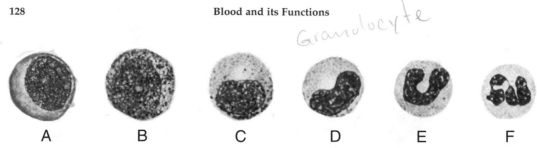

A   B   C   D   E   F

Figure 6.3. Granulocytic (myelocytic) system. **A.** Myeloblast. **B.** Promyelocyte (progranulocyte). **C.** Neutrophilic myelocyte. **D.** Neutrophilic metamyelocyte. **E.** Neutrophilic band. **F.** Neutrophilic segmented. From Diggs LW, Sturm D, Bell A. Morphology of human blood cells. Abott Park, IL: Abbott Laboratories, 1985. Reproduction of morphology of human blood cells has been granted with approval of Abbott Laboratories, all rights rserved by Abbott Laboratories.

as a curved or coiled band without segmentation; these are known as band cells.

Life Span and Numbers

After their development, leukocytes are circulated in the blood until the (relatively short) time they leave the circulation to perform their extravascular function. Granulocytes can be present in the blood for 6 to 10 hours and are constantly leaving. Granulocyte time in the tissues varies considerably but can be 2 or 3 days. Once granulocytes leave the blood, they do not normally return. They leave the body either from inflammatory sites or by way of the gastrointestinal, urinary, respiratory, or reproductive tracts. These organs are normally lined by neutrophils, which help prevent entry of organisms or foreign particles. Monocytes have a circulation time similar to that of granulocytes (6 to 10 hours), but can remain in the tissues for several months. Many monocytes become fixed macrophages in the sinusoids of the liver, spleen, bone marrow, and lymph nodes; in this way, they continue to function in the blood and lymph.

Lymphocytes recirculate repeatedly from the blood to the tissues, to the lymph, and back to the blood. The lymphocyte population is comprised of T cells and B cells. Their life span varies according to species. Generally, T cells are long-lived (100 to 200 days), B cells are short-lived (2 to 4 days), and memory T and B cells are very long-lived (years).

The circulating leukocytes are considerably less numerous than erythrocytes. In general, they number about 10,000/µl among the domestic animals (Table 6.1). The percentage distribution of the various types of leukocytes is not the same among the domestic species. There is a higher percentage of lymphocytes than neutrophils among the cloven-hooved animals (e.g., pig, cow, sheep, goat). The reverse (higher percentage of neutrophils than lymphocytes) is true for the horse, dog, and cat.

Function

NEUTROPHILS The cell membranes of certain cells can engulf particulate matter (e.g., bacteria, cells, degenerating tissue) and extracellular fluid and bring them into their cytoplasm. The ingestion of particulate matter is known as phagocytosis, the ingestion of extracellular fluid is pinocytosis, and both are forms of endocytosis.

Neutrophils are highly phagocytic and this, coupled with their mobility, provides for an effective body defense mechanism. Their numbers increase rapidly during acute bacterial infections. The mechanism for their movement from the blood to an inflammatory site has been hypothesized as follows (Fig. 6.4):

TABLE 6.1.   Total Leukocytes per Microliter of Blood and Percentage of Each Leukocyte

Species	Total Leukocyte Count (Range; no./µl)	Percentage of Each Leukocyte				
		Neutrohil	Lymphocyte	Monocyte	Eosinophil	Basophil
Pig						
1 day	10,000–12,000	70	20	5–6	2–5	<1
1 week	10,000–12,000	50	40	5–6	2–5	<1
2 weeks	10,000–12,000	40	50	5–6	2–5	<1
6 weeks and older	15,000–22,000	30–35	55–60	5–6	2–5	<1
Horse	8000–11,000	50–60	30–40	5–6	2–5	<1
Cow	7000–10,000	25–30	60–65	5	2–5	<1
Sheep	7000–10,000	25–30	60–65	5	2–5	<1
Goat	8000–12,000	35–40	50–55	5	2–5	<1
Dog	9000–13,000	65–70	20–25	5	2–5	<1
Cat	10,000–15,000	55–60	30–35	5	2–5	<1
Chicken	20,000–30,000	25–30	55–60	10	3–8	1–4

From Swenson MJ. Physiological properties and cellular and chemical constituents of blood. In: Swenson, MJ, Reece WO, eds. Dukes' physiology of domestic animals. 11th ed. Ithaca, NY: Cornell University Press, 1993.

1. Degenerative products of inflamed tissue or bacterial cells can be chemotactic (chemically attracting) and diffuse through interstitial spaces to capillaries and venules.
2. Chemotactic substances increase porosity of these vessels and also provide for adhesion of neutrophils to endothelium (margination).
3. Neutrophils squeeze through capillary pores (diapedesis).
4. Neutrophils proceed to inflammatory site by ameboid movement.

This mechanism probably applies to the other leukocytes as well. When the neutrophils arrive at the inflamed site, they phagocytize bacteria and cell debris. The neutrophil life span is relatively short; dead neutrophils and their liquid is known as pus. The accumulation of pus within a connective tissue capsule is known as an abscess.

The comparable leukocyte in birds is known as the heterophil. Whereas the granules in mammals are neutrophilic, those in birds are acidophilic. Also, many of the granules are rod- or spindle-shaped instead of spherical. The nucleus is polymorphic with varying degrees of lobulation.

MONOCYTES   Monocytes are usually the largest leukocyte seen on a stained blood film. Compared to other leukocytes, they have a copious cytoplasm. Circulating monocytes phagocytize bacteria, viruses, and antigen-antibody complexes from the bloodstream. Their circulatory phagocytic function is not as pronounced, however, as that which occurs in the tissues. The movement of neutrophils from capillaries and venules is accompanied by similar margination and diapedesis of monocytes. On entering the tissues, monocytes are transformed into macrophages (large phagocytic cells) and initially participate in the phagocytosis of bacterial cells. Macrophages eventually predominate at the inflammatory site because of their longer life span. Also, they are attracted to some organisms that neutrophils ignore and they phagocytize the cellular debris that remains when inflammation subsides.

Monocyte numbers increase in chronic infections. They are especially valuable in the defense against long-term inflammation because of their larger size and longer life span. Lysosomes within the cytoplasm of the neutrophils and monocytes help in the digestion of the phagocytized materials.

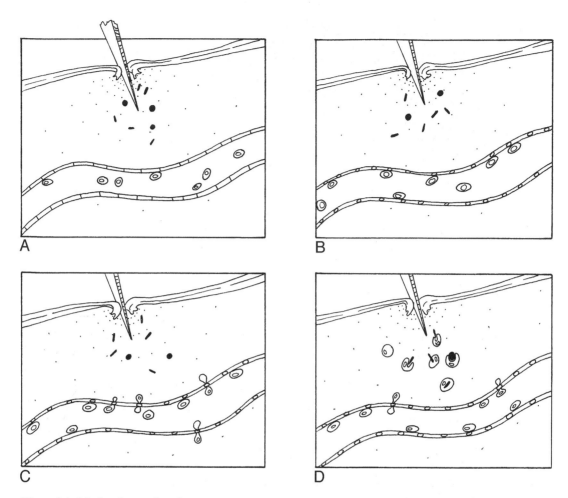

Figure 6.4. Mechanisms whereby neutrophils are attracted to sites of injury. **A**. Tissue injury and introduction of bacteria causes diffusion of a chemotactic substance to capillaries. **B**. Chemotactic substance increases capillary porosity and adhesion of neutrophils to capillary endothelium. **C**. By a process known as diapedesis, the adhered neutrophils squeeze through capillary pores. **D**. Neutrophils proceed to injury site by amoeboid movement and phagocytize bacteria and other debris.

Monocytes are the cells that comprise the mononuclear phagocytic system (MPS). The MPS was formerly known as the reticuloendothelial system. Its cells are either monocytes (intravascular) or derived from monocytes (extravascular). The cells are mobile (macrophages) or become fixed in position (e.g., the Küpffer cells in the liver sinusoids and others in the spleen and lymph nodes). The fixed cells are also phagocytic.

Monocytes in birds are comparable in morphology to avian large lymphocytes,

but in general they have relatively more cytoplasm than large lymphocytes.

EOSINOPHILS On a stained blood film, eosinophils can be seen to have cytoplasmic granules that are red or reddish-orange (eosinophilic). These are about the same size as neutrophils. The granules contain several enzymes (e.g., histaminase) that dampen and terminate local inflammatory reactions of allergic origin. Eosinophils become more numerous in certain types of parasitism. The parasitic forms are opsonized (attacked by antibodies) and the eosinophils discharge their granular contents onto the surface of the opsonized parasite, inflicting lethal damage.

In Cushing's disease, there is an over-secretion of adrenocorticosteroid hormones. When cortisol (an adrenocorticosteroid) is injected, this condition is simulated, and the number of circulating eosinophils decreases. Cortisol reduces the eosinophil count by enhancing eosinophil diapedesis and by diminishing the release of eosinophils by the bone marrow. Cortisol production increases during stress, and lowered eosinophil blood counts have been associated with stress.

Because of their eosinophilic granules and polymorphic nuclei, avian eosinophils have similarities to avian heterophils. However, the eosinophil granules are spherical and are dull red instead of the heterophil granule brilliant red. Also, the nucleus is most often bilobed and stains a richer blue than the heterophil.

BASOPHILS Basophils of the blood are somewhat similar to the mast cells that are present in the interstitial spaces outside the capillaries. Basophil granules contain histamine, bradykinin, serotonin, and lysosomal enzymes, substances that initiate an inflammatory response. Basophils and mast cells have receptors on their cell membranes for IgE antibodies (those associated with allergies). When the antibody on the cell membrane contacts its antigen, the basophil ruptures, releasing its granular contents, and the local vascular and tissue reactions of allergies are manifested. Basophils are rare in normal blood and their distribution in blood is usually considered to be less than 1%.

Basophils enhance allergic reactions, whereas eosinophils tend to dampen them. There is a balance between their functions in that inflammatory reactions proceed quickly (basophils) and then are modified (eosinophils), so that overreaction does not occur.

Avian basophils are about the same size and shape as heterophils. The nucleus is usu-ally round or oval and weakly basophilic. Deeply basophilic granules are numerous in cytoplasm that is devoid of color.

LYMPHOCYTES Lymphocytes can be classified morphologically as small or large lymphocytes. It is believed that the large lymphocytes represent immature lymphocytes, whereas the small lymphocytes represent more mature forms. Lymphocytes are involved in immune responses and on this basis are classified as T cells or B cells. Both T and B cells are derived from hematopoietic stem cells that differentiate to form lymphocytes. Before their general distribution to lymphatic tissue, they are preprocessed in the thymus gland (T cells) or in the bone marrow (B cells). T cells are involved in cell-mediated immunity, which involves the formation of large numbers of lymphocytes to destroy foreign substances (antigens). The three different groups of T cells are (1) cytotoxic T cells, (2) helper T cells, and (3) suppressor T cells. Cytotoxic T cells are sometimes called killer cells. T-cell receptors bind to specific antigens, and cytotoxic substances are released into the foreign cell (e.g., bacteria, virus, tissue cell; Fig. 6.5). Helper T cells are the most numerous of the T cells. When helper T cells are activated, they assist in the activation of cytotoxic T cells, suppressor T cells, and B cells. Antigens ordinarily activate these cells, but activation is more intense when assisted by helper T cells. Suppressor T cells are sometimes called regulatory T cells because they suppress the action of cytotoxic and helper T cells and prevent an excessive immune reaction. Suppressor T cells can help prevent an animal's immune system from attacking its own body tissue (autoimmune disease).

B lymphocytes were first discovered in birds and were found to be preprocessed in the bursa of Fabricius, from which the name was derived (B for bursa). Mammals do not have a bursa of Fabricius, and it is believed that preprocessing occurs in the bone marrow. B cells do not attack foreign

Figure 6.5. Mechanism whereby sensitized cytotoxic T lymphocytes destroy a foreign cell. The attacked cell is killed by the release of cytotoxic and digestive enzymes from the T lymphocytes directly into the cytoplasm of the attacked cell. The T lymphocytes can proceed to other cells following their attack on a cell.

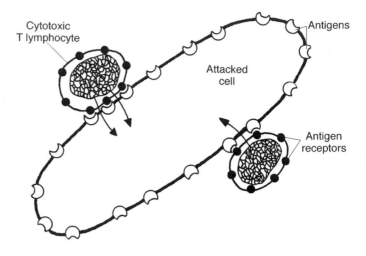

substances directly, but instead produce antibodies (globulin molecules) that inactivate the foreign substance. This type of immunity is known as humoral immunity. Antibodies can produce inactivation by causing agglutination, precipitation, neutralization (antibodies cover toxic sites), or lysis (rupture of the cell).

Agglutination and precipitation reactions are shown in Figure 6.6.

A more common humoral method of immunity is represented by the complement system, which is comprised of a number of enzyme precursors that are activated successively. From a small beginning, a large reaction occurs. Examples of complement reactions are 1) opsonization, in which foreign substances are covered by antibody and become vulnerable to phagocytosis by neutrophils and macrophages, and 2) chemotaxis, in which the complement product attracts neutrophils and macrophages into the local region of the antigenic agent. Several other complement products can be formed and result in lysis, agglutination, inflammation, and activation of mast cells and basophils, which produce a number of inflammatory effects in an effort to incapacitate the antigenic agent.

Lymphocytes comprise about two-thirds f the leukocytes in birds and in this regard are similar to the cloven-hooved animals. There are large and small lymphocytes as in mammals, with varying amounts of cytoplasm (meager in small lymphocytes and abundant in large) that is weakly basophilic.

PLASMA CELLS AND MEGAKARYOCYTES Two other cell types are sometimes considered to be white blood cells: plasma cells and megakaryocytes. Plasma cells are usually not considered to be blood cells because they are rarely found in circulating blood; rather, they are produced in the lymph tissue of the body and stay in this location. They are derived from B lymphocytes and produce the antibodies for humoral immunity.

Megakaryocytes are found in the bone marrow and are large cells which give rise to many platelets that are about 3 μm in diameter. Platelets circulate in the blood and number about 400,000/μl. The principal function of platelets is assisting in hemorrhage control.

Diagnostic Procedures

Diagnostic procedures related to white blood cells include determination of their total number and distribution of the leukocyte types. The total number can be determined by dilution and subsequent counting, either manually in a hemocytometer or

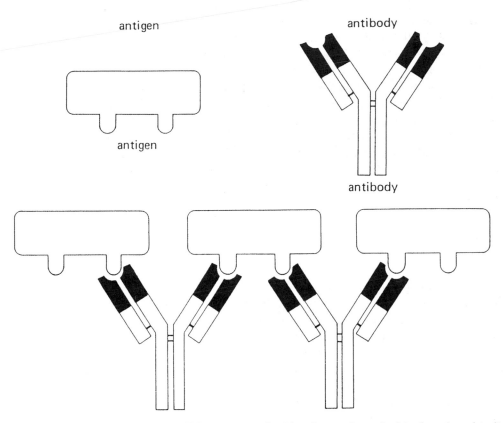

Figure 6.6. Antigens (molecules or cells) are grouped with other antigens by bivalent (two binding sites) antibodies. This causes them to agglutinate or precipitate. From Vander AJ, Sherman JH, Luciano DS. Human physiology: the mechanisms of body function. 4th ed. New York: McGraw-Hill, 1985.

with an electronic counter. An increase in leukocyte numbers is called leukocytosis; this usually occurs in bacterial infections. A decrease in numbers is called leukopenia; this is usually associated with the early stages of viral infections. Leukemia is a cancer of white blood cells and is characterized by leukocytosis. The determination of the percentage distribution of WBCs is known as a differential white blood cell count. In this procedure, a smear is made of a blood drop and is subsequently stained. The cells are observed under a microscope, and the different types are counted and classified until a total of 100 have been tallied. The number for each type is then esti-

mated as the percentage distribution in the blood (Table 6.1).

The absolute number of leukocytes is calculated after the total number and differential count have been determined. The absolute number refers to the number per microliter for each leukocyte type. Determination of the absolute number can prevent misinterpretation of the differential count. For example, the total WBC count for a normal cow might be 9,000/μl. This number could be comprised of 30% neutrophils and 60% lymphocytes, in which the absolute numbers would be 2,700/μl (0.3 × 9,000) and 5,400/μl (0.60 × 9,000), respectively. If traumatic gastritis is present, this same cow might have a total WBC count of 27,000/μl and a differential count of 70% neutrophils and 20% lymphocytes. A first interpretation might be that a lymphopenia exists (60% lymphocytes decreased to 20%). Further calculation shows, however, that the absolute number of lymphocytes remains the same (27,000/μl × 0.20 = 5400/μl), whereas the absolute number of neutrophils increases (27,000/μl × 0.70 = 18,900/μl). The neutrophil increase would indicate inflammation.

Erythrocytes

Numbers

The number of erythrocytes can be determined by making known dilutions and counting the number of RBCs in a known volume using the counting chamber of a hemocytometer with the aid of a microscope. Using various multiplication factors (which allow for dilution and for the limited volume that is counted), the number of RBCs/microliter (μl) of blood can be determined (Fig. 6.7). Formerly, RBC numbers were reported as number/cubic millimeter (mm^3). Cubic millimeter and microliter are the same, as are cubic centimeter (cc) and milliliter (ml). More accurate determinations can be made by using electronic counting equipment (Fig. 6.8). Generally, there are about 7,000,000 RBCs/μl blood in the cow, pig, and dog (Table 6.2). More RBCs are shown for sheep (11,000,000 RBCs/μl). Values for the goat are not given in Table 6.2, but they average about 13,000,000 RBCs/μl blood.

Shape

Erythrocytes are generally considered to be discocytes, with some degree of concavity. The dog's RBCs have typical biconcave disks, whereas the goat's RBCs are more spherical. The camel has elliptic RBCs and the deer has RBCs that are somewhat sickle-shaped. The advantages of a discoid shape are 1) the provision of a larger surface area: volume ratio, 2) minimal diffusion distance, and 3) greater osmotic swelling (water intake) possible without threatening the integrity of the membrane.

The characteristic shape of erythrocytes is maintained by the molecular constitution

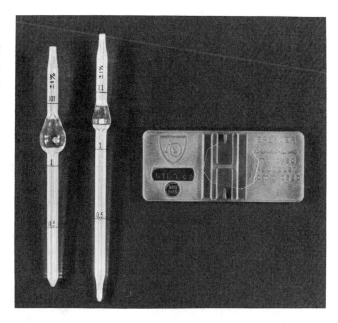

Figure 6.7. Hemocytometer for manually counting erythrocytes and leukocytes. The hemocytometer consists of (left to right): a red blood cell diluting pipet, a white blood cell diluting pipet, and a counting chamber.

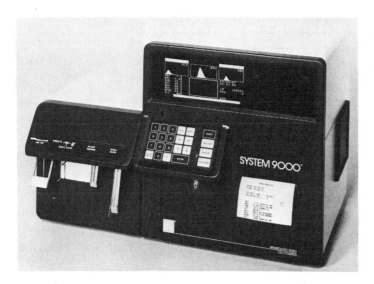

Figure 6.8. An automated cell counter for counting erythrocytes, leukocytes and platelets electronically. The cells are counted as they stream by a photoelectric cell in single file. (System 9000 Automated Cell Counter, Baker Instruments Corp., Allentown, PA.)

of hemoglobin and by certain contractile proteins of the cell membrane. An altered shape, because of a difference in hemoglobin constitution, can result in disease, such as sickle cell anemia in humans. A genetically induced substitution of the amino acid valine for the usual glutamic acid in the amino acid sequence of hemoglobin causes RBCs to assume a sickle shape, rather than the usual biconcave disk shape, when hemoglobin is deoxygenated. The altered shape makes the cells more vulnerable to destruction, and the anemia results.

Erythrocytes are tolerant of shape changes as they circulate. Many variations are noted as they pass through the small lumen (duct) of capillaries or rebound from a collision with a vessel bifurcation (branch). This property of tolerance for shape change is known as plasticity.

Size

Among the domestic animals, dogs have erythrocytes with the largest diameter (7 micrometers, μm) and sheep and goats have those with the smallest (4 to 4.5 μm). It appears that this was an adaptive feature, because even though they have RBCs of the smallest size, they are greater in number.

Because the sheep and goat were commonly found in regions of high altitudes with lower oxygen concentrations, the available hemoglobin was placed in a greater number of smaller packages so that a greater surface area would be available for diffusion.

Erythropoiesis

The production of erythrocytes is known as erythropoiesis. Before birth, erythrocyte formation occurs in the liver, spleen, and bone marrow. During the postnatal, growth, and adult periods, erythropoiesis is restricted almost exclusively to the bone marrow. It appears that most bones are involved in erythropoiesis, and the axial and appendicular skeletons account for about 35 and 65% of RBC production, respectively. This pattern has been observed in 1-year-old beagle dogs and can vary in other animals. The axial skeleton includes almost all bones except those of the limbs, which belong to the appendicular skeleton (Chapter 4). The erythrocytes are continually formed and destroyed. Considering the large number of RBCs in the blood, one should appreciate the dynamic aspect of this phenomenon. For

TABLE 6.2. Average Values for Several Blood Variables[1]

Variable	Animal					
	Horse	Cow	Sheep	Pig	Dog	Chicken
Total RBC/µl blood ($\times 10^6$)	9.0	7.0	12.0	6.5	6.8	3.0
Diameter of RBC (µm)	5.5	5.9	4.8	6.0	7.0	elliptic 7×12
PCV (%)	41.0	35.0	35.0	42.0	45.0	30.0
Sedimentation rate (mm/min)	2–12/10	0/60	0/60	1–14/60	6–10/60	1.5–4/60
Hemoglobin (g/dl)	14.4	11.0	11.5	13.0	15.0	9.0
Coagulation time (capillary tube method; min)	2–5	2–5	2–5	2–5	2–5	**
Specific gravity	1.060	1.043	1.042	1.060	1.059	1.050
Plasma protein (g/dl)	6–8	7–8.5	6–8	6.5–8.5	6–7.8	4.5
Blood pH (arterial)	7.40	7.38	7.48	7.4	7.36	7.48
Blood volume (% of body weight)	8–10	5–6	5–6	5–7	8–10	7–9
Mean corpuscular volume (MCV; fl)	45.5*	52.0	34.0	63.0	70.0	115.0
Mean corpuscular hemoglobin (MCH; pg)	15.9*	14.0	10.0	19.0	22.8	41.0
Mean corpuscular hemoglobin concentration (MCHC; %)	35.0*	33.0	32.5	32.0	34.0	29.0

[1] Data compiled from Dukes' Physiology of Domestic Animals and from Essentials of Veterinary Hematology by Jain NC.

* Hot blooded

**See Differences in Blood Coagulation Among Species.

example, approximately 35,000,000 erythrocytes/second are formed in a 454.5-kg horse.

Erythrocytes are formed in the bone marrow from a beginning cell known as a rubriblast. Several intermediate forms are recognized in the genesis of the erythrocyte (Fig. 6.9). The distribution of these forms can be studied by preparation and by examination of bone marrow smears. Just before the developing erythrocyte's entrance into the circulation, the nucleus is expelled (see the following section). The polyribosomes and ribosomes are retained and might still be apparent on stained smears for a day or so after their arrival in the circulation. If they are present, they are identified as reticulocytes because of the netlike appearance of the polyribosomes and ribosomes. Polyribosomes (polysomes) consist of several ribosomes joined together by the same messenger RNA molecule. During periods of rapid RBC production, reticulocyte numbers can increase. Reticulocytes are seldom present in the circulating blood of horses. The nuclei of avian erythrocytes are not expelled before entry into the circulation, and they persist throughout the life of the erythrocytes.

The life span of erythrocytes in domestic animals is approximately 110 days. It is shorter in some laboratory animal species (e.g., rabbit, rat, mouse). In chickens the life span is considerably shorter—about 30 days.

The rate of erythropoiesis appears to be controlled by the tissue need for oxygen. The reduced oxygen concentration at the tissue level results in the secretion of a hormone by the kidneys known as

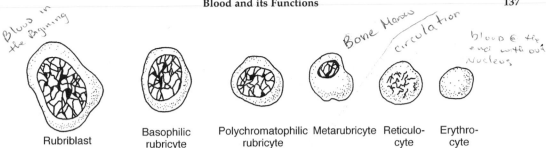

Blood in the Beginning *Bone Marrow circulation* *blood & tie end without Nucleus*

Rubriblast Basophilic rubricyte Polychromatophilic rubricyte Metarubricyte Reticulo-cyte Erythro-cyte

Figure 6.9. The stages of erythrocyte development.

erythropoietin. Erythropoietin stimulates the bone marrow to begin formation of new erythrocytes. The life span of erythropoietin is less than 1 day; this short life span helps provide greater flexibility in the adjustment of erythrocyte numbers to regulate the tissue need for oxygen more precisely. New erythrocytes do not appear in the circulation until about 5 days after their formation begins. Thus, additional erythropoietin can be formed to allow for continued production during the interim. When the new erythrocytes appear in the circulation, the tissue need for oxygen begins to be met and erythropoietin is no longer secreted.

Hemoglobin and its Forms

The principal component of erythrocytes is hemoglobin (Hb), which comprises about one-third of the erythrocyte content, the remainder being water and stroma (structural components). The hemoglobin molecule (Fig. 6.10) has a molecular weight of about 66,000 and is composed of four heme groups combined with one molecule of globin (the protein component). Globin is composed of four polypeptide chains, each containing one of the heme groups. Each heme group contains an iron atom that combines loosely and reversibly with one oxygen molecule. Therefore, one molecule of hemoglobin contains four iron atoms and can carry four molecules of oxygen. The iron atom of heme has a valence of +2 (Fe^{2+}, ferrous) regardless of whether molecular oxygen is combined with it.

Because of the presence of hemoglobin, blood can transport about 60 times more oxygen than would be possible by its simple solution. Certain conditions cause the ferrous iron of heme to be oxidized to its ferric state. In one such condition, nitrate poisoning, the hemoglobin formed is known as methemoglobin, and it cannot transport oxygen. Another abnormal form of hemoglobin is carbonmonoxyhemoglobin (sometimes called carboxyhemoglobin). As the name implies, carbon monoxide occupies the site normally occupied by oxygen. Hemoglobin has an affinity for carbon monoxide that is about 200 times greater than it has for oxygen. Thus, small concentrations of carbon monoxide compete more favorably for sites on Hb than normal concentrations of oxygen.

The hemoglobin of muscle is known as myoglobin. It differs from hemoglobin in that it has only one polypeptide chain and one associated heme group, so it can only combine with one molecule of oxygen instead of four. The concentration of hemoglobin in the blood of domestic animals averages about 12 g/dl (Table 6.2).

Destruction

As erythrocytes age, several metabolic changes occur: the membrane becomes more rigid and fragile, and the discocyte converts to a poorly deformable spherocyte. Accordingly, some intravascular hemolysis of erythrocytes occurs (10%), and the remainder of the RBCs (about 90%) is selectively removed from the circulating

Figure 6.10. Schematic representation of one heme group and its associated polypeptide chain. Four of these combinations, at different orientations to each other, comprise hemoglobin. The heme is held to its specific polypeptide chain (one of four in the protein globin) by cysteine (an amino acid) bridges and by bonding of the iron to imidazole groups of histidine (an amino acid). Molecular oxygen binds with iron. Modified from Conn EE, Stumpf PK. Outlines of biochemistry. New York: John Wiley & Sons, 1963. © 1963, John Wiley & Sons, Inc.

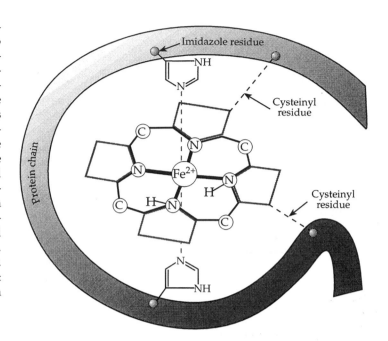

pool by cells of the MPS, mostly the fixed cells in the spleen, liver, and bone marrow.

When erythrocytes are phagocytized by MPS cells they undergo hemolysis within the phagocytic cell (extravascular or intracellular hemolysis), and the Hb, other proteins, and membrane lipids of the phagocytized RBCs are catabolized. A summary of Hb degradation begun in this way is shown in Figure 6.11. The iron and globin are separated from heme, globin is degraded to its amino acids, and they are reutilized. Iron is stored in the MPS cells in the form of ferritin and hemosiderin or is transferred to plasma, where it combines with a plasma protein, apotransferrin, to become transferrin. Transferrin circulates to the bone marrow, where the iron is used for the synthesis of new hemoglobin. During Hb synthesis, iron released from decomposing RBCs is used in preference to storage iron.

Heme is converted to biliverdin (a green pigment) and then reduced to bilirubin (a yellow pigment). Free bilirubin (water-insoluble) is released into the plasma, where it becomes bound to albumin (a plasma protein) and is transported to the liver and is "dumped." In the liver, the insoluble bilirubin conjugates with glucuronic acid to form bilirubin glucuronide, mainly diglucuronide, which is water-soluble. It is secreted into the bile in this form and enters the intestine. Bacteria within the large intestine reduce bilirubin glucuronide to urobilinogen. Most urobilinogen is excreted with the feces in the oxidized forms of urobilin or stercobilin, which are pigments that give feces its normal color. Part of the urobilinogen is reabsorbed into the enterohepatic circulation, from which most is re-excreted into the bile. Some of the absorbed urobilinogen bypasses the liver, enters the general circulation, and is excreted in the urine to become the normal pigment of the urine (urobilin). Carbon monoxide (CO) is formed when the porphyrin ring of heme is opened. This is the only reaction in the body in which CO is formed and is excreted by the lungs.

Because of liver disease, free bilirubin combined with albumin might not be

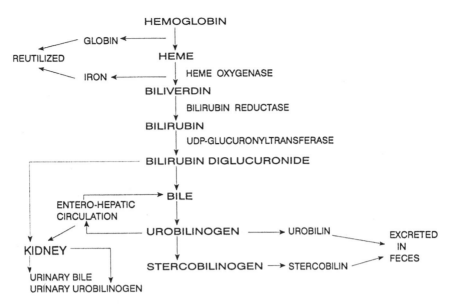

Figure 6.11. Summary of hemoglobin degradation with its beginning in mononuclear phagocytic system cells. The lighter line from bilirubin diglucuronide to the kidneys indicates an insignificant or abnormal direction for its excretion. From Jain NC. Essentials of veterinary hematology. 6th ed. Philadelphia: Lea & Febiger, 1993.

"dumped" and would continue to circulate and appear in high concentration in the plasma and interstitial fluids. Also, if the bile duct becomes blocked, the bilirubin glucuronides could spill over into the plasma. Both these conditions can produce a yellow color in the tissues known as icterus, or jaundice. ← Read →

When erythrocytes are hemolyzed intravascularly, the Hb is first bound to haptoglobin (a plasma protein). This complex is removed rapidly by cells of the MPS, and the Hb is degraded as previously described for extravascular hemolysis. Because the complex is a large molecule, it is not filtered through the kidney glomeruli. Excessive intravascular hemolysis (hemolytic disease) can occur, however, and sufficient haptoglobin might not be available. The plasma takes on a reddish appearance, and the condition is known as hemoglobinemia. The free Hb is then filtered at the glomeruli and enters the kidney tubules. Much of it is reabsorbed from the tubules but can surpass the renal threshold for reabsorption and continue into the urine to give it a reddish color, a condition known as hemoglobinuria.

Iron Metabolism

A large proportion of ingested iron is reduced to ferrous iron (Fe^{2+}) in the stomach. Within the duodenum and jejunum, most of the ferrous iron is absorbed into the intestinal epithelial cells. Iron absorption, transport, storage, and usage is summarized in Figure 6.12. From the intestinal cell it enters the blood or can combine with a cellular protein (apoferritin) to become ferritin, a storage form of iron. Within 2 or 3 days, the ferritin is either converted back to its free form (Fe^{2+}) and absorbed into the blood or is cast into the intestinal lumen. The latter situation would be a result of the normal turnover of intestinal epithelial cells as they migrate from the crypts to the tips of the villi, from which they are exfoliated (passed off into the lumen). The iron

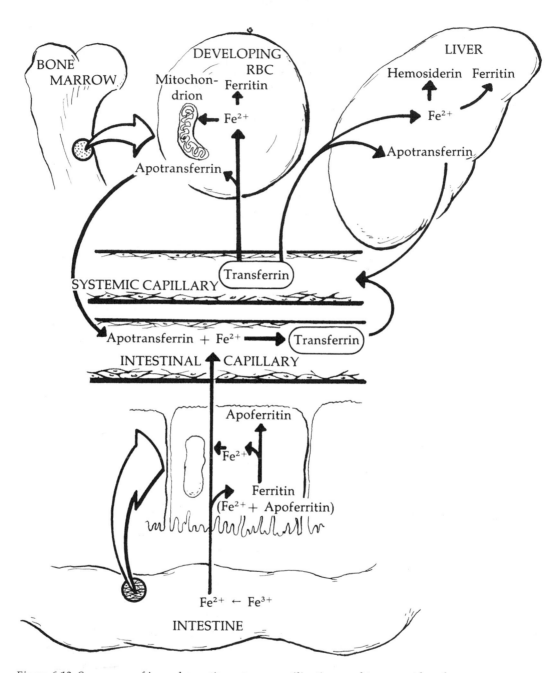

Figure 6.12. Summary of iron absorption, storage, utilization, and transport by plasma.

that enters the blood combines with apotransferrin (a plasma protein) to form transferrin. Combining with a protein prevents it from being excreted by the kidneys (the combination is poorly filtered at the glomerulus).

Within the bone marrow, all the erythroid forms, including reticulocytes, have surface membrane receptors for transferrin. Plasma transferrin binds to these receptors, becomes internalized by endocytosis, and releases its iron, and the apotransferrin is returned to the plasma. The internalized iron is transported into the mitochondria of the developing erythrocyte, where it is incorporated into the heme molecule, or it combines with apoferritin to be stored as ferritin.

Two factors generally affect the absorption of iron from the intestinal epithelium into the blood: (1) the extent of the iron stores in the body, and (2) the rate of erythropoiesis. If the requirement for iron increases and the iron stores are empty, absorption increases. If the requirement for iron decreases and the iron stores are adequate, absorption of iron from the intestine decreases. It appears that there is a self-limiting mechanism for iron absorption based on need. Excess iron can be ingested and subsequently absorbed, however, inducing iron toxicity. The excretion of iron is minimal so that the regulation is unidirectional—that is, controlled absorption. Iron with transferrin can be released to tissue cells anywhere so that excess iron can be deposited in all cells, especially those of the liver. Ferritin is a storage form of iron (see previous text). In addition, a more insoluble form, hemosiderin, accumulates in times of excess. The liver is the principal organ for iron storage. When liver stores are adequate the production of apotransferrin decreases, and when they are depleted the production of apotransferrin increases. Animals with iron deficiency anemia have high concentrations of apotransferrin.

Anemia and Polycythemia

A reduction in the number of erythrocytes, the concentration of hemoglobin, or both is referred to as anemia, which can have several causes. It is considered functional if the tissues do not become hypoxic because of lack of exertion and because erythropoietin is not formed. Blood loss for any reason (e.g., trauma, parasitism) can also cause anemia. A common type of anemia in baby pigs is iron deficiency anemia. This type is common to baby pigs because of their rapid growth and consequent need for greater blood volume, and also because of the lack of iron in their normal diet, which is sow's milk. Because of iron deficiency, an insufficient quantity of hemoglobin is produced. Anemia can also occur from poor erythrocyte production, such as when certain nutritional factors are missing, or if the bone marrow has been poisoned. This latter type is known as aplastic anemia.

A condition opposite to anemia is polycythemia. In this condition, the erythrocyte numbers are greatly increased. This is seldom recognized in animals but does occur.

PREVENTION OF BLOOD LOSS

The effectiveness of blood function depends on its circulation within a closed system of vessels. The vessels might open because of disease or accident, and blood loss can be minimized by hemostasis.

Hemostatic Summary

When a blood vessel is damaged, endothelial cells are separated, the underlying collagen is exposed, and the surface loses its usual smoothness and nonwettability. Often the vessel is torn, cut, or separated and the hemostatic crisis is exacerbated. Regardless of the severity, platelets begin to contact the damaged surface. This initiates the adhesion process because the platelets develop projections (pseudopods) and become sticky (Fig. 6.13). The adhered platelets undergo a reaction in which aggregating agents are released and cause

Figure 6.13. Platelet adhesion. This is the first response to blood vessel injury. The platelets lose their discoid shape and form sticky projections (pseudopods) for their continued adherence to the injured vessel and entrapment of other platelets.

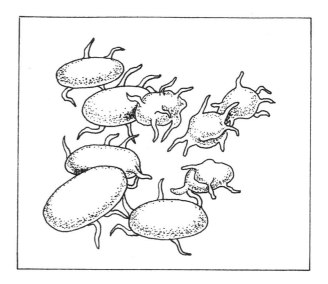

the accumulation of more platelets; a loose platelet plug is formed that impedes blood loss. Blood coagulation soon becomes evident at the damaged site, and the platelet plug is strengthened by the formation of a fibrin meshwork. Finally, the damaged vessel is repaired by connective tissue and endothelial cell growth, and there is a return to normal when the platelet-fibrin complex and other cell debris is removed (Fig. 6.14).

Hemostatic Components

VASCULAR ENDOTHELIUM   The entire cardiovascular system is lined by a single layer of flattened cells known as the endothelium. It not only lines the heart but also the vessels. At the capillary level, all that remains is the endothelial layer. Regardless of its location, it is underlaid with a basement membrane that contains collagen. Collagen fibers are also present throughout the interstitial space. Collagen is a potent platelet activator. In addition to collagen, the subendothelial tissue contains von Willebrand factor (vWF) and fibronectin. These are proteins that have adhesive properties serving to enhance the aggregation of platelets.

As long as the endothelium is intact, the platelets and the proteins that are associated with blood coagulation (procoagulants) are not activated. The properties of the endothelium that prevent activation include (1) the negative charge on the endothelial cell surface that repels the negatively charged platelets, (2) synthesis of inhibitors of platelet function (e.g., prostacyclin) and of fibrin formation (e.g., thrombomodulin), and (3) the generation of activators of fibrin degradation (e.g., tissue plasminogen activator [t-PA]).

PLATELETS   Platelets are also known as thrombocytes. An appreciation for the complexity of the platelet can be obtained from Figure 6.15. The band of microtubules that encircle the platelet contract when platelets are activated and results in change of shape and in extrusion of platelet granule contents into the open canalicular system and subsequent release from the platelet to its exterior. The granules contain many of the coagulation factors, other proteins, calcium, serotonin, ADP, and ATP, all of which assist or potentiate the coagulation process. Release of the granule contents requires energy from the mitochondria and glycogen particles and ionized calcium from the dense tubular system, a component of the membrane system of the platelet.

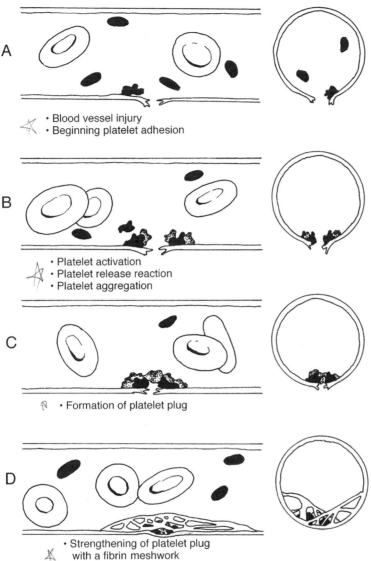

Figure 6.14. A schematic representation of the events leading to the formation of a blood clot. The panel on the left provides a longitudinal view of a blood vessel and the panel on the right a cross-section of that vessel at the injury site. Specific events are described when proceeding from A through D.

A
• Blood vessel injury
• Beginning platelet adhesion

B
• Platelet activation
• Platelet release reaction
• Platelet aggregation

C
• Formation of platelet plug

D
• Strengthening of platelet plug with a fibrin meshwork

CLOTTING FACTORS The elements essential for blood coagulation are present in the blood or tissues and simply await an activation mechanism. The elements are identified as factors, and many of those first discovered were identified further by Roman numerals I to V and VII to XIII (number VI was initially described, but was found later not to exist). Calcium is factor IV and is required for nearly all of the coagulation reactions. The other factors are proteins and nearly all are synthesized in the liver. A listing of the protein factors involved in coagulation is shown in Table 6.3. Vitamin K is required for the liver production of prothrombin (factor II) and of factors VII, IX, and X.

Sequence of Platelet Reactions

Platelets can be activated by their contact with collagen in the endothelial cell

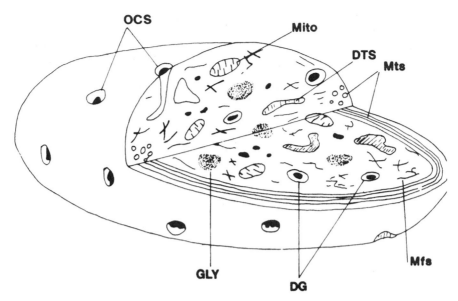

Figure 6.15. Diagrammatic representation of a platelet sectioned through two planes (*DG*, dense granules (amine storage); *DTS*, dense tubular system; *GLY*, glycogen particle; *OCS*, open canalicular system; *Mfs*, microfilaments; *Mito*, mitochondria; *Mts*, microtubules). From Gentry PA, Downie HG. Blood coagulation. In: Swenson MJ, ed. Dukes' physiology of domestic animals. 10th ed. Ithaca, NY: Cornell University Press, 1984.

basement membrane or in the interstitial tissues. They can also be activated by substances released from damaged cells such as ADP, serotonin, and thromboxane A_2 (TXA_2).

PLATELET ADHESION The first response of platelets to disrupted endothelium and contact with subendothelial tissues is their adhesion or attachment to surfaces. When this happens, a monolayer of platelets adhere to the site, lose their discoid shape, and form pseudopods as shown in Figure 6.13. The pseudopods permit greater contact with other platelets flowing by the site of damage and also with those already adhering to the subendothelium. The initial adhesion requires the factors vWF and fibronectin that are present in the subendothelium. Continued adhesion results from vWF and fibronectin presence in platelet granules that are extruded from the platelets.

PLATELET ACTIVATION. This is the means whereby platelets are stimulated to begin their further role in assisting hemostasis. Stimulation involves the formation of an intracellular messenger that will release ionized Ca^{2+} from granule storage into the cytoplasm. The principal messenger, TXA_2, is produced from platelet membrane phospholipids when collagen or ADP make contact with the membrane receptors. Aspirin blocks the formation of TXA_2, thus preventing the major messenger from mobilizing Ca^{2+} from the granules to the cytoplasm.

PLATELET RELEASE REACTION This event is mediated by Ca^{2+}s released from granules in response to TXA_2 formation. It involves clustering of granules into the center of the platelet after microtubular contraction and, finally, granule content extrusion to the exterior from the open canalicular system. The mechanisms of release are illustrated in Figure 6.16.

PLATELET AGGREGATION The exterior presence of the granule contents provides high concentrations of fibrinogen (needed to

TABLE 6.3.   Proteins involved in blood coagulation

Factor	Synonym	Site of synthesis
Fibrinogen	Factor I	Liver
Prothrombin	Factor II	Liver
Tissue factor	Thromboplastin, factor III	Tissues
Factor V	Proaccelerin	Platelets
Factor VII	Proconvertin	Liver
Factor VIII	Factor VIII: C, antihemophilic factor	Vascular endothelium
Factor IX	Christmas factor	Liver
Factor X	Stuart factor	Liver
Factor XI	Plasma thromboplastin antecedent	Liver
Factor XII	Hageman factor	Liver
Factor XIII	Fibrin stabilizing factor	Liver
von Willebrand factor	VWF	Megakaryocytes, endothelial cells
Prekallikrein	Fletcher factor	Liver
High-molecular-weight-kininogen	HMWK	Liver
Fibronectin	Cold-insoluble globulin	Liver

From Gentry PA, Downie AG. Blood coagulation. In: Swenson MJ, Reece WO, eds. Dukes' physiology of domestic animals. 11th ed. Ithaca, NY: Cornell University Press, 1993.

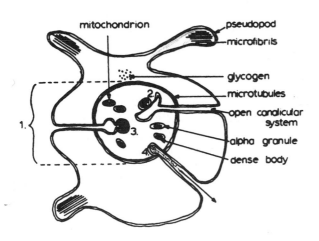

Figure 6.16. Platelet cross section showing how microtubular contraction results in extrusion of platelet granule contents into the open canalicular system and release from the platelet. *1*, Clustering of granules into center of platelet after microtubular contraction; *2*, contact of granule membrane with open canalicular system membrane; *3*, fusion of granule membrane with open canalicular system membrane; *4*, granule content extruded from open canalicular system. From MacIntyre DE. The platelet release reaction: association with adhesion and aggregation and comparison with secretory responses in other cells. In: Gordon JL, ed. Platelets in biology and pathology, Vol. 1. Amsterdam: Elsevier, 1976.

form fibrin), fibronectin and vWF (needed for adhesion), and factor V (needed for conversion of prothrombin to thrombin) at the platelet surface which, by piling platelets upon each other, can lead to the formation of the primary platelet plug. After the release reaction, the platelets lose their individual integrity, lipoprotein membranes are fused, receptors are exposed for coagulation proteins (factors), and thus a highly reactive surface is exposed (platelet aggregation) for the formation of thrombin and fibrin.

Blood Coagulation

Thrombin formation is the penultimate (next to last) stage in the formation of fibrin, which is insoluble; that stabilizes the platelet plug. The stabilized platelet plug is known as the secondary hemostatic plug or thrombus. Once the platelet plug is formed, blood loss through the damaged endothelium is completely stopped. It was recognized previously that, after the platelet reactions, the stage was set for blood coagulation. Most of the proteins that participate in the hemostatic process circulate in plasma as inactive proenzymes and each undergoes activation in sequence as coagulation proceeds. The sequence is referred to as a cascade phenomenon—each reaction represents an amplification point, whereby a small stimulus results in a larger response.

Two mechanisms are recognized as activators of blood coagulation. These depend on whether coagulation proceeds from the contact of blood with a foreign surface, such as disrupted blood vascular endothelium (intrinsic mechanism), or from the contact of blood with extravascular tissue (extrinsic mechanism). The intrinsic mechanism would be independent of the extrinsic mechanism if only the integrity of the vascular endothelium were involved or if blood were drawn into a glass tube. However, most disruptions involve trauma where tissues are also injured. When tissues contact blood, the extrinsic mechanism becomes involved in coagulation as well as the intrinsic mechanism, and the two pathways are interrelated by a number of enzymatic reactions that function to enhance fibrin formation. The initiator of the extrinsic mechanism is tissue factor, also known as tissue thromboplastin and as factor III. A simplified representation of these two mechanisms of blood coagulation is illustrated in Figure 6.17. The extrinsic mecha-

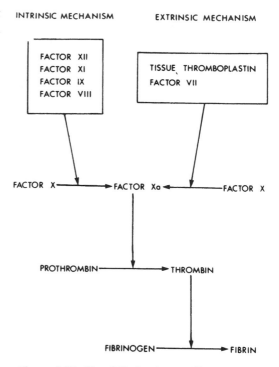

INTRINSIC MECHANISM   EXTRINSIC MECHANISM

FACTOR XII
FACTOR XI
FACTOR IX
FACTOR VIII

TISSUE THROMBOPLASTIN
FACTOR VII

FACTOR X ———→ FACTOR Xa ←——— FACTOR X

PROTHROMBIN ———→ THROMBIN

FIBRINOGEN ———→ FIBRIN

Figure 6.17. Simplified scheme illustrating the intrinsic and extrinsic pathways that lead to the generation of fibrin. From Gentry PA, Downie HG. Blood coagulation. In: Swenson MJ, ed. Dukes' physiology of domestic animals. 10th ed. Ithaca, NY: Cornell University Press, 1984.

nism provides for a more direct activation of factor X and therefore produces thrombin and fibrin at a faster rate than the intrinsic mechanism. The greater efficiency is needed when blood vessels are torn and surrounding tissue is damaged.

A more detailed scheme of blood coagulation is shown in Figure 6.18. This illustration shows the necessity of blood contact with an unusual surface, the contact phase, for the initiation of the intrinsic mechanism. Also shown are the factors involved in both the intrinsic and extrinsic mechanisms for the activation of factor X ($X \rightarrow X_a$). After activation of factor X, there is a common pathway to the formation of thrombin after which fibrin is formed from fibrinogen. Once factor X is activated, it promotes

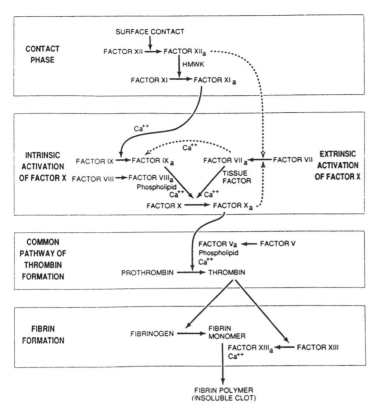

Figure 6.18. The intrinsic and extrinsic pathways for the activation of factor X and subsequent formation of fibrin. Note the necessity of the contact phase for initiation of the intrinsic mechanism. The broken lines represent interactions that link the two pathways. From Gentry PA, Downie HG. Blood coagulation. In: Swenson MJ, Reece WO, eds. Dukes' physiology of domestic animals. 11th ed. Ithaca, NY: Cornell University Press, 1993.

the activation of factor VII, which forms the VII-tissue factor complex that is associated with the activation of factor X.

The formation of fibrin in blood in a test tube can be observed when the blood loses its flow characteristics. The coagulum that appears consists of a homogeneous mass, and there is no identifiable liquid (serum). The thrombin that causes the conversion of fibrinogen to fibrin monomer also activates factor XIII (fibrin-stabilizing factor), which is released from entrapped platelets. Activated factor XIII (XIII_a) results in the formation of cross-linking bonds between adjacent fibrin monomers to produce a fibrin polymer, which has greater strength. Clot retraction (shrinking of the clot) is provided by the direct action of a platelet contractile protein known as thrombosthenin. This protein is exposed when platelets are stimulated and it interacts with fibrin. The presence of Ca^{2+} and thrombin causes the thrombosthenin to contract, and the clot retracts (serum is squeezed from the coagulum). Clot retraction permits greater blood flow in the damaged area while the tissue is being repaired. Failures of clot retraction might be associated with reduced platelet numbers.

Once blood coagulation has been initiated, the process extends into the surrounding blood; this is known as clot growth. Clot growth stops when blood flows fast enough to remove the thrombin that has been generated; this thrombin has not been otherwise absorbed by the fibrin that is formed and by the other activated factors. The thrombin and activated factors washed away by the blood are not effective because they have been diluted and because natural anticoagulant substances (such as antithrombin III) are present.

These can prevent unwanted coagulation when procoagulants (substances favoring coagulation) are present in small quantities.

After hemostasis has been established, the damaged vascular area is repaired by new tissue growth. The fibrin that was formed to assist in the hemostatic process undergoes degradation (fibrinolysis) by a proteolytic enzyme called plasmin. Plasminogen, a protein that is present in plasma, becomes entrapped within the clot when it is formed. Plasminogen is activated to become plasmin by substances in blood and tissues known as plasminogen activators. The principal endogenous plasminogen activator is tissue plasminogen activator (t-PA) that is released from endothelial cells when they are stimulated by the presence of thrombin or by stasis of blood. Plasmin degrades the fibrin molecule into protein fragments known as fibrin degradation products (FDPs). When the outer surface of the fibrin clot is removed, fresh surfaces are exposed and degraded until clot removal is complete. The FDPs, platelets, and other cell debris are removed from the circulation by the MPS. Tissue plasminogen activator is produced commercially for human medical use to dissolve clots that are lodged in vessels and that block blood flow (e.g., coronary arteries).

Prevention in Normal Circulation

The formation of thrombin occurs through a series of chemical reactions, so it is normal to have a small amount of thrombin in the circulation. The thrombin that is present could cause the conversion of fibrinogen (a normal plasma protein) to fibrin except that another protein, antithrombin III, blocks the action of thrombin on fibrinogen and also inactivates the thrombin that it binds.

In addition to antithrombin III action, coagulation in the normal vascular system is prevented by the smoothness of the endothelium. This prevents contact activation of factor XII in the intrinsic mechanism. Also, a monomolecular layer of protein is adsorbed to the surface of the endothelium that repels clotting factors and platelets. When endothelial damage occurs, both the smoothness and protein layer are lost at the damaged site.

Heparin, an anticoagulant, is produced by mast cells that reside in the pericapillary connective tissues. Mast cells are particularly abundant in the lungs because of the vulnerability of the lungs to emboli, which are clots that have broken loose from their original site and flow freely in the blood. The plasma concentration of heparin is normally low. The effectiveness of heparin in preventing normal intravascular clotting depends on its combining with antithrombin III to form a complex that removes not only thrombin but also factors IX, X, XI, and XII.

Prevention in Withdrawn Blood

It is often desirable to prevent blood coagulation when blood is withdrawn from an animal for later examination and analysis. Anticoagulants are used for this purpose. Chelating agents are used most frequently; they bind the calcium ions so that they are not available for the coagulation process. Trisodium citrate, sodium oxalate, or sodium EDTA (ethylenediaminetetraacetic acid, disodium salt) is added in an appropriate quantity to the collection container and mixed with the withdrawn blood. Heparin is also available commercially and can be used to prevent coagulation of withdrawn blood. It is also used to prevent coagulation of blood in the body in certain conditions.

Tests for Coagulation

Tests for blood coagulation are used to determine the adequacy of coagulation in an animal. Several techniques are available. Blood is withdrawn and subjected to standard methods, and the time interval is observed from withdrawal to coagulation. A prolonged time interval indicates an inadequate mechanism in the body. Because platelets supply various factors to the coagulation mechanism, in addition to forming a platelet plug, an estimation of their number is also helpful in assessing coagulation adequacy.

Knowledge of the coagulation process is helpful in understanding coagulation defects when they occur. Vitamin K deficiency results in hemorrhage because of inadequate formation of prothrombin and factors VII, IX, and X. Also, it was discovered that dicumarol interferes with the utilization of vitamin K and hence with prothrombin production.

Differences in Blood Coagulation among Species

The interaction of activated platelets with damaged endothelium and coagulation proteins is a requirement among all animals for a normal hemostatic mechanism, even though platelet numbers and morphology may vary. The absence of factor XII (a factor of the intrinsic mechanism) from the blood of marine mammals and reptiles prolongs the clotting time of their withdrawn blood. Serum harvest is not productive in birds when blood is collected from vessels where trauma to extravascular tissues has not occurred. The contact phase of the intrinsic mechanism is absent in birds, and reliance for blood coagulation depends upon the extrinsic mechanism (needs tissue thromboplastin). A coagulum will form in withdrawn blood but serum is extracted with difficulty. For this reason, when chemical analysis for blood components is desired, one should use an appropriate anticoagulant and harvest plasma (assuming plasma compatibility with the analysis).

PLASMA AND ITS COMPOSITION

Plasma, the liquid part of blood, can contain all those substances that exist in chemical form in the body because it provides the medium of exchange between the blood vessels and the cells of the body. The major constituent of plasma is water, which comprises about 92%. The most abundant substances dissolved or suspended in the water are proteins; their concentration varies but usually ranges from 5 to 8 g/dl. The albumins account for about 80% of the proteins; they represent the major contribution to the intravascular effective osmotic pressure and have an important transport function. The globulin protein fraction is the next most abundant. There are three globulin types: alpha, beta, and gamma. The alpha and beta globulins serve as substrates for new substances and also carry out transport functions. The gamma globulins form the antibodies that are associated with immunity. Fibrinogen is the least abundant protein fraction in plasma, and its role in blood coagulation has been discussed (see previous section). Oxygen, carbon dioxide, and nitrogen are the major gases of the atmosphere and are found in plasma. Their concentration in plasma depends on their concentration in the atmosphere and on their solubility in plasma. The major types of lipids in plasma are triglycerides, phospholipids, and cholesterol. The principal nonprotein nitrogen (NPN) compounds are amino acids, urea, uric acid, creatine, creatinine, and ammonium salts. Inorganic substances in the plasma are presented mainly by the electrolytes, including cations (Na^+, K^+, Ca^{2+}, Mg^{2+}) and anions (Cl^-, HCO_3^-, HPO_4^{-2}).

Values and concentrations for many plasma constituents are listed in Table 6.4 for the domestic animals.

STUDY AIDS—BLOOD AND ITS FUNCTIONS

Composition of Blood

1. What are the components of the hematocrit?

TABLE 6.4.   Values of Some Constituents of Blood from Mature Domestic Animals

Constituents	Horse	Cow	Sheep	Pig	Dog	Chicken
			Value (Range)			
Glucose (mg/dl)	60–110	40–80 80–120 (calf)	40–80 80–120 (lamb)	80–120	70–120	130–270
Nonprotein nitrogen (mg/dl)	20–40	20–40	20–38	20–45	17–38	20–35
Urea nitrogen (BUN) (mg/dl)	10–24	10–30	8–20	8–24	10–30	0.1–1.0
Uric acid (mg/dl)	0.5–1	0.1–2	0.1–2	0.1–2	0.1–1.5	1–2 1–7 (laying hen)
Creatinine (mg/dl)	1–2	1–2	1–2	1–2.5	1–2	1–2
Amino acid nitrogen (mg/dl)	5–7	4–8	5–8	6–8	7–8	4–10
Lactic acid (mg/dl)	10–16	5–20	9–12	–	8–20	47–56 20–98 (laying hen)
Cholesterol (mg/dl)	75–150	80–180	60–150	60–200	120–250	125–200
Bilirubin						
Direct (mg/dl)	0–0.4	0–0.3	0–0.3	0–0.3	0.06–0.1	
Indirect (mg/dl)	0.2–5	0.1–0.5	0–0.1	0–0.3	0.01–0.5	
Total (mg/dl)	0.2–6	0.2–1.5	0.1–0.4	0–0.6	0.10–0.6	
Electrolytes (mEq/L)						
Sodium	132–152	132–152	139–152	135–150	141–155	151–161
Potassium	2.5–5.0	3.9–5.8	3.9–5.4	4.4–6.7	3.7–5.8	4.6–4.7
Calcium	4.5–6.5	4.5–6.0	4.5–6.0	4.5–6.5	4.5–6.0	4.5–6.0 8.5–19.5 (laying hen)
Phosphorus	2–6	2–7	2–7	3–6	2–6	3–6
Magnesium	1.5–2.5	1.5–2.5	1.8–2.3	2–3	1.5–2.0	
Chlorine	99–109	97–111	95–105	94–106	100–115	119–130

From Swenson MJ. Physiological properties and cellular and chemical constituents of blood In: Swenson MJ, Reece WO, eds. Dukes' physiology of domestic animals. 11th ed. Ithaca, NY, Cornell University Press, 1993.

2. What accounts for the color of blood and for the color of plasma?
3. A dog weighs 10 kg, has a PCV of 42%, and a plasma volume of 500 ml. What is its blood volume expressed as percent of body weight?
4. Why is venous blood more acidic than arterial blood?
5. If the blood pH is measured to be 7.1 and the H^+ concentration has doubled, what is an approximate pH of that blood before the H^+ increase? Has the blood become more alkaline or more acidic?
6. How are leukocytes classified? Where are the various cells produced? What do segmented and band cells refer to?
7. Which one of the leukocytes appears to have the longest life span?
8. Do erythrocytes or granulocytes have the longest life span?
9. How do the numbers of RBCs and WBCs compare?
10. Which WBC predominates in horse, dog, and cat? In pig, cow, sheep, and goat?
11. Define phagocytosis, pinocytosis, and endocytosis.
12. Describe the movement of neutrophils from the circulation to sites of inflammation.
13. What is a principal function for each of the leukocytes?

14. What are plasma cells and megakaryocytes?

15. Differentiate between leukopenia, leukocytosis, and leukemia.

16. What is meant by absolute numbers of leukocytes?

17. If there are 7 million RBCs in each microliter of cow blood, how many would there be in one milliliter?

18. What are advantages of a discoid RBC shape? What is tolerance to RBC shape change known as?

19. Which domestic animal has the largest RBC? The smallest?

20. What is the physiologic name for the production of erythrocytes?

21. Where does RBC production occur during the postnatal, growth, and adult periods?

22. Do reticulocytes normally appear in the circulation?

23. What substance controls the rate of erythropoiesis? Where is it produced?

24. How long does it take for new RBCs to enter the circulation after their formation begins?

25. What chemical atom associated with hemoglobin binds loosely and reversibly with oxygen? How many molecules of O_2 can be transported by one molecule of hemoglobin?

26. What is the valence of iron before and after its binding with oxygen?

27. What is methemoglobin, myoglobin, and carbonmonoxyhemoglobin, and how do they differ from hemoglobin?

28. What is the average concentration of hemoglobin in the blood of domestic animals?

29. What cell accounts for removal of about 90% of aged RBCs? What are the organs where this occurs?

30. What is the name of the transport form of iron?

31. How can icterus (jaundice) occur during the degradation of hemoglobin?

32. How can hemoglobinemia and hemoglobinuria occur as a result of RBC destruction?

33. What are the normal limitations to iron absorption? Can iron toxicity occur as a result of excess ingestion and subsequent absorption?

34. Define anemia and polycythemia.

Prevention of Blood Loss

1. What is the substance contained in the basement membrane of capillaries and throughout the interstitial space that is a potent platelet activator?

2. What proteins in subendothelial tissues have adhesive properties and serve to enhance the aggregation of platelets?

3. What properties of vascular endothelium prevent activation of platelets and procoagulants?

4. What is another name for platelets?

5. Study the fine structure of the platelet (Fig. 6.15) and relate its structure to the release of the granular contents.

6. What is the principal chemical composition of the clotting factors? Where is the major site of their synthesis?

7. What vitamin is required for the synthesis of prothrombin (Factor II)?

8. What is the first response of platelets to disrupted endothelium and contact with subendothelial tissues?

9. What factors are required for the initial adhesion of platelets?

10. What is the principal messenger that is formed after platelet stimulation that will release Ca^{2+} from granule storage?

11. What is the role of aspirin in the blood coagulation scheme?

12. What is the platelet release reaction and how is it initiated?

13. What is accomplished by platelet aggregation?

14. What determines whether blood coagulation will proceed via the intrinsic mechanism or the extrinsic mechanism?

15. What coagulation factor is considered the initiator of the extrinsic mechanism?
16. In what way is the activation of Factor X a focal point in the blood coagulation scheme?
17. What is the significance of factor XIII and thrombosthenin? What is their origin?
18. What is the role of plasmin? How is it generated?
19. What are some preventatives against coagulation in the normal vascular system?
20. What is the significance of mast cells? Why are there great numbers in the lung?
21. Why does blood coagulate with difficulty when it is withdrawn from birds?

Plasma and Its Composition

1. What is the concentration of plasma protein?
2. What plasma substance represents the major contribution to intravascular effective osmotic pressure?
3. What are the major functions of the globulins and fibrinogen?
4. Which cation is most abundant in plasma? Which anion?
5. What is the concentration of glucose in the pig and dog? Is it lower in the ruminants and horse?

SELF-EVALUATION— BLOOD AND ITS FUNCTIONS

1. What is an approximate value for hemoglobin concentration in a normal healthy dog?
   a. 5 g/dl
   b. 20 g/dl
   • c. 15 g/dl
   d. 10 g/dl
2. An erythrocyte just entering the blood stream and having a net-like appearance because of polyribosomes and ribosomes is known as a/an:
   • a. reticulocyte
   b. rubriblast
   c. polychromatophilic rubricyte
   d. eosinophil
3. Where is erythropoietin produced?
   a. bone marrow
   b. lungs
   c. spleen
   • d. kidneys
4. What is the name of the transport form of iron?
   a. hemosiderin
   • b. transferrin
   c. ferritin
   d. granola
5. Which WBC is most numerous in pigs, cows, sheep, and goats?
   a. eosinophil
   b. neutrophil
   • c. lymphocyte
   d. monocyte
   e. basophil
6. What substance is formed during the coagulation process that converts fibrinogen to fibrin?
   a. thromboxane A_2
   b. thromboplastin
   • c. thrombin
   d. prothrombin
7. Which one of the following best describes plasma?
   a. about 40% of blood composition, contains no protein
   b. the cellular part of blood, about 40% of blood composition
   • c. about 60% of blood composition, contains fibrinogen
   d. about 60% of blood composition, clot removed
8. The PCV of a hematocrit determination refers to the:
   a. white cells and thrombocyte layer between the erythrocyte mass and plasma
   • b. the erythrocyte mass at the bottom
   c. the yellowish liquid layer at the top of the hematocrit
   d. the total length of the hematocrit tube content

9. Which one of the following most accurately approximates the amount of blood in an animal?
   a. 2 percent of body weight
   b. 16 percent of body weight
   . c. 8 percent of body weight
   d. 24 percent of body weight
10. Erythropoiesis refers to:
    a. blood coagulation
    b. the recycling of iron
    c. the disintegration scheme for RBCs
    . d. RBC production
11. Which one of the following time periods would approximate the life span of erythrocytes in most domestic mammals?
    a. 100 hours
    b. 60 days
    . c. 100 days
    d. 35 seconds
12. Which one of the following best describes the hemoglobin molecule of blood?
    a. has ferric iron (Fe^{3+}), combines with 1 molecule of oxygen
    b. has 1 heme group and 1 globin molecule
    - c. has ferrous iron (Fe^{2+}), combines with 4 molecules of oxygen
    d. has ferrous iron (Fe^{2+}) when unoxygenated and ferric iron (Fe^{3+}) when oxygenated
13. When an erythrocyte is disintegrated, the hemoglobin remains intact and is incorporated into new RBCs.
    a. true
    · b. false
14. A reddish color of plasma which may be coupled with a red color of urine is caused by:
    ⸳ a. hemoglobin
    b. bilirubin
    c. iron
    d. bilinogen
15. The neutrophil is the most numerous leukocyte in all of the domestic species.
    a. true
    ⸳ b. false

16. Which leukocyte will become a macrophage when it enters tissue spaces or becomes attached to certain blood channels?
    a. neutrophil
    b. basophil
    c. eosinophil
    · d. monocyte
17. A term which refers to a reduced number of leukocytes is:
    a. anemia
    · b. leukopenia
    c. leukocytosis
    d. polycythemia
18. Which one of the following cells assists in hemostasis (hemorrhage control)?
    a. basophil
    ⸳ b. platelet
    c. erythrocyte
    d. lymphocyte
19. The mesh of the blood clot is:
    a. thrombin
    · b. fibrin
    c. fibrinogen
    d. prothrombin
20. Which one of the following represents the number of erythrocytes for most domestic species?
    a. 7,000,000
    . b. 7,000,000/microliter of blood (mm^3)
    c. 7,000,000/milliliter of blood
    d. 7,000,000/pound of body weight
21. Arterial blood changes from a bright red color to a darker purplish color when it becomes venous blood. Which one of the following causes this?
    · a. loss of oxygen
    b. gain of carbon dioxide
22. A normal value for arterial blood pH would be closest to which one of the following values?
    a. 3.8
    b. 6.5
    ˋ c. 7.4
    d. 8.2

23. A differential WBC count and a total WBC count have been determined. Sixty of the 100 WBCs counted in the differential were determined to be neutrophils. The total WBC count (per standard unit) was 10,000. What is the absolute number of neutrophils?
    a. 6,000/standard unit
    b. 10,000/standard unit
    c. 60 percent
    d. 60/standard unit

24. Someone tells you that the hemoglobin concentration in a baby pig is 4 gm/dl. What would you say is the status of that pig?
    a. normal
    b. anemic
    c. leukopenic
    d. polycythemic

25. Which one of the following leukocytes has as their function to provide immunity to antigens (foreign substances)?
    a. monocytes
    b. eosinophils
    c. lymphocytes
    d. basophils
    e. neutrophils

26. Which one of the following cations plays an important role in blood coagulation?
    a. Na^+
    b. Mg^{2+}
    c. K^+
    d. Ca^{2+}

27. Which one of the following substances provides for the breakdown of fibrin to fibrin degradation products?
    a. plasmin
    b. thromboxane A_2
    c. fibrinogen
    d. EDTA

28. The blood volume of a 25 kg dog is 2000 ml, of which the plasma volume is 1200 ml. What is the PCV of this dog?
    a. 8%
    b. 60%
    c. 40%
    d. Towser

29. What is the stimulus for the production of erythropoietin?
    a. tissue need for oxygen
    b. iron deficiency
    c. no stimulus, but constantly produced
    d. sympathetic division of ANS

30. Which body organ is the site whereby insoluble bilirubin that is released from MPS cells is made soluble before its transport to the intestine?
    a. kidney
    b. liver
    c. bone marrow
    d. spleen

31. Which one of the blood coagulation mechanisms is activated when blood escapes from the vessels into the surrounding tissues?
    a. extrinsic
    b. intrinsic
    c. the curdler

32. Nearly all of the clotting factors are:
    a. carbohydrates
    b. proteins
    c. lipids
    d. minerals

33. Nearly all of the clotting factors are produced in the:
    a. kidney
    b. lung
    c. liver
    d. intestinal epithelium

34. Loss of individual integrity, fusion of lipoprotein membranes, and exposure of receptors for coagulation factors is characteristic for:
    a. platelet adhesion
    b. platelet activation
    c. platelet release reaction
    d. platelet aggregation

35. Tissue plasminogen activator (t-PA) is associated with:
    a. heparin production
    b. initiation of the extrinsic mechanism of blood coagulation
    c. erythrocyte production
    d. fibrin degradation

SUGGESTED READINGS

Conn EE, Stumpf PK. Outlines of biochemistry. New York: John Wiley & Sons, 1963.

Diggs LW, Sturm D, Bell A. The morphology of human blood cells. Abbott Park, IL: Abbott Laboratories, 1985.

Gentry PA, Downie HG. Blood coagulation and hemostasis. In: Swenson MJ, Reece WO, eds. Dukes' physiology of domestic animals. 11th ed. Ithaca, NY: Cornell University, 1993:49–63.

Jackson ML. Platelet physiology and platelet function: Inhibition by aspirin. Compend Contin Educ Pract Vet 1987;9:627.

Jain NC. Essentials of veterinary hematology. Philadelphia: Lea & Febiger, 1993.

Swenson MJ. Physiological properties and cellular and chemical constituents of blood. In: Swenson MJ, Reece WO, eds. Dukes' physiology of domestic animals. 11th ed. Ithaca, NY: Cornell University Press, 1993:22–48.

Vander AJ, Sherman JH, Luciano DS. Human physiology: the mechanisms of body function. 6th ed. New York: McGraw-Hill, 1993.

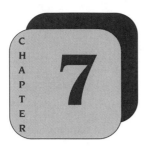
The Cardiovascular System

During early embryonic growth, dividing cells receive their nutrients and expel their wastes by diffusion from the uterine fluids that surround them. With continued development, the innermost cells become too distant from the fluids for diffusional exchange efficiency. The cardiovascular system develops to meet the needs of distant cells for nutrition and excretion. The system consists of a network of joined vessels (arteries, veins, and capillaries) for circulating the nutrient fluid (blood) and a pump (the heart) to propel the fluid through the vessels. An auxiliary system of vessels (the lymphatics) also develops to assist the return of fluids from the interstitial spaces to the blood.

STRUCTURE AND FUNCTION

Heart and Pericardium

The heart is a cone-shaped, hollow, muscular structure located in the thorax (Fig. 7.1).

The large arteries and veins are continuous with the heart at its base. Its base is directed upward (dorsal) and forward (cranial). The opposite end of the cone is known as the apex. During early embryonic development, the heart is pushed into a serous sac known as the pericardium. The part of the sac next to the heart becomes fused to the muscle of the heart and is known as the visceral pericardium, or epicardium (Fig. 7.2). The outer part of the sac is continuous with the epicardium and extends outward from its fusion at the base to envelop the heart completely. The apex of the heart is free (unattached) within the pericardium. This outer layer is known as the parietal pericardium. The pericardial sac is a potential space and contains a small amount of fluid to provide lubrication for the outer surface of the heart during its near-continuous motion. It is referred to as a potential space because it can increase its fluid volume during times of inflammation. A major cause of inflammation in the cow is traumatic pericarditis, such as when a foreign

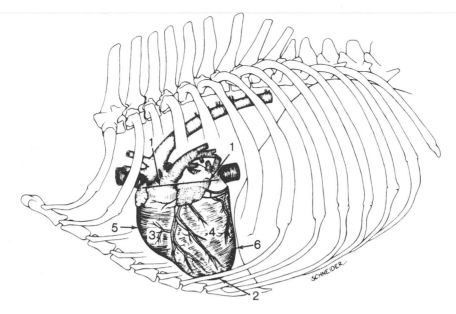

Figure 7.1. The canine heart and its major vessels in the thorax (left view). **1.** Flattened base. **2.** Apex. **3.** Right ventricle. **4.** Left ventricle. **5.** Right ventricular margin. **6.** Left ventricular margin. From Adams DR. Canine anatomy: a systemic study. Ames, IA: Iowa State University Press, 1986.

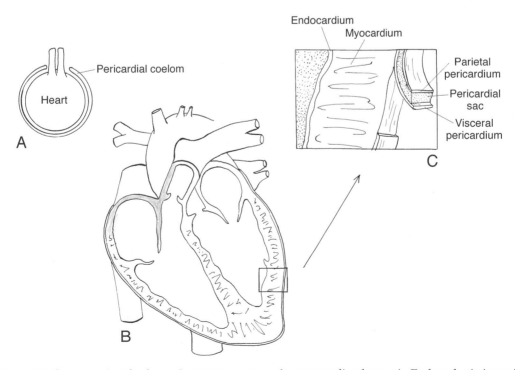

Figure 7.2. Cross-sectional schematic representation of a mammalian heart. **A**. Embryologic invagination of heart into pericardial coelom (becomes pericardial sac). **B**. Sagittal section of heart with pericardial sac. **C**. Details of the heart wall and pericardium.

object (e.g., nail, wire) penetrates from the forward compartment (reticulum) of the bovine stomach (Fig. 7.3). A splashing sound, similar to water in a washing machine, can sometimes be heard with each beat of the heart because of the increased fluid.

Myocardium

The muscular part of the heart is known as the myocardium, which forms the walls for the compartments (chambers) of the heart. The muscle fibers are arranged so that, when they contract, the blood is ejected from the chambers (Fig. 7.4). The heart chambers are divided into those on the right side of the heart and those on the left side (Fig. 7.5); each side has an atrium and a ventricle. To conserve space each atrium

has an extension known as an auricle, with a shape that conforms to that of adjacent parts. The atria receive blood from veins and the ventricles receive blood from the atria. The right and left ventricles pump blood from the heart through the pulmonary artery and aorta, respectively.

Heart Valves

The valves located between the atria and ventricles are known as the atrioventricular (A-V) valves (Fig. 7.6A). The valve on the right side has three cusps (flaps) and is called the tricuspid valve; the left A-V valve has two cusps and is called the bicuspid or sometimes the mitral valve. The A-V valves prevent expulsion of ventricular blood into the atria when the ventricles contract. Because of the pressure associated

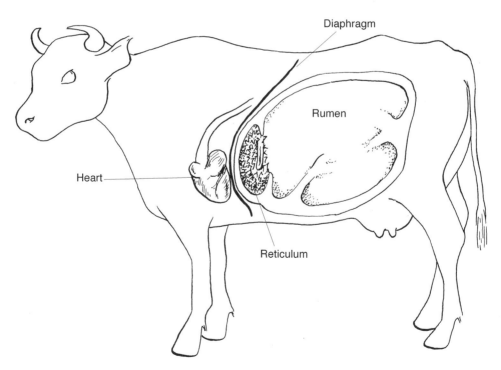

Figure 7.3. Left view of bovine thorax and abdomen showing location of the heart relative to the stomach. Foreign objects (nails, wire), sometimes ingested by cattle, accumulate in the reticulum (one of the bovine forestomachs). Contraction of the reticulum can force pointed objects through the reticulum wall and the diaphragm, causing final penetration of the pericardium and subsequent inflammation (pericarditis).

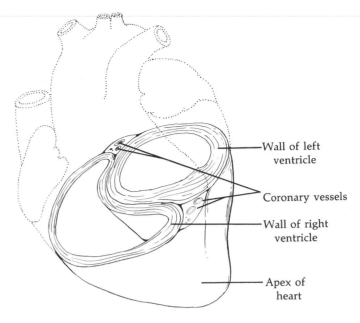

Wall of left
ventricle

Coronary vessels

Wall of right
ventricle

Apex of
heart

Figure 7.4. Cross-sectional view of horse heart at the ventricular level showing the relative thickness of the myocardium and the orientation of the muscle fibers.

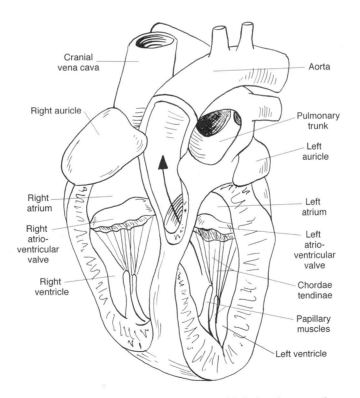

Cranial
vena cava

Aorta

Right auricle

Pulmonary
trunk

Left
auricle

Right
atrium

Left
atrium

Right
atrio-
ventricular
valve

Left
atrio-
ventricular
valve

Right
ventricle

Chordae
tendinae

Papillary
muscles

Left ventricle

Figure 7.5. A sagittal section of the canine heart. The right and left chambers are shown with separation of the atria and ventricles by atrio-ventricular valves. The auricles are extensions of the atria. The aorta is seen to be arising from the left ventricle. The pulmonary trunk arises form the right ventricle (not visible) and divides into right and left pulmonary arteries just beyond the pulmonary semilunar valve. The cranial vena cava and caudal vena cava (not visible) deliver venous blood (unoxygenated) into the right atrium.

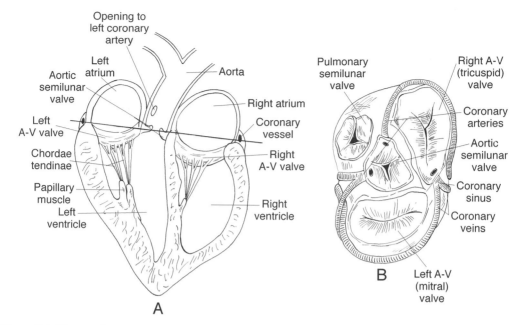

Figure 7.6. Heart valves. **A**. Location relative to the chambers and the aorta. The pulmonary trunk and its semilunar valve are not shown. **B**. A view of the heart from above the ventricles (at the level of the straight line shown in **A**) to show the semilunar and atrioventricular valves. The first branches from the aorta are the coronary arteries. The coronary sinus opens into the right atrium and receives blood from the heart wall through the coronary veins.

with the expulsion of blood from the ventricles, the A-V valves could be everted into the atria. This is prevented by cords (chordae tendineae) attached to the free margin of the cusps at one end and to small muscles (papillary muscles) at the other end that extend from the myocardium. Backflow of blood that has just been ejected from the ventricles is prevented by valves located at the exits of the arteries from the ventricles (Fig. 7.6B). The valves on both the right and left sides have three cusps and are known as the semilunar valves. The valve on the right side is known as the pulmonary semilunar valve because of its location with the pulmonary trunk, and the valve on the left side is known as the aortic semilunar valve because of its location relative to the aorta.

Blood Flow Through the Heart

Blood that originally enters the heart and is finally ejected follows a specific route

(Fig. 7.7). Blood that circulates to the tissues returns to the heart through the cranial vena cava (blood from forward parts of body) and the caudal vena cava (blood from rear parts of body). This is the venous blood. It has lost oxygen to the tissues, gained carbon dioxide, and must now be directed to the lungs, where it becomes arterial blood by gaining oxygen and losing carbon dioxide. The venous blood enters the right atrium during the atrial relaxation phase of the cardiac cycle. At the appropriate time in the cardiac cycle, the blood is directed through the right A-V valve into the right ventricle. The ventricles contract and the blood goes through the pulmonary semilunar valves to the lungs through the pulmonary arteries. These are called arteries, even though they transport venous blood, because they transport blood away from the heart. After the blood has circulated through the lungs, it reenters the heart through the

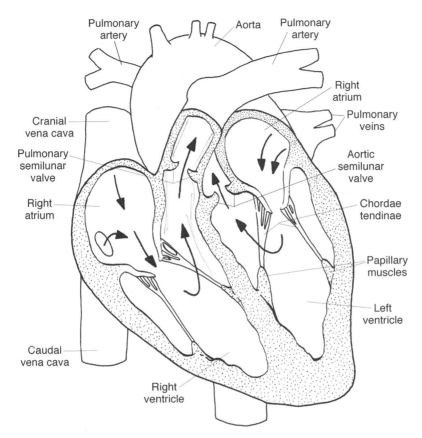

Figure 7.7. Functional parts of the mammalian heart and directions of blood flow through its chambers. Venous blood enters the right atrium from the cranial and caudal venae cavae. It then enters the right ventricle and is pumped via the pulmonary arteries to the pulmonary circulation where it is oxygenated. Arterialized blood enters the left atrium via the pulmonary veins. The left ventricle is then filled and blood is pumped to the systemic circulation via the aorta.

pulmonary veins (contain arterial blood). It enters the left atrium; from here the blood is directed to the left ventricle, from which it is pumped to the systemic (whole body) circulation through the aorta.

Blood Vessels

The inner aspect of the pericardium is described as the outer cell layer of the heart (because of fusion) and is known as the epicardium. The cardiac muscle cells of the heart occupy the middle layer of the heart and the innermost cell layer is known as the endocardium. The endo-

cardium is described here because it continues as the lining (endothelium) for all the blood vessels. Endothelial cells are classified as simple (single-layered), squamous (platelike) epithelium (a primary type of tissue that also covers the body surfaces and forms active parts of glands). Simple squamous epithelium is found wherever a smooth surface is required to reduce friction. In this regard, it is ideal for lining the inner aspects of the heart, its valves, and the inner coat of the blood vessels to minimize the resistance (and hence the energy requirement) for blood flow. Inflammation of the endothelial

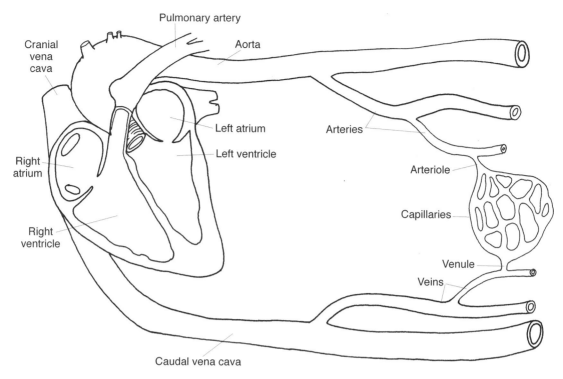

Figure 7.8. Schematic representation of the functional circulatory system. A network of arteries, arterioles, capillaries, venules, and veins exist between the aorta and cranial and caudal venal cavae.

lining in the heart is called endocarditis; if it involves the lining of valves it is called valvular endocarditis.

The blood vessels provide for a continuous route for blood leaving the heart to return to the heart. From the ventricles back to the atria they are, in order, the arteries, arterioles, capillaries, venules, and veins. An overview of the functional circulatory system is shown in Figure 7.8. The large arteries have a greater proportion of their mass composed of elastic tissue than do the small arteries. This elastic tissue provides for expansion as blood is pumped into them, and the expanded fibers serve as a source of energy for continuing the circulation of blood when the ventricles relax. The small arteries have some portion of their elastic fibers replaced by smooth muscle. Contraction of the smooth muscle con-

stricts these vessels and permits reduced blood flow to a particular part and diversion of blood flow to other parts. The arterioles are muscular just before emptying into the capillaries. Changes in their muscle tone (degree of contraction) regulate blood flow to capillary beds (Fig. 7.9).

Capillaries are merely endothelial tubes. Where the endothelial cells border each other, a thin slit (slit pore) or intracellular cleft is provided for the diffusion of dissolved substances in plasma (Fig. 7.10). The limited size of the slit pores inhibits the passage of large molecules. Pinocytotic vesicles are also present in the endothelial cells. These are formed at one surface of the cell and migrate to the opposite surface, where they discharge their contents. Many of the protein molecules are probably transported through the endothelial cells in this

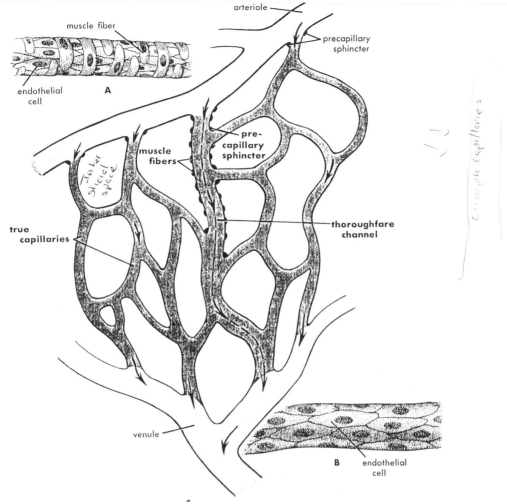

Labels in figure (A, top): muscle fiber, endothelial cell, A

Labels (main figure): arteriole, precapillary sphincter, pre-capillary sphincter, muscle fibers, Inter stitial space, true capillaries, thoroughfare channel, venule, B, endothelial cell

Figure 7.9. Schematic representation of a capillary bed. **A.** Some of the muscle fibers of the proximal part of a thoroughfare channel. **B.** Part of a true capillary. From Crouch JE. Functional human anatomy. 4th ed. Philadelphia: Lea & Febiger, 1985.

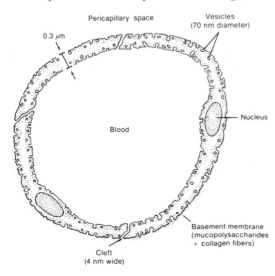

Labels: Pericapillary space, Vesicles (70 nm diameter), 0.3 µm, Blood, Nucleus, Basement membrane (mucopolysaccharides + collagen fibers), Cleft (4 nm wide)

Figure 7.10. Schematic representation of a cross section through the endothelial wall of a muscle capillary. Portions of three endothelial cells are shown; these are separated from each other by intercellular clefts. Many pinocytotic vesicles are also shown. From Eckert R, Randall D, Augustine G. Animal physiology: mechanisms and adaptations. Copyright © 1978, 1983, 1988 by WH Freeman and Co. Reprinted by permission.

manner. The capillaries unite with one another to form larger vessels known as venules, and the venules unite with other venules to form the veins. The largest veins are the venae cavae, which return the blood to the right atrium of the heart.

The veins are thin-walled tubes reinforced by connective tissue, and they also contain smooth muscle fibers. Contraction of the muscle fibers increases resistance to blood flow and helps regulate the circulation. Venous constriction increases the blood pressure in all vessels that precede the veins. Valves are present in veins at irregular intervals that are directed (or opened) toward the heart (Fig. 7.11). External pressure on veins causes blood to advance only in a cranial direction because backflow is prevented by valve closure. Similarly, backflow does not occur when external pressure is released.

The pressures within the veins are the lowest of the vessel pressures (Fig. 7.12). This follows from the physical law of pressure dissipation as distance from the source (heart) increases. The pressure noted for capillaries might seem to be greater than what could be tolerated for a single-celled tube but, because of their extremely small diameter, the tension exerted on the capillary wall is extremely low. For a given pressure within the vascular system, the wall tension increases with the radius of the vessel, according to Laplace's law:

$$T = Pr/2$$

where T = wall tension, P = pressure in the vessel, and r = radius of the vessel.

Blood Circulatory Systems

The blood vessels that have been described serve two separate circulatory systems (Fig. 7.13). The pulmonary system circulates blood through the lungs (Fig. 7.14). The pressure providing for this circulation originates from the right ventricle. The capillaries of the pulmonary system are associated

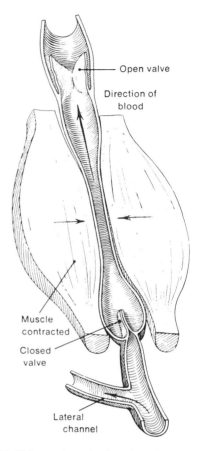

Figure 7.11. Valves of a vein showing the pumping action of adjacent muscles. From Grollman S. The human body: its structure and physiology. 4th ed. New York: Macmillan, 1978.

intimately with the smallest terminations of the air passages, the pulmonary alveoli. Blood from this system is returned to the left atrium.

The systemic circulation carries blood that has returned from the lungs to all areas of the body. The pressure necessary for this circulation originates from the left ventricle. Blood that traverses this system leaves the left ventricle through the aorta and is returned to the right atrium through the venae cavae. The first branches of the aorta supply the heart muscle through the coronary arteries (Fig. 7.15). Within the systemic circulation are a few portal systems. A portal system departs from the usual

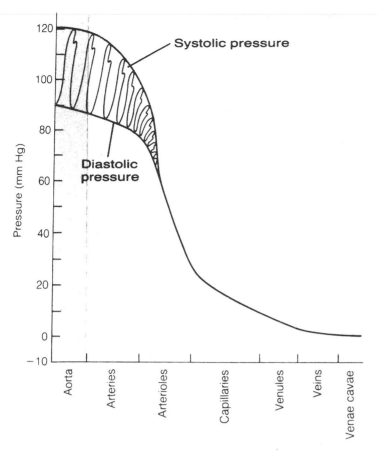

Figure 7.12. Graphic comparison of blood pressures in the different vessels of the systemic circulatory system. From Spence AP, Mason EB. Human anatomy and physiology. 2nd ed. Menlo Park, CA: Benjamin/Cummings, 1983.

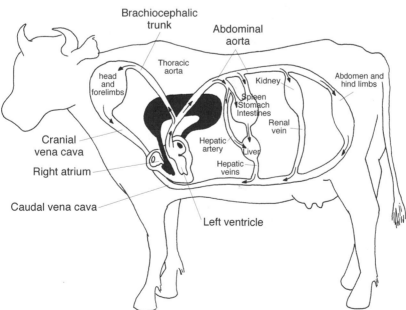

Figure 7.13. General scheme of mammalian circulation showing the pulmonary system, which serves the lungs, and the systemic system which serves the remainder of the body. The pulmonary circulation is shown in black.

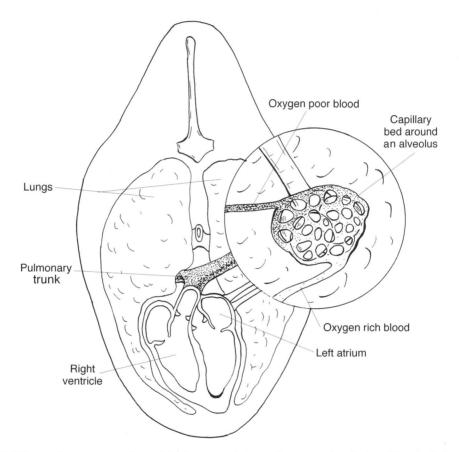

Figure 7.14. Schematic representation of the lungs and the pulmonary circulation. The circled inset represents a functional unit of the lung, the alveolus. Mixed venous blood leaves the right ventricle through the pulmonary trunk and is oxygenated at the level of the alveoli. Oxygenated blood returns to the left atrium through the pulmonary veins.

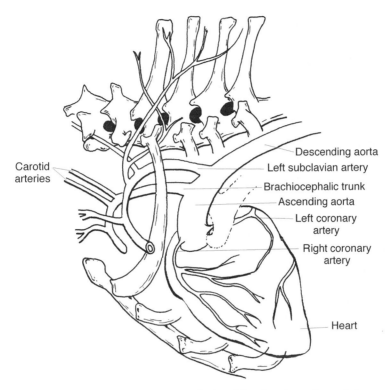

Carotid arteries

Descending aorta
Left subclavian artery
Brachiocephalic trunk
Ascending aorta
Left coronary artery
Right coronary artery

Heart

Figure 7.15. Cranial aspects of the systemic circulation. The first branches of the aorta supply the heart muscles through the coronary arteries. The descending aorta is comprised of the thoracic and abdominal aorta. The main arteries to the forelimbs arise from the left subclavian artery on the left side and from the brachiocephalic trunk on the right side. The carotid arteries ascend to the head.

pattern of circulation in that a vein returning blood to the heart branches to reform capillaries, which reunite to form veins. The primary example of a portal system is the hepatic portal system in the liver (Fig. 7.16). The reformed capillaries are the sinusoids of the liver, which are lined by cells involved in many liver functions and by those that assist in the cleansing of blood or the removal of harmful substances by macrophages (Küpffer cells).

Lymphatic System

An important adjunct to the circulatory system is the lymphatic system. The lymphatic vessels have blind beginnings (lymph capillaries) in the interstitial spaces (the spaces between cells and outside of the blood vessels) and the continuation vessels tend to parallel the veins (Fig. 7.17). Lymph vessels join with each other and eventually form a few large lymph vessels that empty directly into the large veins. The fluid of the lymph vessels is called lymph. There is little difference between the composition of lymph and that of interstitial fluid. Although blood capillaries permit most plasma constituents to diffuse through their endothelium, protein molecules are somewhat restrained because of their size. It is essential for proteins to enter the interstitial fluid, however, because they act as carriers for cell products or for substances needed by cells. In addition, antibodies (protein substances) are needed in the interstitial space for more intimate association with an antigen. It is believed that there is a complete turnover (from capillaries and return to blood) of plasma protein once every 12 to 24 hours. Because the concentration of protein is higher in the plasma than in the interstitial space, the gradient for diffusion is to the interstitial space. Protein in the interstitial space does not diffuse back to the plasma; it can only return to the plasma through the lymphatic vessels. The blind beginnings of the lymph vessels are adapted for the intake of large molecules, and concentration and pressure gradients favor this route (Fig. 7.18). Anchoring filaments prevent collapse of the vessels when the tissue swells with excess fluid (edema). Also, the overlap of endothelial cells with each other permits easy access of interstitial fluid, but because of their valve-like arrangement, backflow is prevented. The return of protein that has leaked or that is otherwise transported from the blood capillaries back to the systemic circulation is one of the most important functions of the lymphatics.

Lymph nodes are nodular structures of varying size located along the course of lymph vessels. They contain clusters of germinal cells that reproduce to form lymphocytes (Fig. 7.19). The lymphocytes in turn can be of a type that produce antibodies or they can be sensitized lymphocytes. In both cases, they are highly specific against substances (antigens) that are foreign to the body. The antibodies and sensitized lymphocytes leave the lymph nodes with the lymph in the vessels and enter the blood, where they can be circulated throughout the body.

Lymph nodes also contain fixed macrophages that are attached to the reticulum (inner framework) of the lymph nodes. Lymph circulating through the nodes thus is in intimate contact with the macrophages and, because the macrophages are highly phagocytic, foreign materials in lymph (e.g., bacteria, cellular debris) are engulfed and prevented from progressing further. Infection or inflammation of a body part often results in enlarged lymph nodes serving that part because of the entrapment and because of lymphocyte proliferation stimulated by the presence of these antigenic materials. Cancer cells might be routed from their origin and be entrapped by lymph nodes, where they can proliferate and continue into the next lymph node in

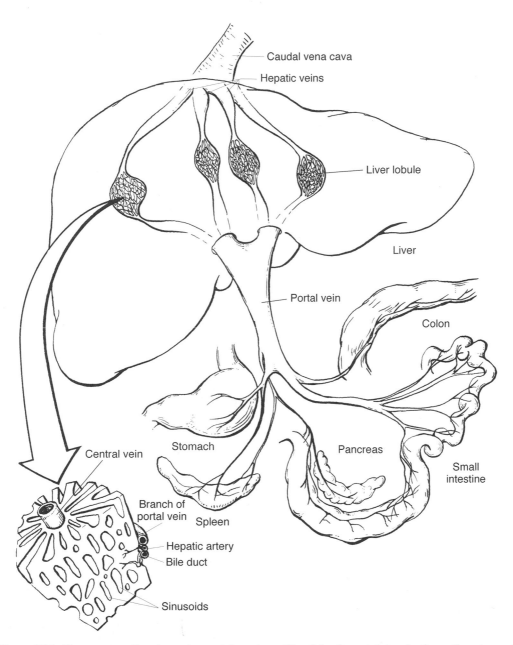

Figure 7.16. The mammalian hepatic portal system. Blood in the portal vein from the stomach, spleen, pancreas, and intestines goes to the liver, where it flows through the sinusoids and is reformed by the central vein of each lobule. It finally enters the caudal vena cava through the hepatic veins.

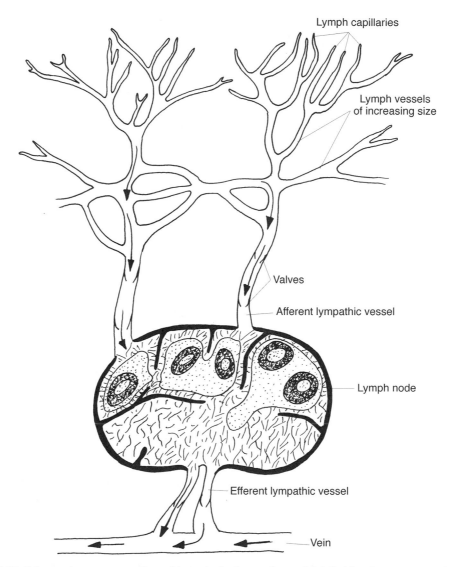

Figure 7.17. Schematic representation of lymph drainage. Interstitial fluid gains access to the blind beginnings of lymph capillaries and proceeds centrally through lymph vessels of increasing size. Lymph nodes are located along the course of lymph vessels. Lymph is returned to blood by drainage into veins.

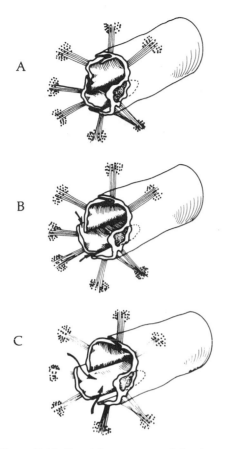

A

B

C

Figure 7.18. Special structure of the lymphatic capillaries that permits passage of high-molecular-weight substances into the lymph. The structures radiating from the capillaries are anchoring filaments that give support to portions of endothelial cells where the capillaries begin. The unsupported portion of the endothelium allows fluid to flow into the capillary (arrows) as shown in **B** and **C**. Raised pressure in the capillary closes the flap against the overlapping supported endothelium as shown in **A.** From Leak LV. The fine structure and function of the lymphatic vascular system. In: Meessen H, ed. Handbüch der allgemeinen pathologie. New York, Springer-Verlag, 1972.

the chain. Inspection of lymph nodes for enlargement is an important part of the postmortem carcass examination procedure for animals that are slaughtered for food consumption.

The lymph vessels are one-way channels that contain valves similar to those in veins, which prevent backflow of lymph once it has progressed toward the veins. Lymph progresses through the channels by contractions of the lymph vessels and by a massaging action of muscles that overlie lymph vessels. Forward movement of lymph lowers the pressure in the part of the vessel evacuated and, because there is no backflow of lymph, entry of lymph from the backward parts is favored. There is no central pump, such as the heart, to facilitate lymph circulation, and disturbances in lymph flow can cause accumulation of interstitial fluid in low-lying body parts. The return of lymph is assisted by elevation of these parts, such as the limbs, to a level higher than the centrally located veins and by muscle movement from exercise.

Spleen

The spleen is the largest lymphoid organ of the body (Fig. 7.20). It is unlike the lymph nodes in that the circulating fluid is blood instead of lymph. It is the only organ specialized to filter blood. A section cut from the spleen (Fig. 7.21) shows that it is surrounded by a capsule that has connective tissue and smooth muscle cells. The amount of smooth muscle varies with species and is quite pronounced in carnivores. Trabeculae extend from the capsule that are composed of elastic fibers, collagen, and smooth muscle. Arteries, veins, lymph vessels, and nerves are contained within the trabeculae. The parenchyma (splenic pulp) of the spleen is comprised of red and white pulp and is supported by the capsule, trabeculae, and reticular fibers. Most of the splenic pulp is red because of the blood that is held within the reticular fiber mesh, which represents the part of the spleen that acts as a filter; it has numerous fixed macrophages. The white pulp is lymphatic tissue distributed throughout the spleen as lymphatic nodules and sheaths of

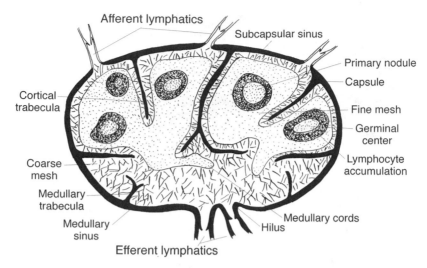

Figure 7.19. Internal structure of a lymph node. Lymph enters through afferent lymphatics and leaves through efferent lymphatics. The lymph percolates through the coarse mesh on which many fixed mononuclear phagocytic cells are located. Lymphocytes are produced in the primary nodules and accumulate throughout the fine mesh (a fine mesh holds small lymphocytes better than a coarse mesh).

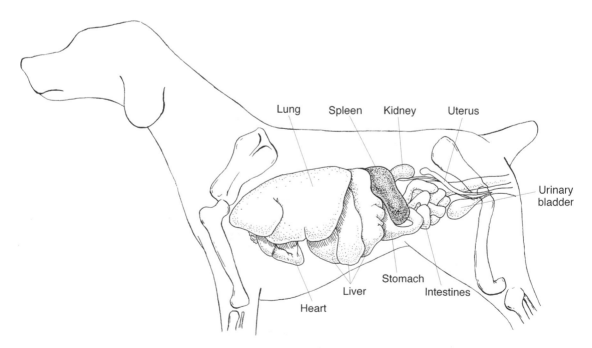

Figure 7.20. Projection of viscera on the left body wall of the female dog showing the location of the spleen relative to other body organs. Except for the dorsal tip, the dog spleen is somewhat variable in position, and its long axis can be almost longitudinal.

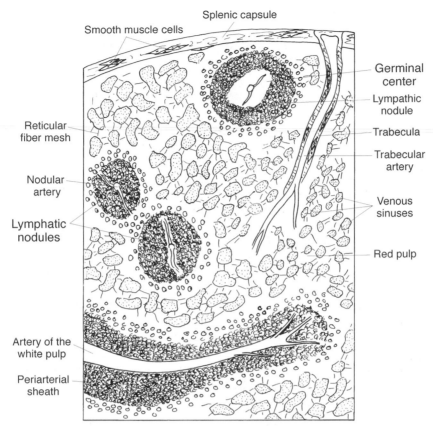

Figure 7.21. Schematic representation of the pig spleen. Multiple branches of the splenic artery enter the capsule and extend into the trabeculae. The lymphatic nodules and periarterial sheaths comprise the white pulp that produces lymphocytes. The red pulp is the reticular fiber mesh that acts as a filter because of its fixed macrophages. Smooth muscle cells are present in the capsule and in the trabeculae. The venous sinuses collect filtered blood and drain into venules and finally trabecular veins (not shown).

lymphatics around arteries and arterioles that produces lymphocytes. Blood enters the spleen via the trabeculae and is distributed either to the lymph nodes via nodular arteries or to the red pulp or venous sinuses via terminal capillaries. Blood entering the red pulp (reticular spaces) via the terminal capillaries is then able to enter the venous sinuses through slits in the venous sinus walls. Blood entering the reticular spaces provides for greater exposure to cells of the mononuclear phagocytic system (MPS). The venous sinuses collect filtered blood and drain into venules and finally trabecular veins.

Because blood circulates through the spleen, it is active in the destruction of aged and abnormal erythrocytes by the numerous MPS cells. Also, the spleen is a storage depot of iron obtained from the destruction of erythrocytes. The spleen is an important reservoir of blood, especially of red blood cells, which accumulate within the venous sinusoids. Contraction of the spleen is possible because of the smooth muscle and occurs when more red blood cells are needed. Splenic contraction that accompanies excitement in the dog can increase their packed cell volume from a value of 40% to a value of more than 50%.

Cardiac Contractility

Origin of the Heartbeat

All muscles appear to have an inherent rhythmicity of contraction. If the three muscle types (cardiac, skeletal, smooth) are removed from the nerve and blood supply and placed into physiologic fluids, contraction begins in a rhythmic manner. The frequency of contraction is greatest in cardiac muscle, followed by skeletal muscle and finally by smooth muscle. When considering only cardiac muscle, the atria have a higher frequency of contraction than the ventricles. In addition, a small area of specialized cardiac muscle fibers near the junction of the cranial vena cava with the right atrium has a contraction frequency higher than that of the atria. These specialized muscle fibers constitute what is known as the sinoatrial (S-A) node. Impulses originating in the S-A node spread throughout the musculature of the atria and the impulse is conducted to the ventricles by way of internodal pathways. Because the contraction frequency for the S-A node exceeds that of the atria and ventricles, the S-A node impulse becomes the stimulus for contraction of the atria and ventricles, and the contraction frequency of the S-A node becomes the contraction frequency of the atria and ventricles. The S-A node therefore serves a pacemaker function.

Conduction of the Impulse

The muscle fibers of the atria and those of the ventricles are arranged to form an atrial and a ventricular syncytium. A syncytium is an arrangement of muscle fibers in which the fibers fuse to form an interconnected mass of fibers. The atrial syncytium is sep-

arated from the ventricular syncytium by a fibrous ring that surrounds the A-V valves. The fibrous ring acts as an insulator between the two syncytia. An impulse that spreads throughout the atria does not spread to the ventricles and an impulse from the ventricles does not spread to the atria. This permits independent contraction and provides an opportunity for the atria and ventricles to coordinate their function of emptying, so the ventricles are filled during their relaxation by the contraction and emptying of the atria.

It is desirable for the muscle fibers in each syncytium to contract as simultaneously as possible. All fibers thereby contribute to the pressure increase needed for evacuation of the blood from the chambers of the syncytium. Fibers contracting at different times could not attain sufficient pressure for efficient evacuation. Because the function of the atria is to fill the ventricles before they contract, impulse conduction is completed first throughout the atria. After a slight delay, the impulse is then conducted throughout the ventricles.

To facilitate rapid conduction (and coordinated contraction), the heart has a specialized conduction system comprised of specialized conduction tracts and fibers called Purkinje fibers (Fig. 7.22). The S-A node conducts the impulse throughout the atria through several small tracts of fibers called internodal pathways. Depolarization of these pathways provides the stimulus for depolarization of adjacent muscle fibers; the transmission of impulses and subsequent depolarization of other muscle fibers is facilitated by the intercalated disks interposed between muscle fibers. Impulse conduction by the internodal pathways is received by the A-V node, which is located at a point between the atria and ventricles. The A-V node is continued through the fibrous ring by the A-V bundle. A-V bundle fibers are smaller in diameter than the other Purkinje fibers, and impulse conduction is slowed to about 10% of the velocity

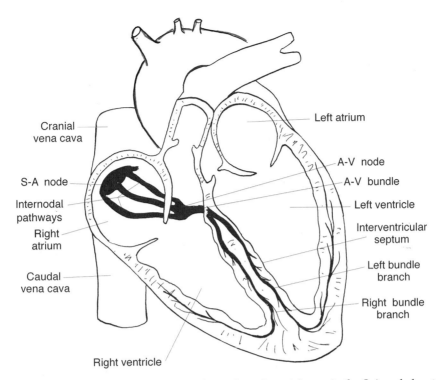

Figure 7.22. Conduction system of the mammalian heart. Impulse originates in the S-A node located near the junction of the venae cavae with the right atrium. The internodal pathways conduct the impulse throughout the atria, and the left and right bundle branches of Purkinje fibers conduct the impulse throughout the ventricles. The A-V node and bundle conduct the impulse from the atria to the ventricles.

of cardiac muscle fibers. This permits a delay of impulse to facilitate complete emptying of the atria before the ventricles contract. Conduction fibers are continued from the A-V bundle in the wall dividing the right from the left ventricles as Purkinje fibers distributed to the right ventricle (right bundle branch) and as fibers distributed to the left ventricle (left bundle branch). These large fibers transmit impulses about two to three times faster than cardiac muscle fibers. The muscle in the walls of the ventricles is thicker than the muscle in the walls of the atria, and the distance of conduction is greater. Therefore, to achieve coordinated contraction of muscle fibers of the ventricles, it is essential to have a greater velocity of conduction that is provided by the Purkinje fibers.

Not only does cardiac muscle contract more slowly than skeletal muscle, but it also has a longer refractory period. A refractory period is the period during repolarization when a stimulus cannot evoke another depolarization. This is advantageous for the heart because, when the impulse completes its travel through each syncytium, the impulse is stopped because all the previously stimulated fibers are refractory to further stimulation. When the impulse is stopped, the muscle fibers are allowed to relax and the chambers fill with blood in preparation for the next cycle.

During this discussion about impulse conduction, it should be noted that both atria contract at the same time, which completes the filling of the ventricles, and that both ventricles contract at the same time, thus pumping blood to the pulmonary circulation and systemic circulation simultaneously. Contraction and relaxation of the muscle fibers within a syncytium are synchronized. When contraction of muscle fibers and relaxation of other muscle fibers occur at the same time in the same syncytium, the condition is referred to as fibrillation. Electrical current conducted through the heart during defibrillation causes simultaneous depolarization of all fibers; the heart can then start a new cycle with impulses that begin in the S-A node.

Cardiac Cycle

The cardiac cycle refers to the sequence of events that occurs during one complete heartbeat. These events are continuous, and the assigned periods are arbitrary for descriptive purposes. Diastole refers to relaxation of a heart chamber before and during filling of the chamber. Systole refers to contraction of a heart chamber in the process of emptying. During atrial diastole, the atria are filled with blood. After ventricular systole, and during ventricular diastole, the following sequence of events occurs (Fig. 7.23):

1. Volume and pressure increase in the atria as they fill by receiving blood from the venae cavae and pulmonary veins (occurs during ventricular systole); A-V valves open when atrial pressure exceeds the ventricular pressure (occurs at beginning of ventricular diastole)
2. Blood flows into relaxed ventricles (accounts for up to 70% of ventricular filling)
3. Atria contract (accomplishes complete filling or priming of ventricles)
4. Atria relax and begin refilling
5. Ventricles begin contraction and A-V valves are closed because ventricular pressures exceed atrial pressures

6. Continued contraction of ventricles creates sufficient pressure to exceed arterial pressures
7. Semilunar valves are opened
8. Blood is ejected from ventricles
9. Ventricles begin to relax
10. Arterial pressures begin to exceed the ventricular pressures, and the semilunar valves close

The cycle ends and is repeated at a frequency consistent with the heart rate for each species. The process of recording these changes is called electrocardiography, and the record obtained is known as the electrocardiogram (ECG).

Electrocardiogram

When impulse conduction was explained for nerve and muscle fibers (see previous section), it was noted that voltage changes occur across the nerve and muscle membranes during waves of depolarization and repolarization. The changes are relatively small and are measured in millivolts. Similar voltage changes occur when heart muscle depolarizes and repolarizes. Voltage changes that occur locally are conducted through the body fluids because body fluids are good conductors. With appropriate amplification, these voltage changes can be recorded as they occur.

Wave Forms

Connection of the amplifier with wires (known as leads) to selected body parts (usually the limbs) and to a recorder provides a characteristic wave form. The wave form is a recording of the electrical activity of the heart. Because the electrical activity can be changed by alterations in the heart muscle, such as thickening of the chamber walls or interruptions of current flow caused by damaged muscle, it is useful for studying heart activity in conditions of health and disease. The wave form recording is the electrocardiogram (ECG). Several

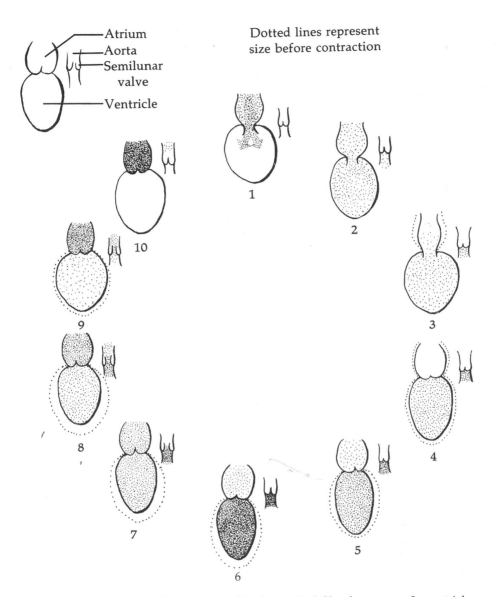

Figure 7.23. The cardiac cycle of the mammalian heart. *1,* A-V valves open; *2,* ventricles receive blood; *3,* atria contract and empty; *4,* ventricles begin contraction and close A-V valves; *5,* atria relax and begin to fill; *6,* ventricular pressure increases; *7,* semilunar valves open; *8,* blood is ejected from ventricles; *9,* ventricles begin relaxation; and *10,* semilunar valves close and atrial filling is complete.

leads and their characteristic wave forms are shown for the dog in Figure 7.24. The ECG for each cycle of the heart has characteristic deflections associated with the depolarization and repolarization of the atria and ventricles as they occur in sequence. An ECG recording, such as that which might be obtained from lead II in the dog, is shown in Figure 7.25. The sequence of deflections and the activity associated with them are as follows:

1. P wave is associated with depolarization of atria; after depolarization, atrial contraction occurs.

Lead	Electrode Placement		Lead Illustration	ECG Example
	Negative	Positive		
I	RA	LA		
II	RA	LL		
III	LA	LL		
aVR	LA-LL	RA		
aVL	RA-LL	LA		
aVF	RA-LA	LL		

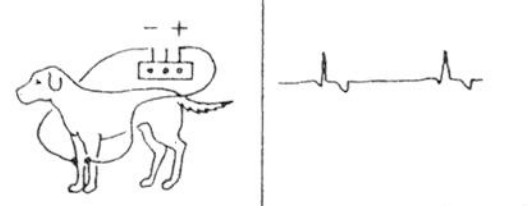

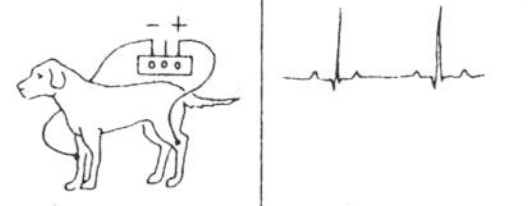

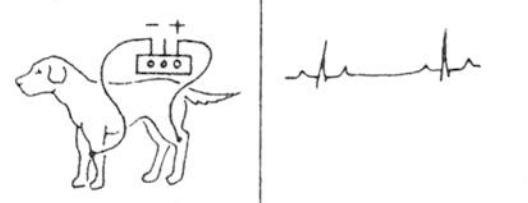

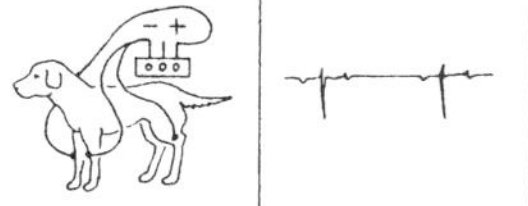

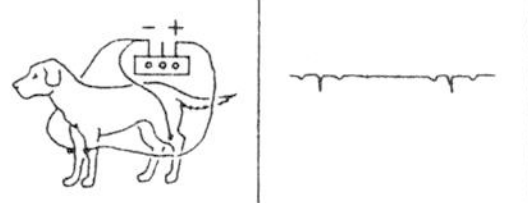

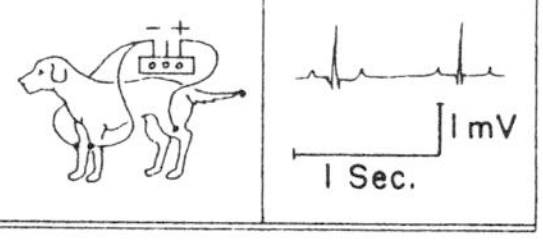

Figure 7.24. Examples of different electrode placements (leads) and their characteristic wave forms for the dog. From Breazile JE. Textbook of veterinary physiology. Philadelphia: Lea & Febiger, 1971.

2. QRS wave complex represents both positive (upward) and negative (downward) deflections associated with ventricular depolarization; ventricular contraction begins after depolarization of fibers.

3. T wave is the last wave for each heartbeat; it represents ventricular repolarization (may be positive or negative).

Because repolarization of the atria occurs during depolarization of the ventricles, a separate wave form is not observed. Instead, the voltage changes of atrial repolarization are algebraically summed into the QRS complex.

It should now be apparent why conduction of the impulse throughout each atrial and ventricular syncytium takes place rapidly. Impulse conduction results in depolarization, which must occur before contraction proceeds. Coordinated contraction of all the muscle fibers, therefore, requires near-simultaneous depolarization.

Isoelectric Line

When viewing an electrocardiogram, it can be seen that deflections of the waves, whether positive (upward) or negative (downward), commence from a common line, known as the isoelectric line. Deviations from the line represent the amplitude of the wave; it is measured in millivolts and can be positive or negative. The interval between waves is measured in hundredths of a second (Fig. 7.25). Hypertrophy of ventricular muscle might require a greater time for depolarization, and the QRS interval (time for depolarization) would be increased. Certain heart conditions can cause the interval segment to be depressed from the isoelectric line. An S-T segment depression is observed when hypoxia (lack of oxygen) occurs in heart muscle.

Heart Sounds

Listening to the heart (cardiac auscultation) enables the listener to hear the sounds that accompany contraction of heart muscle and the sounds associated with closure of the heart valves. These are repeated for each cardiac cycle. The more pronounced sounds are those associated with valve closings, but contracting muscle also makes a sound.

The first heart sound resembles the word "lub" and the second heart sound resembles "dub." They usually occur one after the other—lub-dub, lub-dub, lub-dub, and so on. The first sound is produced when the ventricles contract and the A-V valves close. The second sound is produced when ventricular relaxation begins and the semilunar valves close. The abrupt closing of the valves and their potential for making sounds can be visualized. A third heart sound can sometimes be detected on a

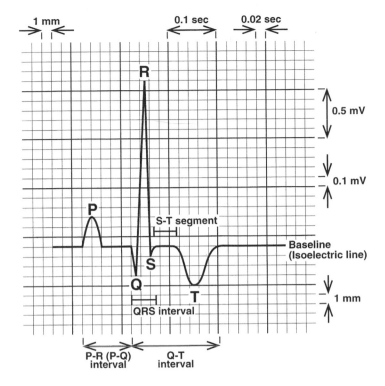

Figure 7.25. Close-up of normal canine lead II P-QRS-T complex. Measurements for amplitude (in millivolts) are indicated by positive and negative movement; time intervals (in hundredths of a second) are indicated from left to right. There is much variation in T wave configuration and it is shown as negative in this illustration. Paper speed, 50 mm/s; 1 cm = 1 mV. Modified from Tilley. Essentials of canine and feline electrocardiography, 3rd ed. Philadelphia: Lea & Febiger, 1992.

phonocardiogram (recording of heart sounds); this occurs toward the end of rapid filling of the ventricles. Heart sounds are useful as diagnostic aids because the heart valves can become diseased and might not close completely. When this happens, blood leaks through the valves, and the turbulence of the leakage is heard as some variation from a "shhh" sound after the lub or dub. Abnormal heart sounds are called murmurs and usually result from valve disorders. A review of the relationship of the ECG waves with ventricular systole and associated pressures and of the resulting valve closings with their associated sounds is illustrated in Figure 7.26.

Heart Rate and Its Control

Metabolic Rate

The heart rate refers to the frequency of cardiac cycles and is usually measured by the number of beats per minute (bpm). Generally, small animals have higher heart rates than larger animals. This is a consequence of the higher metabolic rate (and oxygen consumption) necessitated by their larger surface area per unit of body mass. The inverse relationship between heart rate and body size applies both within a species and among different species. For example, a small dog can have a resting heart rate of 120 bpm, whereas a large dog might show a resting heart rate of only 80 bpm or lower. The resting heart rate of the mouse is about 600 bpm; rat, 400 bpm; guinea pig, 280 bpm; elephant, 30 bpm. Physical conditioning and the cardiac hypertrophy that occurs as a result of physical conditioning lower the resting heart rate in all animals. Young animals have a higher heart rate than mature animals, explained in part by their smaller size. Another factor is that tonic vagal inhibition is less developed in young animals. Resting heart rates for

Figure 7.26. Relationship of the electrocardiogram and phonocardiogram to valve closings, heart sounds, and ventricular pressure. Dashed line **A** correlates ventricular depolarization and beginning contraction with beginning elevation of ventricular blood pressure and A-V valve closure and associated first heart sound (lub). Dashed line **B** associates declining ventricular pressure with semilunar valve closure and the second heart sound (dub).

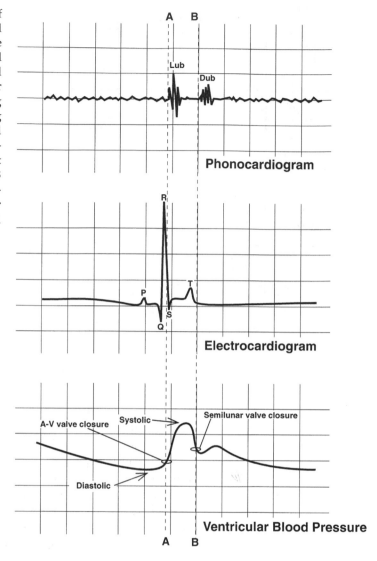

Autonomic Nervous System

Heart rates compared among species are usually obtained with the animals at rest. A number of factors can influence heart rate, including activity, excitement, fever, heart disease, and altitude. The regulation of heart rate is a function of the autonomic nervous system. Sympathetic innervation of the heart occurs by way of efferent fibers from the stellate ganglia of the sympathetic trunk. Parasympathetic innervation is supplied by fibers from the vagus nerves. Sympathetic stimulation increases all heart activities, and parasympathetic stimulation decreases all heart activities. Activities of the heart that are important in this regard are 1) rate of contraction, 2) force of contraction, 3) rate of impulse conduction, and 4) amount of coronary blood flow.

some domestic animal species and for the human are shown in Table 7.1.

TABLE 7.1. Heart Rates in Adult, Resting Animals

Animal	Heart Rate (beats/minute)
Horse	32–44
Horse (thoroughbred)	38–48
Dairy cow	60–70
Sheep and goat	70–80
Pig	60–80
Dog	70–120
Cat	110–130
Chicken	200–400
Human	60–90

Autoregulation

In addition to the nervous regulation of heart function and output, an autoregulation of cardiac output based on the amount of blood received also exists. In other words, the more the heart is filled during diastole, the greater is the volume of blood pumped out. This is known as Starling's law of the heart. The heart can do this because the greater volume of incoming blood stretches the heart muscle fibers, resulting in a greater force of contraction. There are limits, however, to the amount of stretch by which the force of contraction increases. The stretch phenomenon is characteristic of all types of muscle.

Reflexes

Several important reflexes within the cardiovascular system assist in its regulation. In the arch of the aorta and where the carotid artery branches to form the internal carotid (the aortic and carotid sinuses, respectively), there are many receptors that respond to stretching of these vessels. Their stretch is caused by increased blood pressure from within. The receptors fire with greater frequency when stretched. The impulses from the aortic arch are transmitted to the medulla by the vagus nerves, and those from the carotids are transmitted to the medulla by the glossopharyngeal nerves. The responses of the greater number of impulses are directed toward lowering the blood pressure. This is done by greater stimulation of the cardioinhibitory center (which increases parasympathetic stimulation to the heart and decreases its activities) and by inhibition of the vasomotor center (thereby causing dilatation of the systemic blood vessels). The effects of these responses (decreased heart rate and decreased peripheral resistance) lower the blood pressure (Fig. 7.27). A decrease in blood pressure causes fewer impulses to be transmitted from the aortic and carotid sinuses; thus, the cardioinhibitory center receives less stimulation and the vasomotor center receives less inhibition, producing an increase in blood pressure. There are also receptors in the right atrium of the heart that are stimulated by stretch of that chamber, such as during exercise when greater amounts of blood are returned to the heart. The resulting reflex is known as the Bainbridge reflex. Stretch receptors transmit their impulses through the vagus nerves to the medulla of the brain. The effect of this reflex is to increase all activities of the heart to increase the circulatory effort necessary for the increased requirements.

Blood Pressure

Pressure Generation and Flow

Blood pressure has been mentioned briefly without regard for its dynamic aspects. Because there is a pressure gradient within the circulation (highest in aorta and lowest in venae cavae), the blood flows from the left ventricle, through the vessels, and back to the right atrium. The greatest pressure develops within the aorta when the left ventricle contracts. The ventricle relaxes completely after contraction, but blood pressure in the aorta does not diminish entirely. The large arteries contain a higher proportion of elastic connective tissue fibers than muscle fibers. These elastic fibers permit expansion when blood

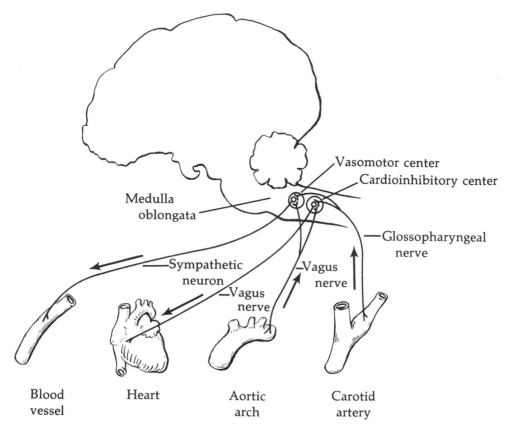

Figure 7.27. Lowering blood pressure. The reflex controlling blood pressure involves receptors in the aortic and carotid sinuses and centers in the medulla oblongata. The vasomotor center is inhibited, resulting in vasodilatation. The cardioinhibitory center is stimulated, resulting in diminished heart activ-

advances into them from the left ventricle, and stretched elastic fibers have a rebound tendency that exerts pressure on the blood in the large vessels after the heart ceases to exert the pressure (Fig. 7.28). The continuous pressure in the arteries permits a continuous rather than an intermittent blood flow through the body.

Systolic and Diastolic Pressures

The high point of the arterial pressure obtained at the peak of left ventricular contraction (systole) is called the systolic blood pressure. The lowest pressure in the arteries occurs while the left ventricle is relaxed (diastole) and before it begins its next contraction. The low point of pressure is called

the diastolic pressure. Blood pressure measurements are often given as two values, one over the other (e.g., 130/70). The upper value is the systolic pressure and the lower value is the diastolic pressure. The term "pulse pressure" refers to the difference between the systolic and the diastolic pressures; in the previous example it would be 60. The appropriate unit for expressing blood pressure values is millimeters of mercury (mm Hg) or torr. The mean blood pressure is not a value halfway between the systolic and diastolic blood pressures; it usually tends to be the diastolic pressure plus about one-third of the pulse pressure. Therefore, in the previous example the mean blood pressure would be about 90

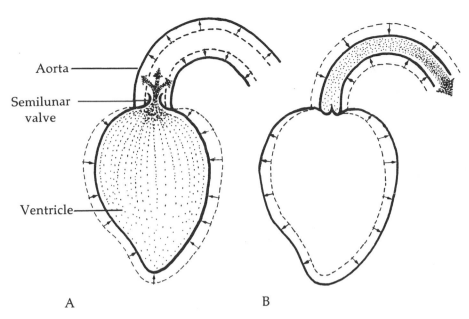

Figure 7.28. Generation of systemic blood pressure during left ventricular systole and maintenance of blood flow and pressure during diastole. **A.** Contraction of ventricle and stretch of elastic aorta. **B.** This is followed by retention of systemic blood in vessels by closed aortic semilunar valve. Continued blood flow provided by elastic recoil of aorta. Solid lines in **A** represent ventricular and aortic size at end of systole. Solid lines in **B** represent ventricular and aortic size at end of diastole. The stippling in the ventricle and aorta represents blood.

mm Hg. Mean blood pressure determines the average rate at which blood flows through the systemic vessels. It is closer to diastolic pressure than systolic pressure because, during each pressure cycle, the pressure usually remains at systolic levels for a shorter time than it remains at diastolic levels.

Measurements

The conformation of the body parts of animals is not conducive to their blood pressure being measured by the same noninvasive sphygmomanometric means used in humans. Therefore, clinical measurements are more difficult to obtain. A most effective method in animals involves actually cannulating arteries and measuring the pressure electronically with appropriate transducers. A blood pressure measurement taken from the carotid artery in a dog

is illustrated in Figure 7.29. The systolic, diastolic, mean, and pulse pressures are also shown, as well as the correlation with the ECG. Values for characteristic blood pressures in several animals are given in Table 7.2.

Blood Flow

There must be a difference in blood pressure between intake and output for blood to flow. Blood pressure alone does not imply blood flow. The flow of blood to a part can be changed by changing the diameter of the vessel supplying the part. Constriction of a vessel reduces the blood flow and dilatation increases the blood flow.

Autoregulation

Generally, there is an autoregulatory mechanism affecting blood flow to a part that is controlled by the amount of oxygen being

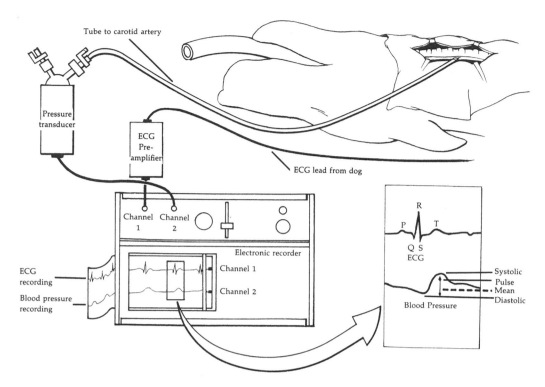

Figure 7.29. Recording blood pressure from a surgically placed cannula and an electrocardiogram from lead II in an anesthetized dog. Note the increase in pressure that follows the QRS waves (depolarization of ventricles and subsequent contraction). Pulse pressure is represented by the double arrow between diastolic and systolic blood pressure.

received by the cells. When the oxygen is reduced in concentration, the blood vessels dilate and more blood is permitted to flow so that oxygen is replenished. It is also thought that more oxygen being supplied than is needed can result in vasoconstriction, which would reduce blood flow and reestablish oxygen at its lower level.

Cardiac Output and Blood Diversion

Cardiac output is defined as the amount of blood pumped by the heart in a unit period of time. It is usually measured in milliliters or liters per minute. Under resting conditions, each body organ or muscle mass receives a rather constant amount. The percentage of the cardiac output that goes to the various organs or tissues changes, however, with the activity condition. At rest, the

muscles might receive only 20 to 25% of the cardiac output, whereas they might receive up to 75% during extreme muscular exertion. At such times there is diversion of blood flow from other organs (e.g., kidneys, intestines) so that it can be used by the muscle. This is accomplished by constriction of the arteries and arterioles supplying the kidneys and intestines and by dilatation of the vessels supplying the muscles. During muscle exertion, the cardiac output is also increased; coupled with vasodilatation, this provides adequate blood flow to the muscle to satisfy the greater oxygen needs of muscle activity (Fig. 7.30).

Breathing and Blood Flow

An assist to blood flow is provided during the inspiratory phase of breathing. The

TABLE 7.2. Characteristic Blood Pressures in Adult, Resting Animals

Species	Systolic/diastolic (mm Hg)	Mean (mm Hg)
Giraffe	260/160	219
Horse	130/95	115
Cow	140/95	120
Swine	140/80	110
Sheep	140/90	114
Human	120/70	100
Dog	120/70	100
Cat	140/90	110
Rabbit	120/80	100
Guinea pig	100/60	80
Rat	110/70	90
Mouse	111/80	100
Turkey	250/170	190
Chicken	175/145	160
Canary	220/150	185

From Detweiler DK. Control mechanisms of the circulatory system. In: Swenson, MJ, Reece WO, eds. Dukes' physiology of domestic animals. 11th Ed. Ithaca, NY: Cornell University Press, 1993:185.

venae cavae course through the thorax on their way to the right atrium. More specifically, they course through the mediastinum, a space shared by the other major vessels of the heart, the large lymph vessels, and the esophagus (Fig. 7.31). The mediastinal space is intimately associated with the intrapleural space, a space that is in the thorax but outside the lungs. When animals inspire (inhale air), a vacuum (negative pressure) develops in the intrapleural space because of enlargement of the thorax. This vacuum provides for lung expansion. The negative pressure in the intrapleural space is also transferred to the mediastinal space because of the thin wall of separation. Any thin-walled structure within the mediastinal space responds to the developing vacuum by expansion, with the result being lowered pressure within the thin-walled structures (venae cavae, lymph vessels, and esophagus). This is helpful for the return of venous blood and lymph to the heart because it increases the pressure gra-

dient to assist blood and lymph flow with every breath.

The above sequence of events is illustrated in Figure 7.32. In this laboratory model, the muscular diaphragm is represented by a rubber glove stretched over the bottom of a bell jar. Downward traction on the glove simulates contraction of the diaphragm. The lung and caudal vena cava are represented by balloons that respond to decreasing and increasing external pressure by expansion and collapse, respectively. During inspiration the diaphragm contracts; this is followed, in order, by (1) increased thoracic volume, (2) decreased intrapleural pressure, (3) increased volume in the lung and vena cava, (4) decreased intrapulmonic and intravenous pressures, and (5) air flow into the lung and blood flow into the thoracic part of the vena cava. During expiration, the diaphragm returns to its original position, so that (1) the volume decreases in the thorax, lung, and vena cava, and (2) the intrapleural, intrapulmonic, and intravenous pressures increase. Backflow of blood is prevented by the cranially directed valves in the vena cava, and air flows out of the lung.

Circulation Time

Circulation time refer to the time required for blood to return to the right atrium after it has been pumped from the left ventricle. This is variable but is approximately 40 to 60 seconds. Circulation time is distinct from mixing time, which is the time required for a substance injected into the blood to be mixed thoroughly, either with the blood or the body fluid compartment with which it is compatible. In any case, the mixing time exceeds the circulation time.

CAPILLARY DYNAMICS

Capillary dynamics refers to the physical factors associated with the exchange of fluid between the blood and interstitial

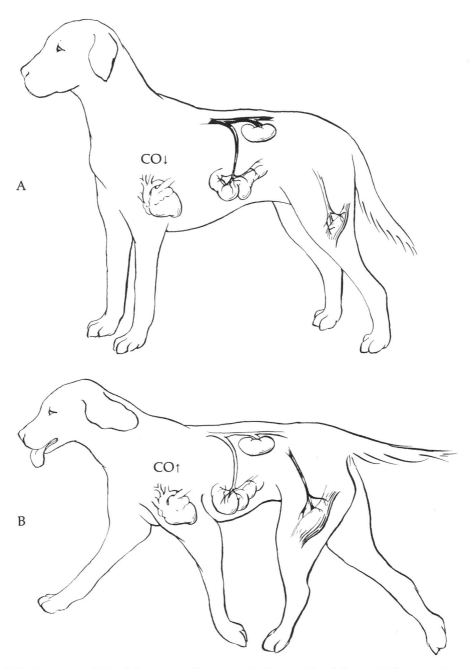

Figure 7.30. Diversion of blood flow according to need. Greater blood flow to kidneys and intestine at rest (**A**) and to muscles during exertion (**B**). Cardiac output (*CO*) is greater during exertion. Blackened vessels indicate locations of greater blood flow.

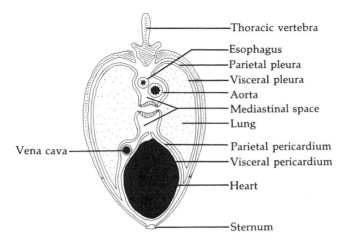

Figure 7.31. Transverse section of equine thorax at a level that shows the esophagus, caudal vena cava, aorta, and heart within the mediastinal space.

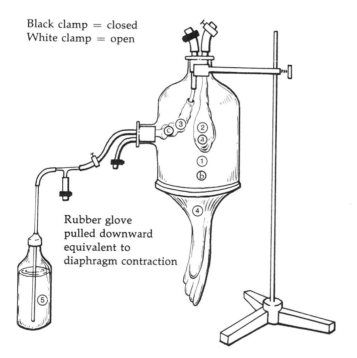

Figure 7.32. Laboratory model of the thorax. This illustrates the mechanics of breathing and the influence of breathing on venous blood return to the heart. Structures: *1*, thorax; *2*, lung; *3*, vena cava; *4*, diaphragm; *5*, venous blood reservoir. Pressures: *a*, intrapulmonic; *b*, intrapleural; *c*, intravenous. During inspiration, the diaphragm (*4*) contracts, resulting in an increase in thoracic volume (*1*) and a decrease in intrapleural pressure (*b*). This is followed by an increase in lung volume (*2*) and a decrease in intrapulmonic pressure (*a*). Air flows into the lung. Also, there is an increase in vena cava volume (*3*) and a decrease of its intravenous pressure (*c*). Blood flow (*5*) to the heart increases. During expiration the diaphragm (*4*) relaxes, resulting in a decrease in the volumes of the thorax (*1*), lung (*2*), and vena cava (*3*), and an increase in intrapleural (*b*), intrapulmonic (*a*), and intravenous (*c*) pressures. Air flows out of the lung. Valves prevent blood from flowing backward. Black clamp, closed; white clamp, open.

fluid at the level of the capillaries. The capillaries have slit-like spaces between adjacent endothelial cells that comprise the capillary wall, known as intercellular clefts. Although water can diffuse through all parts of the endothelium (capillary membrane), it seems to diffuse more freely through the clefts, or pores. Lipid-soluble materials (e.g., oxygen, carbon dioxide) in blood diffuse freely through the lipid portion of the capillary membrane, but lipid-insoluble substances (e.g., electrolytes, glucose, urea) must diffuse through the pores. Large lipid-insoluble molecules (e.g., protein) diffuse through the pores with difficulty.

Diffusion and Bulk Flow

The diffusion of water and its dissolved substances accounts for the greatest degree of interchange between capillaries and interstitial fluid (Fig. 7.33). It is believed that by the time blood traverses the distance of a capillary, the water of the plasma has been exchanged with water of the interstitial fluid about 80 times. Usually the relative proportions of the extracellular water between the plasma and interstitial space are in equilibrium. In addition to diffusional flow of fluid, there is also a bulk flow; this results from osmotic and hydrostatic pressure differences between plasma and interstitial fluid. It should be noted, however, that the volume of interchange occurring by diffusion is 15,000 to 20,000 times greater than the volume of interchange by bulk flow. The volume of bulk flow into the interstitial space from the plasma is usually balanced by the amount returning to the capillaries from the interstitial space, coupled with that returning

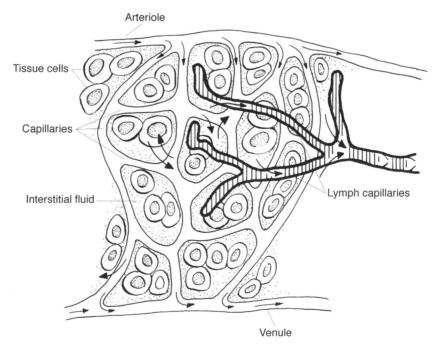

Figure 7.33. A schematic representation of a capillary bed. Blood is supplied to capillaries by arterioles, and it leaves the capillaries through the venules. Tissue cells are surrounded by interstitial fluid (ISF). Water and dissolved substances from blood capillaries are interchanged with ISF and intracellular fluid by diffusion. ISF not returned to the blood capillaries, is returned as lymph through lymphatic capillaries.

through the lymphatics. In certain circumstances, imbalances occur and fluid can accumulate excessively in the interstitial spaces. In such cases, bulk flow into the interstitial space from the plasma exceeds the volume returned to the blood and lymph capillaries.

Mechanism of Bulk Flow

The mechanism of bulk flow is determined by a number of parameters.

CAPILLARY PRESSURE. The capillary pressure (P_c) is the hydrostatic pressure in the capillary. It averages 17 mm Hg (25 mm Hg at the arterial end and 10 mm Hg at the venous end).

INTERSTITIAL FLUID PRESSURE. The interstitial fluid pressure (P_{if}) is the hydrostatic pressure in the interstitial fluid. It averages about -6 mm Hg. It is a negative pressure (vacuum) and is created by the return of interstitial fluids to the venous end of the capillary and to the lymphatics. This can be compared to the attachment of a device to a water faucet to create a vacuum. When water flows through its open end, a vacuum is created at its side port.

PLASMA COLLOIDAL OSMOTIC PRESSURE. The plasma colloidal osmotic pressure (π_p) is the effective osmotic pressure of the plasma. It occurs because of the presence of the protein molecules and cations (positive ions) retained by the net negative charge of the protein. It can also be called the oncotic pressure. It averages about 28 mm Hg.

INTERSTITIAL FLUID COLLOIDAL OSMOTIC PRESSURE. The interstitial fluid colloidal osmotic pressure (π_{if}) is the effective osmotic pressure of the interstitial fluid and, like the π_p, is a result of the presence of protein molecules that have leaked from the plasma and have not yet returned to the blood through the lymphatics. The π_{if} averages about 5 mm Hg.

To understand bulk flow, it is helpful to consider these various pressures and to determine their effects, first at the arterial end of the capillary and then at the venous end. Normally, filtration or net outward flow occurs at the arterial end, and reabsorption or net inward flow occurs at the venous end of the capillary.

The arterial and venous ends of a capillary are shown in Figure 7.34. Each of the

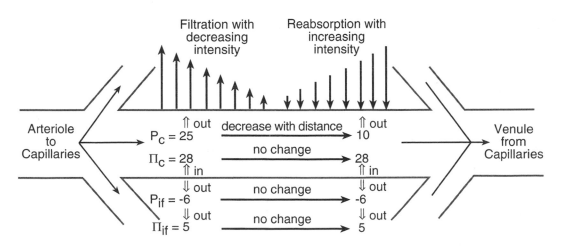

Figure 7.34. Physical factors associated with filtration at the arterial end and reabsorption at the venous end of a capillary. Values are in mm Hg (P_c, capillary pressure; π_c, plasma colloidal osmotic pressure; P_{if}, interstitial fluid pressure; π_{if}, interstitial fluid colloidal osmotic pressure). The open arrows indicate the direction of influence of P_c, K_c, P_{if}, and π_{if}.

four pressures that influence the direction of fluid flow is shown with an arrow pointed in the direction of its influence. Their effects can be summarized as follows:

Arterial end

Pressure Out (mm Hg)		Pressure In (mm Hg)	Summary
P_c =	25	π_c = 28	Pressure out = 36 mm Hg
P_{if}* =	6		Pressure in = 28 mm Hg
π_{if} =	5		
Total	36	28	Filtration pressure = 8 mm Hg

*A negative value of the interstitial fluid pressure favors outward flow and is the same as equivalent positive value in the capillary.

Venous end

Pressure Out (mm Hg)		Pressure In (mm Hg)	Summary
P_c =	10	π_c = 28	Pressure out = 28 mm Hg
P_{if} =	6		Pressure in = 21 mm Hg
π_{if} =	5		
Total	21	28	Filtration pressure = 7 mm Hg

A filtration pressure of 8 mm Hg and an absorption pressure of 7 mm Hg would appear to represent an imbalance, in which fluid would accumulate in the interstitial fluid. Accumulation does not ordinarily occur, however, because the extra filtration represented by these values is removed from the interstitial fluid by the lymphatics. In fact, some of the interstitial fluid bulk flow must be removed by the lymphatics to carry the protein that has leaked from the capillaries back to the blood. Once again, the lymphatics are the only route by which leaked protein can return.

Capillary Imbalances

An imbalance of bulk flow can occur; when this happens, fluid accumulates in the interstitial space. This can be seen when high capillary pressure, low blood protein concentration, lymphatic blockage, and increased porosity (which allows more protein to escape) are each sufficient to favor filtration over absorption and lymphatic drainage (Fig. 7.35). Increases of venous blood pressure are more con-ducive to imbalance caused by high capillary pressure than to increases from the arterial side, because a venous side increase transmits the increase throughout the length of the capillary, whereas the effect of an arterial side increase is minimized by its reduction in going from the arterial to the venous end. Venous constriction or obstruction and the inability of the heart to circulate all the blood returned to it increase blood pressure on the venous side that would be transmitted all the way back throughout the length of the capillary. A reduction of the plasma protein level that is low enough to cause an imbalance can result from severe malnutrition, kidney disease, or leakage from damaged capillaries. Lymphatic blockage increases the P_{if} because protein is not being removed from the interstitial fluid. With increased porosity, there is a loss of protein from the capillary, which in turn reduces the potential for reabsorption. In each of these examples, fluid accumulates in the interstitial space and gives it a swollen appearance, a condition known as edema.

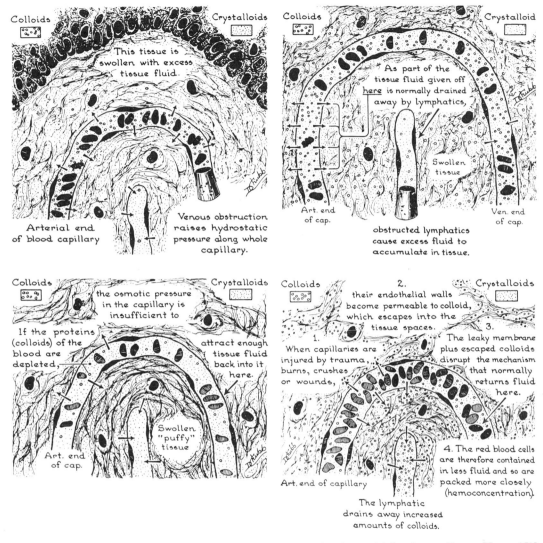

Figure 7.35. Capillary dynamic imbalances as causes for interstitial edema. From Ham AW. Histology. 7th ed. Philadelphia: JB Lippincott, 1974.

STUDY AIDS—THE CARDIOVASCULAR SYSTEM

Structure and Function

1. Know the orientation of the heart within the thorax with regard to its base and apex.

2. What is the pericardial sac and where is it attached to the heart? What is its function?

3. Know the chambers of the heart. Which chamber normally has the greatest thickness?

4. Know the location of A-V and semilunar valves. What prevents eversion of A-V valves when ventricles contract?

5. Follow a drop of blood from its entrance to the heart at the vena cava until its ejection from the heart into the aorta.

6. What is the relationship of the blood vessel linings to the heart?

7. What is the order of blood vessels from the ventricles back to the atria? Which one of the vessel divisions permits exchange with interstitial fluid?

8. What is the function of elastic fibers in arteries?

9. What comprises a capillary? Do they have muscle fibers and elastic fibers in their walls?

10. Is back-flow of blood possible in veins? Do veins have muscle fibers in their walls?

11. Which blood vessels have the lowest pressure within them?

12. Differentiate between the pulmonary and systemic circulations (origin and distribution).

13. What is meant by the lymphatic system? What is the fluid of its vessels known as?

14. Does protein ever "leak" from capillaries? What is its turnover rate?

15. What is the route for return of protein to the blood after it has leaked?

16. What is one of the most important functions of the lymphatics?

17. What is the location and what are the functions of lymph nodes?

18. What are four of the functions of the spleen?

19. What is the S-A node? What is its pacemaker function?

20. What are the two syncytia of the heart and how are they separated?

21. What is the contraction sequence of the two syncytia and what function is thereby served?

22. Describe conduction of the impulse throughout the heart. What purpose is served by fast conduction?

23. Do both atria contract at the same time? Do both ventricles contract at the same time?

24. Define diastole and systole.

25. Describe the events of the cardiac cycle.

26. What is the ECG? What are the wave forms associated with one cardiac cycle? What phase of electrical activity is associated with each wave form?

27. How are amplitudes of waves and intervals between waves measured?

28. What are the heart sounds and with what are they associated?

29. What is a generalization about the relationship between heart rate and size of animal?

30. What are the effects of autonomic stimulation upon the heart?

31. What is Starling's law of the heart?

32. What is the response of the carotid and aortic sinus receptors to increased blood pressure?

33. Why does blood flow continuously rather than intermittently, considering that the ventricles contract intermittently?

34. Define diastolic, systolic, pulse, and mean blood pressure.

35. How is blood flow to body parts autoregulated?

36. Is blood flow to body parts constant regardless of their need?

37. Study "Breathing and Blood Flow" very well. Visualize expansion of the venae cavae that occurs with each inspiration. Translate expansion of the venae cavae to increased blood flow to the heart.

Capillary Dynamics

1. Distinguish between diffusion and bulk flow.

2. What are the four pressures that are associated with bulk flow?

3. What contributes to plasma colloidal osmotic pressure?

4. Consider each of the four pressures and determine the direction of fluid flow caused by each.

5. Study the examples given for the arterial and venous ends of a capillary that determine the extent of filtration and reabsorption.

6. Study the examples of capillary imbalance and relate their causes to the pressure factors.

7. Why are venous side pressure increases more conducive to imbalance caused by increased capillary pressure than to arterial side pressure increases?

SELF-EVALUATION—THE CARDIOVASCULAR SYSTEM

1. A greater amount of ventricular filling results simply from blood flow into relaxed chambers rather than that caused by atrial contraction.
   a. true
   b. false
2. An increase in the resistance to blood flow to the lungs would cause hypertrophy (because of greater work) of which one of the following chambers?
   a. right atrium
   b. left atrium
   c. right ventricle
   d. left ventricle
3. Venous blood (unoxygenated):
   a. enters the left atrium from the vena cava
   b. enters the pulmonary trunk from the left ventricle
   c. enters the pulmonary trunk from the right ventricle
   d. enters the left atrium from the pulmonary veins
4. Which one of the following occurs during expansion of the thorax during inspiration?
   a. decrease in intrapleural, mediastinal, and intravenous (vena cava) pressure with assist to return of blood and lymph to the heart
   b. compression of the lungs upon the vena cava with resistance to return of blood and lymph to the heart
5. The impulse is transmitted throughout the ventricular muscles at a rate 2 to 3 times faster than it would be transmitted through atrial muscle because of the characteristics of the:

a. S-A node
b. A-V node
c. A-V bundle
d. Purkinje fibers

6. The first heart sound, "lub", is caused by:
   a. closure of the semilunar valves
   b. opening of the semilunar valves
   c. closure of the A-V valves and contraction of the ventricles
   d. opening of the A-V valves and contraction of the atria
7. Venous obstruction of blood flow from a body part would tend to increase interstitial fluid volume of that part.
   a. true
   b. false
8. During the time between the measurements for systolic blood pressure and diastolic blood pressure, the energy for the flow of blood is derived from:
   a. the left ventricle
   b. there is no blood flow; it is at a standstill
   c. the right ventricle
   d. arterial elasticity
9. Which one of the following circulatory divisions has the lowest pressure?
   a. capillaries
   b. veins
   c. arterioles
   d. arteries

	Capillary	Interstitial Space
10. Hydrostatic pressure	26	-2
Colloidal osmotic pressure	25	5

Which end of the capillary does this situation represent?
a. arterial (filtration)
b. venous (reabsorption)

11. The QRS wave complex would immediately precede which one of the following events?
   a. atrial contraction
   b. ventricular contraction
   c. the second heart sound
   d. semilunar valve closure

12. Blood pumped from the left ventricle goes through the:
    a. aortic semilunar valve
    b. pulmonary artery semilunar valve
    c. right A-V valve
    d. left A-V valve
13. Blood flow through the arteries is maintained during diastole because of:
    a. contraction of the ventricles
    b. inertia
    c. elastic fibers in large vessels
    d. expansion of the thorax during inspiration
14. Interstitial fluid enters lymph vessels by:
    a. diffusion
    b. inward flow through flap valves
15. The lymphatic system:
    a. is the only route back to the blood for the return of protein that leaks from the capillaries
    b. has a fluid in its vessels known as lymph
    c. has a fluid in its vessels similar to interstitial fluid
    d. has lymph nodes along the course of the lymphatic vessels that phagocytize foreign material and generate lymphocytes
    e. all of the above
16. Which one of the following organs is active in the destruction of erythrocytes, stores iron, acts as a blood reservoir, phagocytizes foreign material, and produces lymphocytes?
    a. lymph nodes
    b. carotid body
    c. spleen
    d. dubissary
17. Which of the following is the correct sequence of contraction for the heart?
    a. simultaneous contraction of both atria followed by simultaneous contraction of both ventricles
    b. right atrium followed by right ventricle followed by left atrium followed by left ventricle

c. simultaneous contraction of right atrium and right ventricle followed by simultaneous contraction of left atrium and left ventricle
18. Which one of the autonomic nervous system divisions is associated with a decrease in all activities of the heart?
    a. sympathetic
    b. parasympathetic
19. Blood pressure is being measured with an electronic recorder. The upper swing of the pen is at 130 mm Hg and the lower swing of the pen is 70 mm Hg. Which one of the following is the pulse pressure?
    a. 130 mm Hg
    b. 70 mm Hg
    c. 60 mm Hg
    d. 90 mm Hg
20. Which one of the following would increase filtration at the capillary and tend to cause edema?
    a. increased plasma colloidal osmotic pressure
    b. increased venous blood pressure
    c. an increase (towards positive) of the interstitial fluid hydrostatic pressure

SUGGESTED READINGS

Adams DR. Canine anatomy: a systemic study. Ames, IA: Iowa State University Press, 1986.

Breazile JE. Textbook of veterinary physiology. Philadelphia: Lea & Febiger, 1971.

Crouch JE. Functional human anatomy. 4th ed. Philadelphia: Lea & Febiger, 1985.

Eckert R, Randall D, Augustine G. Animal physiology: Mechanisms and adaptations. 3rd ed. New York: WH Freeman, 1988.

Evans HE, deLahunta A. Miller's guide to the dissection of the dog. 4th ed. Philadelphia: WB Saunders, 1996.

Frandson RD, Spurgeon TL. Anatomy and physiology of farm animals. 5th ed. Philadelphia: Lea & Febiger, 1992.

Ghoshal NG. Equine heart and arteries. In: Getty R, ed. Sisson and Grossman's The anatomy of the domestic animals, Vol. 1.

5th ed. Philadelphia: WB Saunders, 1975:554–618.

Grollman S. The human body: its structure and physiology. 4th ed. New York: Macmillan, 1978.

Guyton AC. Function of the human body. 8th ed. Philadelphia: WB Saunders, 1991.

Guyton AC. Textbook of medical physiology. 7th ed. Philadelphia: WB Saunders, 1986.

Ham AW. Histology. 7th ed. Philadelphia: JB Lippincott, 1974.

Langley LL, Telford IR, Christensen JB. Dynamic anatomy and physiology. 3rd ed. New York: McGraw-Hill, 1969.

Leak LV. The fine structure and function of the lymphatic vascular system. In: Meessen H, ed. Handbüch der allgemeinen pathologie. New York: Springer-Verlag, 1972:149–196.

Spence AP, Mason EB. Human anatomy and physiology. 2nd ed. Menlo Park, CA: Benjamin/Cummings, 1983.

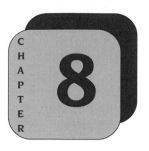

Respiration

Respiration is the means by which animals obtain and use oxygen and eliminate carbon dioxide. In this chapter, the chemical factors involved in oxygen uptake and carbon dioxide production are not discussed. However, the mechanical and physical aspects of respiration presented here are mainly concerned with the provision of oxygen to the cells, where it is taken up by the mitochondria at the end of the electron transport chain. Here, the reduced cofactors of metabolism are reoxidized and, in the process of electron transport, hydrogen combines with oxygen to form water. This water is referred to as metabolic water. Generally, the mechanical and physical aspects of respiration are involved with ventilation of the lungs and with transport of gases between the lungs and blood and between the blood and tissues. The respiratory system also serves nonrespiratory functions, and some of these functions are discussed.

STRUCTURE AND FUNCTION OF THE RESPIRATORY SYSTEM

The respiratory apparatus consists of the lungs and the air passages leading to them, including the nostrils, nasal cavities, pharynx, trachea, pulmonary alveoli, and pleura.

Nostrils

The nostrils (nares) are the paired external openings to the air passages (Fig. 8.1). The nostrils are the most pliable and dilatable in the horse and the most rigid in the pig. Nostril dilatation is advantageous when more air is required, as in running, and in situations in which breathing is not done through the mouth. The horse is a runner and open mouth breathing is not characteristic, so it appears that dilatable nostrils are an adaptation.

Nasal Cavities

The nostrils provide the external openings for the paired nasal cavities. The nasal cavities are separated from each other by the nasal septum and from the mouth by the hard and soft palates. In addition, each nasal cavity contains mucosa-covered turbinate bones (conchae) that project to the interior from the dorsal and lateral walls, separating the cavity into passages

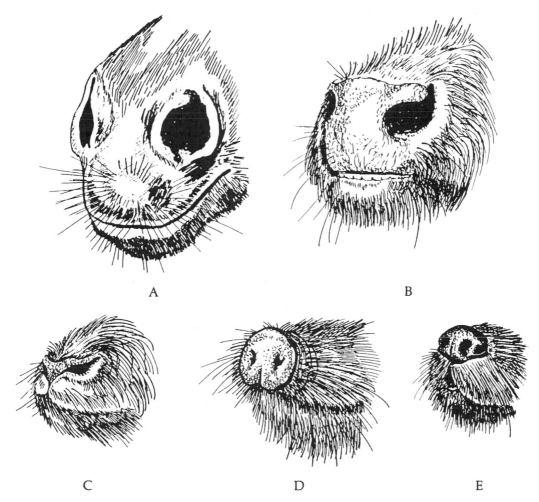

Figure 8.1. The nostrils of several domestic animals. **A.** Horse. **B.** Cow. **C.** Sheep. **D.** Pig. **E.** Dog. From Frandson RD, Spurgeon TL. Anatomy and physiology of farm animals. 5th ed. Philadelphia: Lea & Febiger, 1992.

known as the common, dorsal, middle, and ventral meatuses (Fig. 8.2). The mucosa of the turbinates is well vascularized and serves to warm and humidify inhaled air. Another function, mainly for the conchae, that is often overlooked involves cooling the blood that supplies the brain. Arteries that supply blood to the brain divide into many smaller arteries at its base and then rejoin before entering. These smaller arteries are bathed in a pool of venous blood that comes from the walls of the nasal passages, where it has been cooled. As a result,

brain temperature might be 2° or 3°C lower than body core temperatures. The brain is the most heat-sensitive body organ, so this cooling method is particularly important during times of extreme activity. The mouth breathing that occurs when the environmental air is extremely cold seems to be reflexive, which might prevent the overcooling of the brain that could otherwise occur if all the inhaled air traversed the meatuses and had contact with the conchae. The olfactory epithelium is located in the caudal portion of each nasal cavity, and greater perception of odors (a nonrespiratory function) is achieved by sniffing (i.e., fast, alternating, and shallow inspirations and expirations).

Pharynx

The pharynx is caudal to the nasal cavities and is a common passageway for air and food (Fig. 8.3). The openings to the pharynx include two posterior nares, two eustachian tubes, a mouth (oral cavity), a glottis, and an esophagus. The opening from the pharynx leading to the continuation of the respiratory passageway is the glottis. Immediately caudal to the glottis is the larynx, the organ of phonation (sound production) in mammals. Sound is produced by the controlled passage of air, which causes vibration of vocal cords in the larynx. The organ of phonation in birds is called the

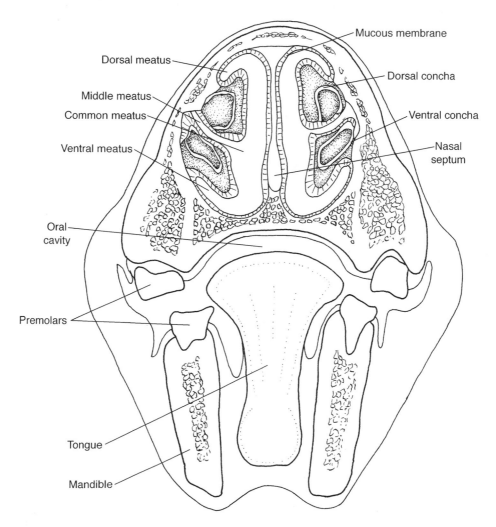

Figure 8.2. Transverse section of the head of a horse showing the division of the nasal cavities. The airways are noted as the dorsal, middle, ventral, and common meatuses. The conchae consist of turbinate bones covered by a highly vascularized mucous membrane. Incoming air is exposed to a large surface area for adjustment of its temperature and humidity.

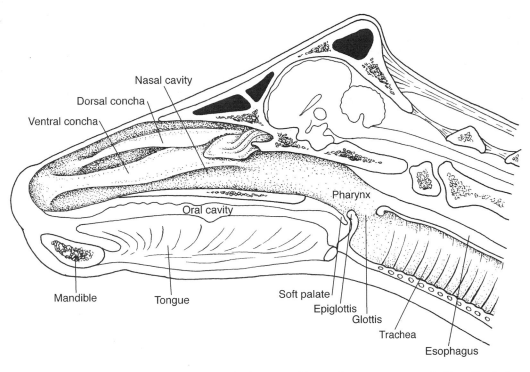

Figure 8.3. Midsagittal section of the head of a cow with nasal septum removed. The stippled area represents the pathway for air through the nasal cavity, pharynx, and trachea. The glottis is the opening to the trachea.

syrinx; this is located where the trachea divides to form the bronchi.

Trachea and Its Subdivisions

The trachea is the primary passageway for air to the lungs. It is continued from the larynx cranially and divides caudally to form the right and left bronchi. The tracheal wall contains cartilaginous rings to prevent collapse of the tracheal airway (Fig. 8.4). Each tracheal ring is incomplete (not joined dorsally), which permits variations in diameter that are regulated by the tracheal muscle. This diameter can increase during times of greater ventilatory requirements.

The right and left bronchi and their subdivisions continue all the way to the alveoli, the final and smallest subdivisions of the air passages (Fig. 8.5). The subdivisions of the trachea to the alveoli, from the largest to the smallest, are the 1) bronchi, 2) bronchioles, 3) terminal bronchioles, 4) respiratory bronchioles, 5) alveolar duct, 6) alveolar sac, and 7) alveoli.

Pulmonary Alveoli

The pulmonary alveoli are the principal sites of gas diffusion between the air and blood. The separation of air and blood, and thus the diffusion distance, is minimal at the alveolar level. The alveolar epithelium and the capillary endothelium are intimately associated (Fig. 8.6). Here, venous blood from the pulmonary artery becomes arterial blood and is returned to the left atrium by the pulmonary veins. The darker purple color of venous blood becomes bright red arterial blood during the resaturation of hemoglobin with new oxygen that has diffused from the alveoli. During the seventeenth century, Richard Lower showed that the change in blood color occurred in the lungs because of the influence of fresh air. The idea that the diffusion of oxygen and carbon dioxide between blood and air was separate from a secretion process was proven by August and Marie Krogh. (August Krogh won the Nobel prize in 1920 for his studies of the capillaries.)

Lungs

The lungs are the principal structures of the respiratory system. They are paired structures and occupy all space in the thorax that is not otherwise filled. When the thorax expands in volume, the lungs also expand; this provides for air flow into the lungs. The lungs have an almost friction-free movement within the thorax because of the pleura, a smooth serous membrane.

Pleura

The pleura consists of a single layer of cells fused to the surface of a connective

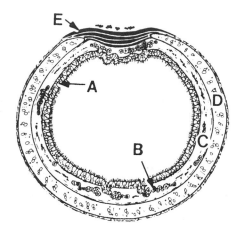

Figure 8.4. Schematic representation of cross section of trachea. **A.** Pseudostratified epithelium lines the lumen. **B.** Glands in the lamina propria and submucosa. **C.** Glands in the submucosa. **D.** Cartilage. **E.** Band of smooth muscle. The tracheal muscle and the cartilage form most of the tracheal wall. From Dellmann H-D. Textbook of veterinary histology. 4th ed. Philadelphia: Lea & Febiger, 1993.

tissue layer. It envelops both lungs (visceral pleura). The pleura for the right and

Figure 8.5. Schematic representation of lung subdivisions. From McNaught AB, Callander R. Illustrated physiology. 3rd ed. Edinburgh: Churchill Livingstone, 1975.

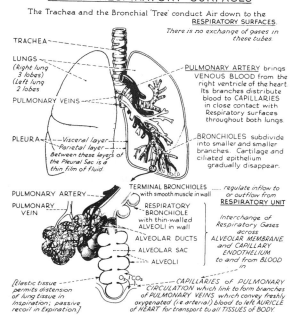

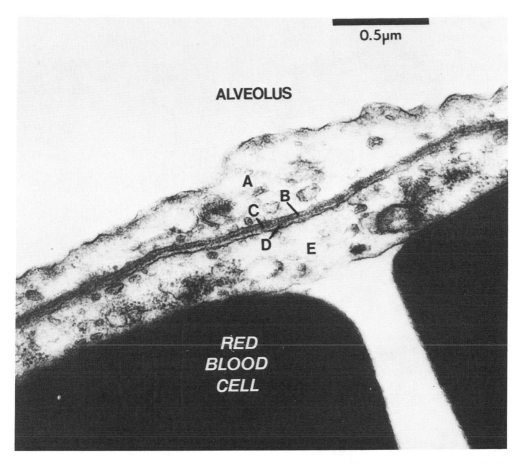

Figure 8.6. Electron micrograph of mouse lung showing attenuated portion of alveolar epithelium and its proximity to capillary endothelium. The respiratory membrane (without alveolar fluid layer) is composed of the following: **A.** Alveolar epithelium; **B.** Alveolar epithelial basement membrane; **C.** Interstitial space; **D.** Capillary endothelial basement membrane; **E.** Capillary endothelium. From Reece WO. Respiration in mammals. In Swenson MJ, Reece WO, eds. Dukes' physiology of domestic animals. 11th ed. Ithaca, NY: Cornell University Press, 1993:263–293.

left lung meet near the midline, and here it reflects upward (dorsally), turns back on the inner thoracic wall, and provides for its lining (parietal pleura). The space between the respective visceral pleura layers as they ascend to the dorsal wall is known as the mediastinal space. Within the mediastinal space are the venae cavae, thoracic lymph duct, esophagus, aorta, and trachea (Fig. 8.7). The mediastinal space is intimately associated with the intrapleural space (space between visceral and parietal pleura); thus, pressure changes in the intrapleural space are accompanied by similar changes in the mediastinal space. Also, pressure changes within the mediastinal space are accompanied by changes within the mediastinal structures, provided that their walls are responsive to relatively low-pressure distensibility.

Figure 8.7. Transverse section of equine thorax showing the relationships of the visceral, parietal, and mediastinal pleura. The aorta, esophagus, venae cavae, and thoracic lymph duct (not shown) are within the mediastinal space. The esophagus, venae cavae, and lymph duct (soft structures) respond by increasing and decreasing pressures within their lumens. They are associated with similar changes in intrapleural and mediastinal spaces.

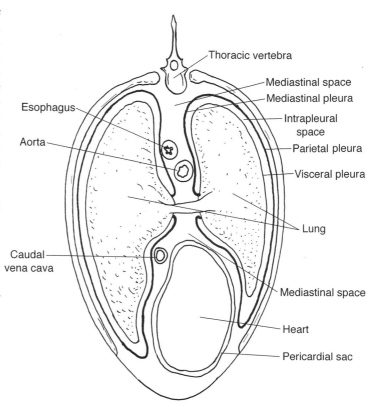

FACTORS AFFECTING RESPIRATION AND VENTILATION

Mechanics of Respiration

Respiratory Cycles

A respiratory cycle consists of an inspiratory phase followed by an expiratory phase. Inspiration involves an enlargement of the thorax and lungs, with an accompanying inflow of air. The thorax enlarges by contraction of the diaphragm (the musculotendinous separation between the thorax and abdomen) and by contraction of appropriate intercostal muscles (muscles located between the ribs) (Fig. 8.8). Diaphragmatic contraction enlarges the thorax in a caudal direction, and intercostal muscle contraction enlarges the thorax in a craniad and outward direction. Under normal breathing conditions, inspiration requires greater effort than expiration, and sometimes expiration might appear to be passive. Expiration can become quite an active process, particularly during times of accelerated breathing and also when there are impediments to the outflow of air. The appropriate intercostal muscles contract to assist in expiration. Other skeletal muscles can aid in either inspiration or expiration, such as the abdominal muscles. When contracted, these muscles force the abdominal viscera forward to press on the diaphragm, which in turn decreases thoracic volume.

Types of Breathing

There are two types of breathing: abdominal and costal. Abdominal breathing is characterized by visible movements of the abdomen, in which the abdomen protrudes during inspiration and recoils during expiration. Normally, the abdominal type of

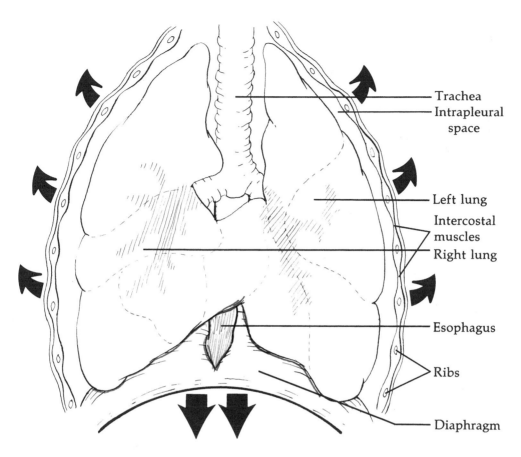

Figure 8.8. Schematic of the thorax during inspiration (ventral view). Shown are the directions of enlargement (*arrows*) when the diaphragm and inspiratory intercostal muscles contract during inspiration.

breathing predominates. The other type is called costal breathing; it is characterized by pronounced rib movements. During painful conditions of the abdomen, such as peritonitis in which movement of the viscera would aggravate the pain, costal breathing can predominate. Similarly, during painful conditions of the thorax, such as pleuritis, abdominal breathing might be more apparent. Binding of the thorax to minimize the outward and craniad expansion of the thorax requires greater diaphragmatic effort, and subsequent movement of abdominal viscera accentuates the abdominal type of breathing.

States of Breathing

In addition to the different types of breathing, there are variations in breathing relating to the frequency of breathing cycles, depth of inspiration, or both. Eupnea is the term used to describe normal quiet breathing, with no deviation in frequency or depth. Dyspnea is difficult breathing, in which visible effort is required to breathe. The animal is usually aware of this breathing state. Hyperpnea refers to breathing characterized by increased depth, frequency, or both, and is noticeable following physical exertion. The animal is not acutely conscious of this state. Polypnea is rapid, shallow breathing, somewhat similar to panting. Polypnea is similar to hyperpnea in regard to frequency but is unlike hyperpnea in regard to depth. Apnea refers to a cessation of breathing. However, as used clinically, it generally refers to a transient state of cessation of breathing. Tachypnea is excessive rapidity of breathing, and bradypnea is abnormal slowness of breathing.

Pulmonary Volumes and Capacities

Conventional descriptions for lung volumes are either associated with the amount of air within them at any one time or with the amount associated with a breath. Tidal volume is the amount of air breathed in or out during a respiratory cycle. It can increase or decrease from normal, depending on ventilation requirements. Tidal volume is probably used more frequently than other terms. Inspiratory reserve volume is the amount of air that can still be inspired after inhaling the tidal volume, and expiratory reserve volume is the amount of air that can still be expired after exhaling the tidal volume. Residual volume is the amount of air remaining in the lungs after the most forceful expiration. Also, some part of the residual volume remains in the

lungs after they have been removed from the thorax during slaughter or for postmortem examination. Because of the remaining residual volume, excised lung sections float in water.

Sometimes it is useful to combine two or more of these volumes. Such combinations are called capacities. Total lung capacity is the sum of all volumes. Vital capacity is the sum of all volumes over and above the residual volume; it is the maximum amount of air that can be breathed in after the most forceful expiration. Inspiratory capacity is the sum of the tidal and inspiratory reserve volumes. Functional residual capacity is the sum of the expiratory reserve volume and the residual volume. This is the lung volume that is ventilated by the tidal volume. It serves as the reservoir for air and helps to provide constancy to the blood concentrations of the respired gases. Relationships of pulmonary volumes and capacities are illustrated in Figure 8.9.

Respiratory Frequency

Respiratory frequency refers to the number of respiratory cycles each minute. It is an excellent indicator of health status, but it

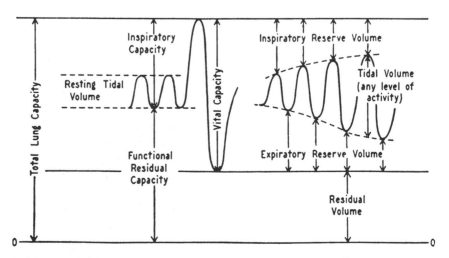

Figure 8.9. Subdivisions of lung volume. From Pappenheimer JR, et al. Standardization of definitions and symbols in respiratory physiology. Proc Soc Exp Biol Med 1950;9:602.

TABLE 8.1. Respiratory Frequency for Several Animal Species Under Different Conditions

| Animal | Number | Condition | Cycles/min | |
			Range	Mean
Horse	15	Standing (at rest)	10–14	12
Dairy cow	11	Standing (at rest)	26–35	29
	11	Sternal recumbency	24–50	35
Dairy calf	6	Standing (52-kg body weight, 3 weeks old)	18–22	20
	6	Lying down (52-kg body weight, 3 weeks old)	21–25	22
Pig	3	Lying down (23 to 27-kg body weight)	32–58	40
Dog	7	Sleeping (24° C)	18–25	21
	3	Standing (at rest)	20–34	24
Cat	5	Sleeping	16–25	22
	6	Lying down, awake	20–40	31
Sheep	5	Standing, ruminating, ½-1½ inch wool 18° C	20–34	25
	5	Same sheep and conditions except 10° C	16–22	19

From Reece WO. In Dukes' Physiology of domestic animals. 11th Ed. Edited by M.J. Swenson and W.O. Reece, Ithaca, NY: Cornell University Press, 1993.

must be interpreted properly because it is subject to numerous variations. In addition to variations observed among species, respiratory frequency can be affected by other factors, such as 1) body size, 2) age, 3) exercise, 4) excitement, 5) environmental temperature, 6) pregnancy, 7) degree of filling of the digestive tract, and 8) state of health. Pregnancy and digestive tract filling increase frequency because they limit the excursion of the diaphragm during inspiration. When expansion of the lungs is restricted, adequate ventilation is maintained by increased frequency. For example, when cattle lie down, the large rumen pushes against the diaphragm and restricts its movement, and the respiratory frequency is seen to increase.

Respiratory frequency usually increases during disease. Thus, frequency is a useful determinant of health status, but the frequency for a species under various conditions must be known so that this parameter can be interpreted properly (Table 8.1). Values are meaningful only when they are obtained unobtrusively from animals at rest.

Respiratory Pressures

Solutes and solvents diffuse from an area of their higher concentration to an area of their lower concentration, and so do gases. The concentrations of gases are usually expressed as pressures. It occasionally helps to think in terms of concentration instead of pressure when determining the diffusion of a single gas within a mixture of gases.

PARTIAL PRESSURE. Usually, gas pressure is considered in terms of total pressure, regardless of whether it is a single gas or a mixture of gases. When considering the equilibrium of two gas mixtures separated by a permeable membrane, however, it is necessary to consider each gas in the mixture separately in terms of its contribution to the total pressure. The term "partial pressure" is therefore used. It is defined as the pressure exerted by a particular gas in a mixture of gases. The sum of the partial pressures of the gases within a mixture equals the total pressure. The physiologic notation for partial pressure is P. Specific gases are noted by their chemical symbol. Accordingly, the partial pressure of oxygen in a gas mixture is denoted by PO_2. The partial pressure of oxygen in arterial blood and venous blood is given by P_aO_2 and P_vO_2, respectively. The particularization of arterial and venous blood is noted by subscript.

ATMOSPHERIC AIR. The total pressure of one atmosphere (1 atm) of air under conditions of standard temperature and pressure is 760 mm Hg. The appropriate composition of dry atmospheric air (and corresponding partial pressures) is as follows: 21.0% O_2 (P_{O_2}; about 159 mm Hg); 0.03% CO_2 (P_{CO_2}; about 0.23 mm Hg); 79.0% N_2 (P_{N_2}; about 600 mm Hg). The total pressure is approximately 760 mm Hg. CO_2 is almost absent in the atmospheric air. This explains the effective diffusion gradient for CO_2 from the body (where it is produced) to the air around us. Note that this is the composition of dry air. Any amount of humidification is represented by a partial pressure value (P_{H_2O}) for water vapor. Its presence would cause a dilution of the other gases and thus their partial pressures would be lowered to maintain the total pressure at 760 mm Hg.

ALVEOLAR AIR. It might be supposed that the composition of alveolar air is the same as atmospheric air because it merely represents the transfer of air from one place to another. The ventilation process does not evacuate the alveoli completely with each breath, but rather it is a gradual replenishment and evacuation. The approximate composition of alveolar air, measured in partial pressure, is as follows (dry atmospheric air partial pressures are in parentheses): P_{O_2} = 104 mm Hg (159); P_{CO_2} = 40 mm Hg (0.23); P_{N_2} = 569 mm Hg (600); P_{H_2O} = 47 mm Hg (0.00). The differences from atmospheric air are apparent. The total pressure of alveolar air is equal to 760 mm Hg, and all its components are diluted by water vapor, which is equal to 47 mm Hg. A P_{H_2O} of 47 mm Hg represents 100% humidification of alveolar air at body temperature (37°C for humans). In addition, the P_{O_2} is lower and the P_{CO_2} is higher than their respective atmospheric pressures because oxygen is continually diffusing from alveolar air to the tissues (where it is used), and CO_2 is continually diffusing from the tissues, (where it is pro-

duced) to the alveolar air (where it is expelled). The P_{N_2} of alveolar air is lower than its value in atmospheric air primarily because of its dilution by water vapor.

Pulmonary Ventilation

Ventilation is generally regarded as the process by which gas in closed places is renewed or exchanged. As it applies to the lungs, it is a process of exchanging the gas in the airways and alveoli with gas from the environment. The main function of breathing is to provide for ventilation. When cattle are stunned before slaughter it has been observed that breathing often stops. The heart continues to beat for 4 to 10 minutes longer, but it also stops when the oxygen available from the functional residual capacity has been depleted.

Dead Space Ventilation

The tidal volume is used to ventilate not only the alveoli, but also the airways leading to the alveoli. Because there is little or no diffusion of oxygen and carbon dioxide through the membranes of the airways, they comprise part of what is called dead space ventilation. The other part of dead space ventilation is made up of alveoli with diminished capillary perfusion. Ventilating these alveoli is ineffective in producing changes in the blood gases. Ventilation of non-perfused alveoli and the airways, because neither accomplish exchange of the respiratory gases, are referred to as physiologic dead spaces. Therefore, the tidal volume (V_T) has a dead space component (V_D) and an alveolar component (V_A), or $V_T = V_D + V_A$.

Dead space ventilation is a necessary part of the process of ventilating the alveoli and is not totally wasted. It assists in tempering and humidifying inhaled air and in the cooling of the body under certain conditions, such as when panting is necessary. Panting is predominantly dead space ventilation. During panting, the res-

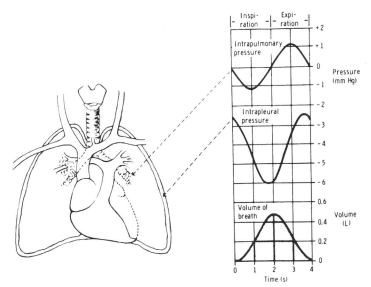

Figure 8.10. Intrapleural and intrapulmonic (intrapulmonary) pressures associated with inspiration and expiration. Reproduced, with permission, from Ganong WF. Rev Med Physiol, 17th ed. East Norwalk, CT: Appleton & Lange, 1995.

piratory frequency increases and the tidal volume decreases, so that alveolar ventilation remains approximately constant.

Pressures That Accomplish Ventilation

INTRAPULMONIC AND INTRAPLEURAL PRESSURES. The pressure within the lungs is referred to as intrapulmonic pressure, and the pressure outside the lungs, but within the thoracic cavity (between the visceral and parietal pleura), is referred to as intrapleural pressure. Air flows into the lungs during inspiration because the pressure within the lung, the intrapulmonic pressure, becomes lower than the atmospheric pressure. Similarly, air flows out of the lungs during expiration because the intrapulmonic pressure exceeds atmospheric pressure at that time. The intrapleural and intrapulmonic pressures associated with inspiration and expiration are shown in Figure 8.10.

GENERATION OF PRESSURE CHANGES. The intrapulmonic pressure decreases during inspiration because the volume of the lungs increases. The lungs can increase in volume because they are elastic structures that can stretch. Also, the pressure around

them, the intrapleural pressure, is being reduced because the volume of the intrapleural space increases in response to contraction of the diaphragm and intercostal muscles (Fig. 8.8). When contraction of the inspiratory muscles ceases, expiration begins.

To permit air to flow out of the lungs during expiration, the intrapulmonic pressure must become positive. Positive pressure is generated primarily by the recoil tendency of the lungs, which were previously stretched during inspiration. The recoil tendency is produced not only by the elastic fibers within the lung, but also by the surface tension of the fluid that lines the alveoli. Retraction of the lungs can also be assisted by expiratory muscles. The diaphragm is an inspiratory muscle, and its contraction assists only inspiration; conversely, its relaxation permits expiration. During eupnea, the intrapulmonic pressure can be about -1 mm Hg (below atmospheric) during inspiration and it can be +1 mm Hg during expiration. During this time, the intrapleural pressure changes from -2 mm Hg at the end of expiration to about -6 mm Hg at the end of inspiration. Thus, the intrapleural pressure changes slightly more than the intrapulmonic pressure changes.

Intrapleural pressure (pressure in a closed space) is normally lower than atmospheric pressure, even at the end of expiration and before inspiration. This is a result of the constant recoil tendency of the lungs and of the absorption of gases from closed spaces caused by the existence of a diffusion gradient between the closed space and venous blood. The total pressure in the intrapleural space is in equilibrium with venous blood. It is lower than atmospheric pressure because the reduction of PO_2 caused by oxygen absorption is greater than the increase in PCO_2. The reduced total pressure of the intrapleural space is comparable to that of a slight vacuum.

PNEUMOTHORAX. If the intrapleural space is opened to the atmosphere (e.g., during certain surgical procedures), it would not be possible for diaphragmatic contraction to generate a greater vacuum in the intrapleural space, and the lungs would not inflate (Fig. 8.11). This condition is known as pneumothorax. A respirator would be necessary to ventilate the lungs or the animal would die. Correction of pneumothorax involves effecting final closure of the unnatural opening simultaneously with full inflation of the lungs. Normal lung retraction could then reestablish the normal negative intrapleural pressure. The next inspiration would generate more negative pressure and the lungs would expand because the trachea would be the only passageway available for air intake.

MEDIASTINAL PRESSURE. During inspiration, when the intrapleural pressure is reduced, the mediastinal space pressure is also reduced. Reduction of the mediastinal space pressure is followed by the expansion of volume and reduction of pressure within the distensible structures of the mediastinal space (venae cavae, thoracic lymph duct, esophagus). This reduction in pressure assists in the return of blood and lymph to the heart. During regurgitation in ruminants (see below), reduced pressure in the esophagus, associated with an exaggerated inspiration with a closed glottis, also assists in this process.

DIFFUSION OF RESPIRATORY GASES

The respiratory gases diffuse readily throughout the body tissues. Because of its greater lipid solubility, carbon dioxide diffuses about 20 times more readily than oxygen through membranes. Also, as the distance of diffusion increases, as in pulmonary interstitial edema, the diffusion rate decreases. Under this condition, one may notice greater ventilation efforts in an attempt to compensate for the hypoxemia (decreased O_2 concentration in arterial blood) that has developed because of the reduced rate of diffusion. Blood-gas analysis shows reduced partial pressures for O_2 and CO_2. Because of the decrease in diffusion rate caused by distance, one might have expected an increase in PCO_2 in view of its reduced elimination. Its diffusion coefficient is much greater than that for O_2, however, so that the increased ventilation overcompensates for diffusion decrease caused by distance. The thicker membrane (and thus greater diffusion distance) does impair O_2 diffusion, however, resulting in reduced arterial PO_2 and hypoxemia.

Table 8.2 presents information to help explain the movement of gases from alveoli to blood to tissues and from tissues to blood to alveoli. Ventilation brings O_2 to the alveoli and removes CO_2. Because O_2 is being consumed in the tissues, a pressure difference exists for its diffusion from alveoli to venous blood (which then becomes arterial) and from arterial blood to the tissues. Because CO_2 is being produced in the tissues, a pressure differ-

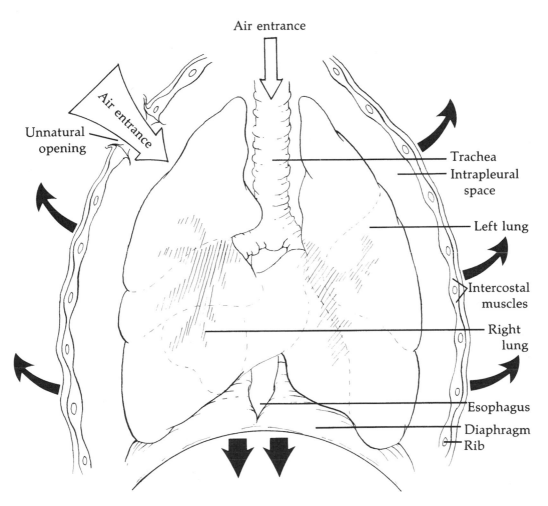

Figure 8.11. Pneumothorax (ventral view). The volume of air that enters at the unnatural opening exceeds that which enters the trachea when the intrapleural volume is increased during inspiration. The intrapleural pressure reduction is then not sufficient to permit lung inflation. The dark arrows show the directions of thoracic enlargement when the diaphragm and inspiratory intercostal muscles contract during inspiration.

TABLE 8.2. Total and Partial Pressures (in mm Hg) of Respirtory Gases in Humans at Rest (sea level)

Gases	Venous blood	Alveolar air	Arterial blood	Tissues
Oxygen	40	104	100	30 or less
Carbon dioxide	45	40	40	50 or more
Nitrogen	569	569	569	569
Water vapor	47	47	47	47
Total	701	760	756	696

From Comroe J. Physiology of respiration, 2nd ed. Chicago, 1974 Year Book.

ence exists for its diffusion from tissue to arterial blood (which then becomes venous) and from venous blood to the alveoli. Table 8.2 indicates that no change occurs in PH_2O and PN_2. The aqueous environment of the body ensures a constant PH_2O and, because N_2 is neither produced nor consumed, its pressure also remains constant. Nitrogen acts only as a filler. The total pressure in venous blood is somewhat less than atmospheric pressure (760 mm Hg) because the volume of CO_2 produced is lower than the volume of O_2 consumed; in other words, the added PCO_2 is less than the subtracted PO_2. This is also true for O_2 and CO_2 in the tissues, but it is only true to a slight degree in arterial blood because not all the blood going to the lungs is arterialized (nonperfused alveoli). The intraperitoneal pressure (pressure in the abdomen, a closed space) is similarly affected. The inrush of air into the abdomen can be heard faintly when an incision is first made.

The direction of diffusion in response to differences in partial pressures is shown for oxygen and carbon dioxide in Figure 8.12.

Oxygen Transport

Under normal circumstances, there are about 20 ml of molecular oxygen in each deciliter of arterial blood (20 ml/dl, or 20 vol-%). Normal activity consumes about 25% of that amount as the blood is circulated to the tissues. The remainder is available as reserve for times of greater activity. The 25% value is referred to as the utiliza-

tion coefficient; with strenuous activity, the utilization coefficient is increased.

Transport Scheme

The transport scheme for oxygen is illustrated in Figure 8.13. The procession of oxygen during its uptake by hemoglobin is from air in the alveolus to successive solution in interstitial fluid (1), in plasma (2), and in erythrocyte fluid (3), and finally to combination with hemoglobin (4). For oxygen yield to the cells, the procession of oxygen is from interstitial fluid (1), followed by that which is from plasma (2), and from erythrocyte fluid (3), which in turn is replenished by the oxygen that is combined with hemoglobin (4). Diffusion of oxygen away from hemoglobin lowers the PO_2 of the erythrocyte fluid and, just as an increased PO_2 increases the saturation of hemoglobin with oxygen, decreased PO_2 causes desaturation of hemoglobin.

Oxygen in Solution and the Oxygen-Hemoglobin Dissociation Curve

Oxygen dissolves in blood only slightly. If blood contained O_2 only in solution, there would need to be about 60 times more blood to transport the 20 vol-% present. Transport is accomplished with the available volume of blood because of the O_2 transport potential of the hemoglobin contained in erythrocytes. Oxygen in solution only needs to diffuse into and out of the erythrocytes to be associated with or dissociated from hemoglobin.

The relationship between the PO_2 of

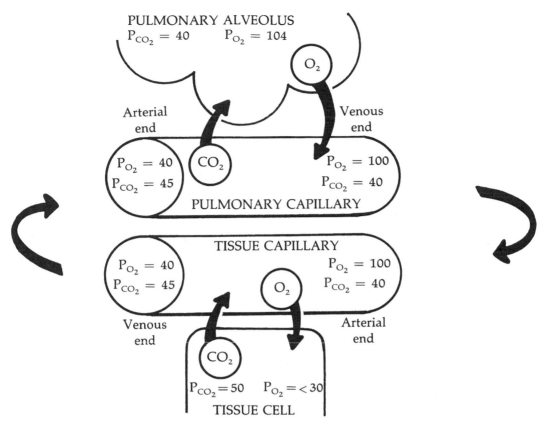

Figure 8.12. Direction of diffusion for oxygen (O_2), and carbon dioxide (CO_2), as shown by arrows. In the pulmonary alveolus the P_{CO_2} is 40 mm Hg and the P_{O_2} is 104 mm Hg; at the arterial end of the pulmonary capillary the P_{O_2} is 40 mm Hg and the P_{CO_2} is 45 mm Hg, whereas at the venous end the P_{O_2} is 100 mm Hg and the P_{CO_2} is 40 mm Hg; at the venous end of the tissue capillary the P_{O_2} is 40 mm Hg and the P_{CO_2} is 45 mm Hg, whereas at the arterial end the P_{O_2} is 100 mm Hg and the P_{CO_2} is 40 mm Hg; and in the tissue cell the P_{CO_2} is 50 mm Hg and the P_{O_2} is <30 mm Hg.

blood and the percentage saturation of hemoglobin with oxygen is shown in Figure 8.14<fig8.14>. Note that hemoglobin is nearly 100% saturated when the P_{O_2} of the blood is 100 mm Hg. This is the normal P_{O_2} of arterial blood. Also, at the P_{O_2} of mixed venous blood (about 40 mm Hg), hemoglobin is still about 75% saturated with oxygen. The 25% that has been lost (dissociated from hemoglobin) corresponds to the utilization coefficient. Regardless of the hemoglobin concentration (15 g/dl or 7.5 g/dl), the percentage saturation of hemoglobin is identical for the same P_{O_2} exposure. The uptake of O_2 by hemoglobin is in equilibrium with the partial pressure of O_2. Figure 8.14 illustrates the effect of a lowered hemoglobin concentration (15 g/dl, normal; 7.5 g/dl, 50% normal) on the volume of O_2 transported. A P_{O_2} analysis does not reveal the amount of oxygen present in blood. There would be twice the amount of oxygen in blood having 15 g/dl hemoglobin than there would be for blood having 7.5 g/dl at any particular P_{O_2}. Figure 8.14 also shows that the rate of oxygen dissociation from hemoglobin increases sharply as the P_{O_2} decrease approaches the middle and lower ends of the P_{O_2} scale. This characteristic of hemoglobin facilitates the provision of oxygen at the capillary level by supplying greater amounts with less lowering of P_{O_2}, thus maintaining an adequate pressure difference for diffusion to the cells.

Carbon Dioxide Transport

The transport of carbon dioxide is facilitated by several reactions that effectively provide other CO_2 forms in addition to that which is in solution. Even though CO_2 is more soluble in water than O_2, the amount produced exceeds the amount that can be carried in solution. The general scheme for CO_2 transport is shown in Figure 8.15.

Hydration Reaction

About 80% of carbon dioxide transport occurs in the form of bicarbonate (HCO_3^-). Its formation results from the hydration reaction (Equation 8.1):

$$CO_2 + H_2O \leftrightarrow H_2CO_3 \leftrightarrow H^+ + HCO_3^-$$

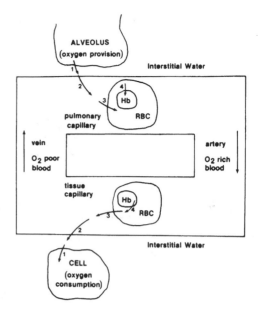

Figure 8.13. General scheme of oxygen transport showing oxygen procession. Procession occurs because of the presence of pressure gradients. In this diagram, blood is oxygenated at the top and deoxygenated at the bottom; blood flow is clockwise. See text for further explanation. From Reece WO. Respiration in mammals. In: Swenson MJ, Reece WO, eds. Dukes' physiology of domestic animals. 11th ed. Ithaca, NY: Cornell University Press, 1993.

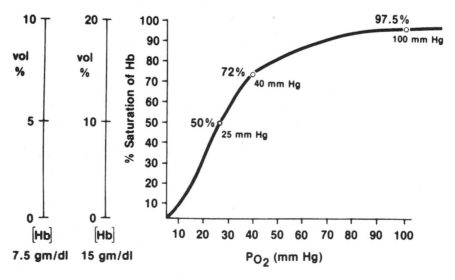

Figure 8.14. The oxygen-hemoglobin dissociation curve. See text for explanation. From Reece WO. Respiration in mammals. In: Swenson MJ, Reece WO, eds. Dukes' physiology of domestic animals. 11th ed. Ithaca, NY: Cornell University Press, 1993.

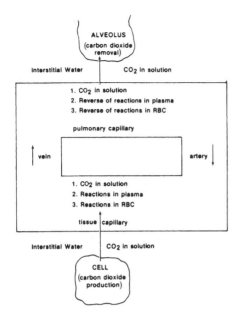

Figure 8.15. General scheme of carbon dioxide transport showing carbon dioxide procession. Procession occurs because of the presence of pressure gradients. In this diagram flow is clockwise; carbon dioxide is taken up from cells at the bottom and removed from blood at the top. Items are numbered in the order of their occurrence. From Reece WO. Respiration in mammals. In: Swenson MJ, Reece WO. Dukes' physiology of domestic animals. 11th ed. Ithaca, NY: Cornell University Press, 1993.

The equilibrium of the hydration reaction is far to the left in plasma, and the plasma reaction accounts for little transport of CO_2. The reaction is favored within the erythrocytes because of the presence of the enzyme carbonic anhydrase, and it proceeds with ease, forming H^+ and HCO_3^-. It would be a rate-limited reaction, however, if the reaction products were not removed. Removal is accomplished by chemical buffering of the H^+ and by diffusion of HCO_3^- out of the erythrocytes into the plasma. Not all the hydrogen ions are buffered, so venous blood has a lower pH than arterial blood. Also, because of the diffusion of HCO_3^- from erythrocytes to plasma, venous blood has a higher HCO_3^- concentration than arterial blood.

The most plentiful compound available for buffering H^+ formed during the hydration reaction is hemoglobin. When hemoglobin is deficient, as in anemia, buffering of H^+ from all sources is jeopardized, and acidemia results during periods of increased H^+ production, such as exertion.

The erythrocyte processes involved in carbon dioxide transport are shown in Figure 8.16.

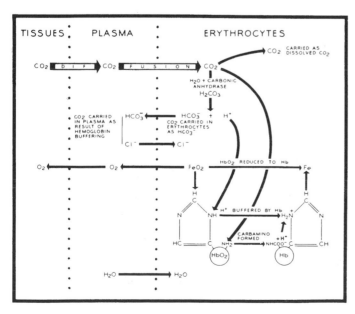

Figure 8.16. Schematic representation of the processes that occur when carbon dioxide diffuses from tissues into erythrocytes. From Davenport HW. The ABC of acid-base chemistry. 6th ed. Chicago: University of Chicago Press, 1974.

Formation of Carbamino Compounds

Another reaction accounting for CO_2 transport involves the combination of CO_2 with terminal amino groups on the proteins of plasma and hemoglobin to form carbamino compounds (Equation 8.2).

$$R\text{-}NH_2 + CO_2 \leftrightarrow R\text{-}N\begin{array}{c}H\\ \diagup\\ \diagdown\\ COOH\end{array} \leftrightarrow R\begin{array}{c}H\\ \diagup\\ \diagdown\\ COO^- + H^+\end{array}$$

The amount produced with hemoglobin exceeds that produced with plasma proteins because there are fewer terminal amino groups on plasma proteins.

Loss of Carbon Dioxide at the Alveolus

When the venous blood reaches the alveoli and the CO_2 pressure difference favors diffusion of CO_2 in solution from the plasma to the alveoli, there is a prompt reversal of the hydration reaction and of the reaction that forms carbamino compounds (return of CO_2 to solution). The effect is loss of the CO_2 that was transported from the tissues.

Regulation of Ventilation

Pulmonary ventilation is regulated closely to maintain the concentrations of H^+, CO_2, and O_2 at relatively constant levels while meeting the needs of the body under varying conditions. If either the H^+ or CO_2 concentration increases or if the O_2 concentration decreases, their levels will be returned to normal by increasing ventilation. Conversely, if either the H^+ or CO_2 concentration decreases or if the O_2 concentration increases, pulmonary ventilation will be decreased. This regulatory mechanism is controlled by changes in tidal volume, frequency of respiratory cycles, or both. The central mediator of these changes is the respiratory center in the brain stem, which has four specific regions (Fig. 8.17):

1. Pneumotaxic center: believed to modulate respiratory center sensitivity to inputs that activate termination of inspiration and facilitate expiration
2. Apneustic center: believed to be associated with deep inspirations, such as the sigh
3. Dorsal respiratory group: group of neurons predominately associated with inspiratory activity (particularly

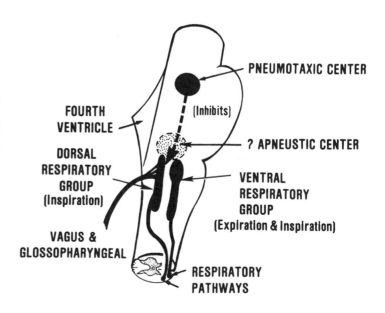

Figure 8.17. Components of the respiratory center. The pneumotaxic and apneustic centers are located in the pons, and the dorsal and ventral respiratory groups are located in the medulla. From Guyton AC. Textbook of medical physiology. 8th ed. Philadelphia: WB Saunders, 1991.

involved in lung inflation-induced termination of inspiration)

4. Ventral respiratory group: group of neurons containing inspiratory and expiratory neurons (assist in inspiration begun by those in the dorsal respiratory group and also provide for assisted expiration)

A central pattern generator has been hypothesized; it is believed to be the neural network that provides for rhythmicity. This central pattern generator is also thought to be in the brain stem. It is influenced by inputs from the vagus and glossopharyngeal nerves and by chemoreceptors.

Neural Control

Impulses going to the respiratory center (afferent impulses) from several receptor sources have been identified. The Hering-Breuer reflexes are probably the most noteworthy. The receptors for these reflexes are located in the lungs, particularly in the bronchi and bronchioles. The nerve impulses generated by the receptors of the Hering-Breuer reflexes are transmitted by fibers in the vagus nerves to the respiratory center. The effect of inflation-receptor stimulation is to inhibit further inspiration (stimulation of neurons in the dorsal respiratory group) and to stimulate expiratory neurons in the ventral respiratory group. Tidal volume can be increased, however, by pneumotaxic center modulation. Another component of the Hering-Breuer reflexes is activated at some particular point of deflation. The deflation receptors might not be activated to bring about the next inspiration during eupnea, but they might be active when deflation is more complete.

In addition to lung receptors, there are other peripherally located receptors that modify the basic rhythm. Stimulation of receptors in the skin are excitatory to the respiratory center, and deeper than usual inspiration can be noted. Their excitation to the inspiratory area might be through the apneustic area because inspiratory gasps are occasionally noted. Advantage is taken of these receptors when breathing stimulation is desired in newborn animals. Rubbing the skin with a rough cloth often initiates the breathing cycles. It is also believed that, when impulses descend from the cerebral cortex to the skeletal muscles, a branch might also go to the respiratory center to increase ventilation. This mechanism could explain changes that occur during exercise, in which increases in ventilation occur that are not explainable merely by observing changes in the CO_2, O_2, and H^+ concentrations in the blood.

Several respiratory reflexes originate from receptors in the upper air passages. Stimulation of the mucous membranes in these regions causes reflex inhibition of breathing. A striking example of this reflex is the inhibition of breathing that occurs during swallowing; also, in diving birds and mammals, there is a reflex inhibition of breathing when they submerge. Stimulation of the laryngeal mucous membrane in the unanesthetized animal causes not only inhibition of breathing, but also usually powerful expiratory efforts (coughing). Similarly, sneezing can be observed after stimulation of the nasal mucous membrane by various mechanisms. The function of all these latter reflexes is protection of the delicate respiratory passages and the alveoli of the lungs from harmful substances (e.g., irritating gases, dust, smoke, food particles) that might otherwise be inspired. To ensure protection, the glottis is closed and the bronchi can be constricted.

Ordinary respirations proceed involuntarily. It is generally true, however, that they can be altered voluntarily within wide limits—they can be hastened, slowed, or stopped altogether, for a while. Phonation and use of the abdominal press in the expulsive acts of defecation, urination, and parturition are all examples of (more or less) complete voluntary control of the respiratory movements. These acts, however, are not concerned with gas exchange between the organism and its environment but represent secondary functions of the respiratory apparatus.

Afferent impulses from pressure receptors in the carotid and aortic sinuses have as their principal function a role in the regulation of circulation, but impulses from these receptors also go to the respiratory center. The impulses are inhibitory in nature—the higher the blood pressure, the greater the inhibition to respiration. Because of the influence of inspiration on return of blood to the heart, the reduction in inspirations would slow down the return flow of blood to the heart and thus help to lower blood pressure.

Humoral Control

Humoral control refers to those factors in the body fluids that influence ventilation: carbon dioxide, hydrogen ion, and oxygen. Because these are constituents of the body fluids, it seems natural that they should exert the greatest influence on ventilation in maintaining constancy. Their concentrations in the blood affect alveolar ventilation in several ways:

1. Carbon dioxide increase causes alveolar ventilation to increase; its decrease causes alveolar ventilation to decrease.
2. Hydrogen ion increase causes alveolar ventilation to increase; its decrease causes alveolar ventilation to decrease.
3. Oxygen decrease causes alveolar ventilation to increase; its increase causes alveolar ventilation to decrease.

The effects of carbon dioxide and hydrogen ions are mediated through bilateral chemosensitive areas beneath the ventral surface of the medulla (Fig. 8.18). Because of the much greater diffusibility of carbon dioxide, as compared to H^+, its concentration in the blood is distributed more quickly to the interstitial fluid of the medulla and to the cerebrospinal fluid than

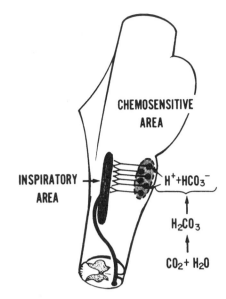

Figure 8.18. The chemosensitive area of the brainstem respiratory center. The chemosensitive area is stimulated by hydrogen ions, which are formed by the conversion of carbon dioxide through the hydration reaction. From Guyton AC. Textbook of medical physiology. 8th ed. Philadelphia: WB Saunders, 1991.

hydrogen ions. It is believed, however, that the H^+ concentration of the interstitial fluid of the brain stem is the deciding stimulus for respiratory drive. The influence of CO_2 is exerted by its conversion to H^+ through the hydration reaction (Equation 8.1; see previous section).

The influence of oxygen is transmitted from the carotid and aortic bodies to the respiratory center. Its receptors also respond to carbon dioxide and hydrogen ion concentration, but the effectiveness of this response is far less than the response from the brain stem. Thus, the carotid and aortic bodies are considered to be the most influential for the regulation of oxygen. These bodies are distinct structures with an abundant blood supply located just outside the aortic arch, at the division of the carotid arteries. They respond to changes in the PO_2 of blood. Blood with reduced amounts of hemoglobin, and consequently less oxy-

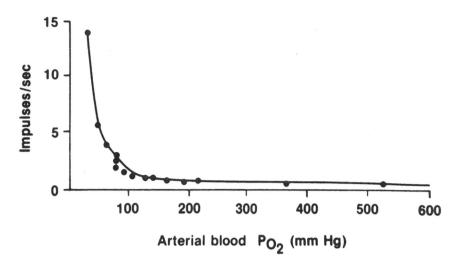

Figure 8.19. Effect of arterial oxygen partial pressure on the number of impulses per second from the carotid body to the respiratory center. The impulses are excitatory. From Reece WO. Respiration in mammals. In: Swenson MJ, Reece WO, eds. Dukes' physiology of domestic animals. 11th ed. Ithaca, NY: Cornell University Press, 1993.

gen, has the same PO_2 as blood with normal hemoglobin and oxygen, and thus no ventilation response would be elicited because there is no change in PO_2. Also, blood in which oxygen has been displaced from hemoglobin by carbon monoxide has the same PO_2 as normal blood, and there would be no increase in ventilation. The PO_2 would remain the same because it is an expression of alveolar PO_2 (which has not changed) and represents the PO_2 of oxygen in solution. In the case of decreased hemoglobin (e.g., as in anemia), ventilation might be increased, not because of less oxygen, but because of greater hydrogen ion concentration caused by reduced buffering associated with the hemoglobin decrease. In the case of carbon monoxide poisoning and lack of oxygen carried by hemoglobin, ventilation is not increased, not only because the PO_2 is normal, but also because there is adequate hemoglobin present for buffering hydrogen ion.

Arterial blood PO_2 must be in the range of 30 to 60 mm Hg for the respiratory center to receive stimulation to ventilation from the carotid and aortic bodies (Fig.

8.19). This appears to be an appropriate range because hemoglobin is still about 90% saturated with oxygen at a PO_2 of 60 mm Hg. Also, the slowing effect of an increased arterial PO_2 is subtle and would not normally be observed in animals breathing atmospheric air because the arterial PO_2 seldom rises above 100 mm Hg. The slowing effect is noted, however, in anesthetized animals breathing an oxygen-enriched atmosphere, in which the arterial PO_2 could increase to 350 to 400 mm Hg (Fig. 8.20).

The regulation of ventilation by oxygen is not ordinarily thought to be important. There is usually no problem in maintaining arterial blood PO_2 in the range of 80 to 100 mm Hg, and it is not advantageous to have it higher than 100 mm Hg, because hemoglobin is almost saturated at that partial pressure. Ventilation could even be reduced to about 50% of normal and hemoglobin still would be considerably saturated. Accordingly, the most important chemical factor in the regulation of ventilation is the concentration of carbon dioxide; relatively small changes can have an effect.

Figure 8.20. Pneumogram showing effect of oxygen enrichment on respiratory frequency. An oxygen atmosphere was provided to a pentobarbital-anesthetized dog. Note the decreased respiratory frequency after administration of oxygen (drawn from actual recording). From Reece WO. Respiration in mammals. In: Swenson MJ, Reece WO, eds. Dukes' physiology of domestic animals. 11th ed. Ithaca, NY: Cornell University Press, 1993.

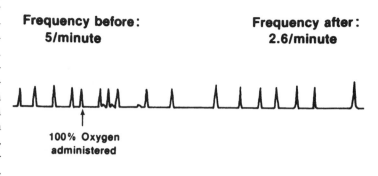

The regulation of ventilation by oxygen becomes more important in such conditions as pneumonia and pulmonary edema, in which gases are not diffused as readily through the respiratory membrane. Decreased diffusion is more noticeable for oxygen than for carbon dioxide (see previous section) because of the smaller diffusion coefficient for oxygen. Hyperventilation caused by oxygen lack can therefore reduce the carbon dioxide concentration (because CO_2 readily diffuses) and thus the consequent formation of hydrogen ions is reduced (see Equation 8.1) so that they become ineffective in stimulating increased ventilation. The oxygen deficiency mechanism (originating from the carotid and aortic bodies) continues to function and provides the drive to increase ventilation.

The effect of decreased concentrations of H^+ and CO_2 and increased concentration of O_2 to slow down ventilation is referred to as a braking effect. The braking effect of O_2 was shown to be unimportant, but it is important for CO_2 and H^+ to decrease ventilation because they are both involved in maintaining the acid-base equilibrium of the body fluids. The uncontrolled lowering of either CO_2 or H^+ would result in some degree of alkalemia. A braking effect can be observed when anesthetized animals being hyperventilated with a respirator are removed suddenly from the respirator. A minute or more might be required for CO_2 and H^+ to accumulate to a level at which they no longer exert their braking effect, and breathing finally resumes. In this example, oxygen lack is apparent, and it could also be a contributory factor in the resumption of breathing.

The factors that influence ventilation are summarized in Figure 8.21.

RESPIRATORY CLEARANCE

The surface area of the inner aspects of the lungs is about 125 times larger than the surface area of the body, and therefore the lungs represent an important route of exposure for many environmental substances. The inhalation of certain agricultural chemicals is a significant health hazard for which precautionary measures to prevent inhalation have been developed. The removal of particles that have been inhaled into the lungs is called respiratory clearance. There are two types, upper respiratory clearance and alveolar clearance, and each depends on the depth to which particles have been inhaled. Inhaled particles that settle out onto a membrane of the respiratory tract are said to have been deposited.

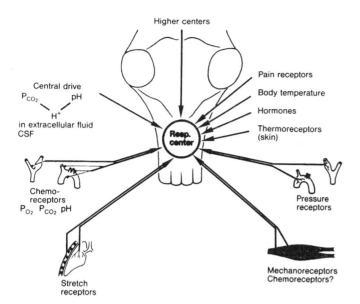

Figure 8.21. Summary of factors that influence pulmonary ventilation. From Schmidt PS, Thews G, eds. Human physiology. Berlin: Springer-Verlag, 1989.

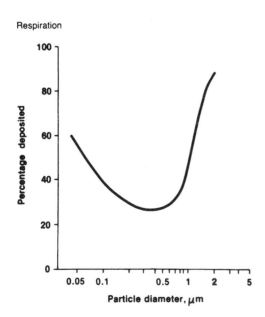

Figure 8.22. Percentage of inhaled particles of unit density deposited in the lung according to their size. Particles in the range of 0.1 to 1.0 μm are those least affected by combined brownian motion, sedimentation, and inertial impaction. Redrawn, with permission, from Morrow PE. Some physical and physiological factors controlling the fate of inhaled substances—I. Health Physics 1960;2:372. Copyright Pergamon Press, Ltd.

Physical Forces of Deposition

The physical forces that affect deposition are gravity, inertia, and brownian movement. Gravitational settling (sedimentation) causes deposition of particles simply because of the force of gravity and the mass of the particle. Particles of greater mass settle out more rapidly than those with lesser mass. Inertia accounts for the deposition of particles when, because of their mass, they continue forward as the air in which they are suspended makes a turn. Considering the branching of the bronchioles, there is considerable opportunity for inertial deposition. Brownian motion accounts for the deposition of submicronic particles (less than 0.3 μm), which show a random motion that is imparted by air molecule bombardment. Deposition by brownian motion is most significant in extremely small airways where the surface area is large relative to the airway diameter. The percentage of particles deposited according to their size is shown in Figure 8.22.

Upper Respiratory Tract Clearance

Removal of particles deposited cranial to the alveolar ducts is accomplished by the

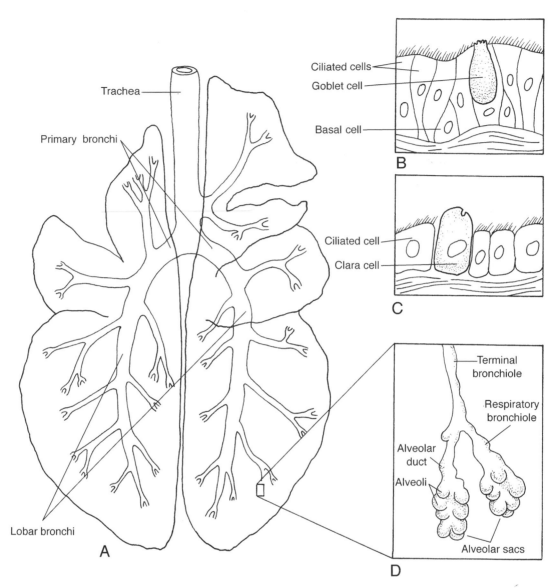

Figure 8.23. Contributors to the moving mucous blanket of the bronchial tree. The moving mucous blanket is directed toward the pharynx by the action of the ciliated cells, and the secretion is provided by the goblet cells of the bronchi, the Clara cells of the bronchioles, and alveolar fluid. **A.** Outline of the bovine lung superimposed over the bronchial tree. **B.** Pseudostratified epithelium of the bronchi, composed of secretory (goblet) cells, ciliated cells, and basal cells. **C.** Cuboidal epithelium of the terminal bronchioles, composed of ciliated cells and secretory (Clara) cells. **D.** The terminal bronchiole is the most distal air passage free of alveoli.

moving mucous blanket. This blanket of mucinous fluid is located on the surface of the epithelial cells lining the airways and is derived from alveolar fluid and mucus-secreting cells along the airways (Fig. 8.23). The mucous blanket contains the deposited particles and is propelled toward the pharynx at a rate of about 15 mm/min by cilia of the epithelial cells. Mammals swallow the mucinous fluid and particles after they reach the pharynx.

Alveolar Clearance

Particles can escape gravitational and inertial forces and be deposited in the alveoli. These particles are usually smaller than 1 μm in diameter. The mechanisms of alveolar clearance of these particles can be summarized as follows:

1. After their deposition in the alveoli, they can be phagocytized by a macrophage or can continue as free particles. The "dust"-laden macrophage or free particles might be directed to the moving mucous blanket along with the alveolar fluid film.
2. Particles might enter the interstitial space of the alveoli and be transported to lymph nodes in series with the lungs.
3. Particles might be dissolved and transferred in solution, either into the lymph or into the blood.
4. Some particles might fail to be phagocytized or might be insoluble. Instead, they could stimulate a local connective tissue reaction and be sequestered (isolated) within the lung. Examples of this include the conditions known as asbestosis and silicosis. Dogs and cats living in highly industrialized areas have shown signs of anthracosis caused by inhalation of coal dust.

The importance of respiratory clearance is apparent when considering the exposure of livestock to the aerosols emanating from feedlot dust or other confinement sources. The aerosols can be combined with bacteria and viruses, so their prompt removal can help prevent diseases caused by them. Similarly, the removal of irritant substances prevents lung disease and protects lung efficiency.

FURTHER CONSIDERATIONS

Nonrespiratory Functions of the Respiratory System

Panting

Panting is prevalent among many animal species and has been best described in the dog. It is probably similar for the other animals in which it is observed.

The respiratory center of the dog responds not only to the usual stimuli, but also to body core temperature. When these inputs are integrated, the dog's body responds to metabolic needs by regulating alveolar ventilation and to dissipation of heat by regulating dead space ventilation. Dead space ventilation is increased by panting, which provides for body cooling by evaporation of water from the mucous membranes of the tissues involved.

Studies have shown that the three patterns of panting are 1) inhalation and exhalation through the nose, 2) inhalation through the nose and exhalation through the nose and mouth, and 3) inhalation through the nose and mouth and exhalation through the nose and mouth. The least amount of cooling is accomplished by inhaling and exhaling through the nose (pattern 1) because the heat and water added to the air during inhalation are partially regained during exhalation. Pattern 2 is more effective because air entering the nose is exposed to a large surface area (nasal conchae) as compared to the mouth, and water is added by the nasal mucosa and nasal glands. This combination picks up a considerable amount of heat, which is then dissipated mainly by exhalation through the mouth. Pattern 3 is somewhat similar to pattern 2, except that inhalation through the mouth and the nose permits a greater tidal volume, which might be required during times of exertion. The advantage of changing the relative amount of air exhaled either through the nose or mouth is that the dog can modulate the amount of heat dissipated without changing the frequency or tidal volume associated with panting. Energy is conserved by not changing the frequency (300 pants/minute), and hyperventilation (and thus alkalemia) is prevented by keeping the tidal volume constant.

Purring

Purring is noted in some members of the feline family and is both audible and palpable in most domestic cats. Studies in the domestic cat have shown that the purr results from a highly regular, alternating activation of the diaphragm and of the intrinsic laryngeal muscles (those within the larynx) at a frequency of 25 times/second during both inspiration and expiration. Contraction of the laryngeal muscles closes the vocal cords. The laryngeal muscles then relax while the diaphragm contracts. Contraction of the diaphragm accomplishes air inflow, which vibrates the vocal cords and results in the purring sound while they are opening (no longer closed by laryngeal contraction), and also contributes to a fraction of the inspiratory phase of the respiratory cycle. The diaphragm then relaxes and the laryngeal muscles contract; this is again followed by their relaxation and diaphragm contraction. The entire process is repeated 25 times/second until inspiration is completed. The accumulation of small sounds produced with each opening of the vocal cords makes the purring sound. The same sequence occurs during expiration, except that the diaphragm does not contract, and air outflow and hence vibration of the vocal cords is accomplished by recoil of the lungs.

The reason for purring in cats is not known. Cats purr when they are contented, sick, and asleep. Purring might provide for more effective ventilation during periods of shallow breathing because of the intermittent inspiration and expiration that is provided.

Descriptive Terms

Many terms associated with respiration have been defined in this chapter. The following terms are also commonly used.

Anoxia literally means without oxygen, and it should not be used to describe conditions of decreased oxygen. In such a case, hypoxia is more appropriate.

Hypercapnia and hypocapnia refer to excess and reduced amounts of carbon dioxide, respectively, in the blood.

Cyanosis refers to a bluish or purplish coloration of the skin and mucous membranes. The intensity of the color is a result of the degree of deoxygenation of hemoglobin. As observed systemically, it relates to inadequate oxygenation of blood. When seen locally, it is probably caused by blood flow obstruction.

Asphyxia is a condition of hypoxia combined with hypercapnia. Hypoxia and hypercapnia can occur as separate entities, but only their combination results in asphyxia. Breathing into a closed space is an example, resulting in what is commonly called suffocation.

Three pathologic conditions often referred to when discussing respiratory physiology are emphysema, pneumonia, and atelectasis. Emphysema is a condition in which destruction of alveolar membranes has occurred, resulting in a smaller area available for gas diffusion. It is often coupled with other conditions, such as chronic bronchitis, that increase the positive pressure within alveoli that is needed for the expiratory phase of the respiratory cycle. Pneumonia is an inflammatory condition of the lungs in which the alveoli fill with fluid and cell debris. Atelectasis is a collapse of alveoli. This can result from airway obstruction and from lack of surfactant. Pulmonary surfactant is a surface tension-reducing substance produced by the alveolar epithelial cells. The alveolar surface is compressed during expiration, which concentrates surfactant at the sur-

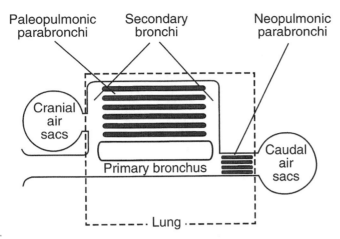

Paleopulmonic parabronchi   Secondary bronchi   Neopulmonic parabronchi

Cranial air sacs

Primary bronchus

Caudal air sacs

Lung

Figure 8.24. A schematic representation of the avian lung and air sacs. The blackened areas correspond to blood capillaries and the white areas adjacent to the blood capillaries correspond to tertiary bronchi (parabronchi). The air sacs are extensions form the lungs, acting as bellows to create air flow. Modified from Fedde, MR: Respiration in birds. In: Swenson MJ, Reece WO, eds. Dukes' physiology of domestic animals. 11th ed. Ithaca, NY: Cornell University Press, 1993.

face. The concentration of surfactant reduces the surface tension and makes beginning inspiration easier. At the end of inspiration the surfactant is spread out because of enlargement of the alveoli, and surface tension increases, which assists expiration.

AVIAN RESPIRATION

General Scheme of Avian Respiratory Morphology

The respiratory apparatus of birds is decidedly different from that of mammals. It was mentioned previously that the organ of phonation, the syrinx, is located at the bifurcation of the trachea, near the lungs, rather than near the pharynx. Also, the tracheal rings are complete rather than incomplete as in mammals. Beyond the trachea, more striking differences are apparent. The lungs continue to be the gas exchange structures, but they do not expand and contract during respiratory cycles. They are relatively small and are fixed in position by their attachment to the ribs. Their ventilation depends on bellows-like extensions from the lungs known as air sacs, which do expand and contract during respiratory cycles, as will be discussed later. The lungs and air sacs are served by airway divisions

from the trachea known as primary, secondary, and tertiary bronchi. The tertiary bronchi are also known as parabronchi. The relationship of the bronchi to each other and to the air sacs is shown in Figure 8.24. There are nine air sacs that are divided among a cranial group (two cervical, two cranial thoracic, and one clavicular) and a caudal group (two caudal thoracic and two abdominal). The air sacs occupy space in the thoracic and abdominal cavities and many have diverticula (extensions) into many of the bones, causing them to be pneumatic. In the domestic species, the most prominent pneumatic bone is the humerus. It is not known what function is served by pneumatic bones.

The parabronchi give rise to outpocketings (atria), extensions from the atria (infundibuli), and finally extensions from the infundibuli known as air capillaries (Fig. 8.25). The structures arising from the parabronchi are known as its mantle. The blood capillaries make intimate contact with the air capillaries and provide for the gas exchange that occurs in the mantle of the lung. In most avian species, there are two sets of parabronchi and they are known as the paleopulmonic parabronchi and the neopulmonic parabronchi. The latter set is caudal to the former and exists just prior to the caudal air sacs (Fig. 8.24).

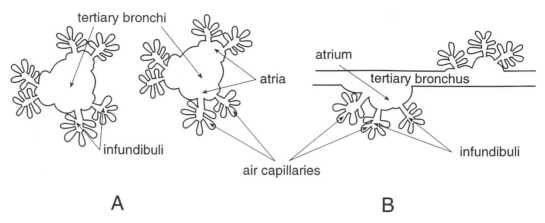

Figure 8.25. Schematic representation of tertiary bronchi and their extensions. **A.** Cross-section. **B.** Longitudinal section. The atria are outpocketings from the tertiary bronchi. The infundibuli extend from the atria and they have a number of extensions known as air capillaries. The air capillaries are in intimate contact with the blood capillaries. The association of air capillaries with blood capillaries is known as the parabronchial mantle.

The air sacs are mucoserous sacs regarded as continuations of secondary bronchi beyond the lungs. Their walls are thin and have a poor blood supply. There is no significant gas exchange taking place in the air sacs. They do change volume during respiratory cycles and thereby function to increase pulmonary ventilation.

Mechanics of Respiration and Air Circulation

Birds have no diaphragm; therefore, no separation exists between the abdominal and thoracic cavities. Accordingly, the entire body volume is changed during each respiratory cycle. The energy for the body volume change is derived from skeletal muscles in the body wall. During expiration, the body wall muscles contract, causing the body volume to decrease. The decrease in body volume increases air sac pressure, forcing the air within to flow back through the lungs and into the environment. Inspiration follows when the body wall muscles relax and body volume increases. Body volume increase is followed by a decrease in its pressure that is

followed by expansion of the air sacs and a decrease in their pressure. The decreased pressure allows air to flow through the lungs and into the air sacs. Air flows through avian lungs during both phases of the respiratory cycle. During inspiration, air moving to cranial air sacs goes through a large set of parabronchi (paleopulmonic) before getting to the sacs. Air moving to the caudal air sacs goes through a smaller set of parabronchi (neopulmonic) before getting to the sacs. During expiration, gas from the caudal air sacs passes again through the neopulmonic parabronchi and then through paleopulmonic parabronchi (directed to cranial air sacs). Gas from the cranial air sacs moves into secondary bronchi and out of lungs through primary bronchi and trachea without passing through gas exchange surfaces (parabronchial mantles). Air flow as described previously is illustrated in Figure 8.26. One bolus of air is followed through two respiratory cycles from its entrance during inspiration of the first cycle to its exit during expiration of the second cycle. Notice that air entering the caudal air sacs during inspiration has already been subjected to

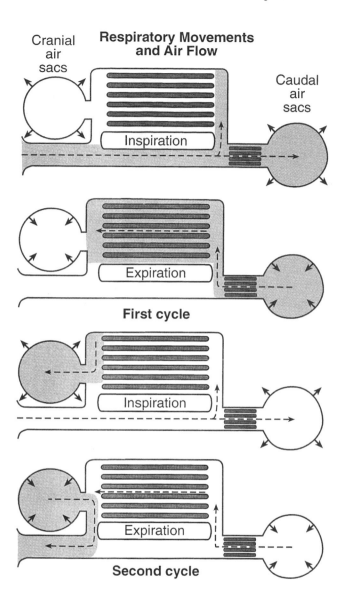

Figure 8.26. Pathway of air flow associated with inspiration and expiration in birds. The same bolus of air (darkened area) is followed through two respiratory cycles. It can be seen that ventilation of the parabronchial mantle is accomplished during inspiration and during expiration. Air going to the caudal air sacs ventilates the neopulmonic mantle and as it leaves it ventilates both neopulmonic and paleopulmonic mantles. When the cranial air sacs expand during inspiration, they are filled by air that has passed through the parabronchial mantles. Cranial air sac air is then directed to the exterior during expiration without ventilating parabronchial mantles. Modified from Scheid P, Slama H, Piiper J. Respir Physiol 1972;14:83–95.

gas exchange and it is again aerating the lungs during expiration. The cranial air sacs receive gas that has passed through the parabronchial mantles during inspiration and expel the gas into the environment during expiration without sending it through the parabronchial mantles.

Gas exchange between blood capillaries and air capillaries is illustrated in Figure 8.27. Air moves through the parabronchi by convection and into the air capillaries by diffusion. Blood perfusing a parabronchial mantle is partitioned so that each increment perfuses separate air capillaries throughout the length of the parabronchus. This arrangement whereby the gas flows through a parabronchus at right angles to the flow of blood is known as cross-current flow. As gas flows through the parabronchus, CO_2 is continuously diffusing from the blood and O_2 is continuously diffusing to the blood. Even though the air

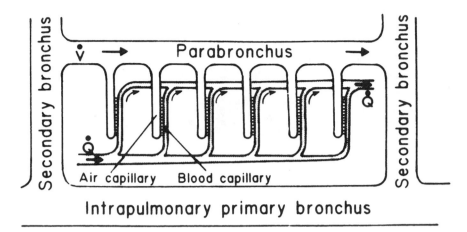

Figure 8.27. Schematic model of the cross-current gas exchange system in the avian lung. $\dot{Q}$ is the blood perfusion of the parabronchial mantle, and $\dot{V}$ represents the convective flow of gas through the parabronchus. Because of this arrangement, blood leaving the parabronchial mantle has a higher PO_2 and a lower PCO_2 than air leaving the parabronchus. From Fedde MR. Respiration in birds. In: Swenson MJ, Reece WO, eds. Dukes' physiology of domestic animals. 11th ed. Ithaca, NY: Cornell University Press, 1993.

capillaries that progress to the parabronchial outflow have an increasing PCO_2 and a decreasing PO_2, the potential for gas diffusion is maintained because each increment of blood perfusing the air capillaries has the same high PCO_2 and low PO_2. Because of this arrangement, the continuous loss of CO_2 and gain of O_2 causes the PCO_2 of arterial blood leaving the lung to be lower and the PO_2 to be higher than the gas leaving the parabronchus. The cross-current arrangement is more efficient than gas exchanges in the mammalian lung and is most apparent when ventilation is increased in response to low oxygen (i.e., high altitude). Under these conditions, arterial PO_2 may be only a few mm Hg less than air entering the parabronchi.

General Considerations

1. Valves to direct air flow have not been found in birds, and it is believed that airflow dynamics are in response to smooth muscle contraction that constricts bronchi.

2. Birds have a respiratory center and, similar to mammals, have chemoreceptors for CO_2 and O_2 that influence the response of the respiratory center.

3. Unlike mammals, birds have CO_2 receptors in their lungs which detect the CO_2 levels in lung air. There is maximum receptor activity when CO_2 is low and this causes inhibition to respiration.

4. Oxygen saturation of hemoglobin of arterial blood (approximately 90%) and of venous blood (approximately 40%) in the chicken is lower than in mammalian blood (arterial blood approximately 97.5% and venous blood approximately 72%).

5. The PCO_2 of avian blood is lower than for mammals (28–34 mm Hg vs 40–45 mm Hg, respectively).

6. Utilization coefficient for most birds is about ½ versus about ¼ for mammals.

7. Diving ducks (not dabbling) have respiratory centers sensitive to pos-

tural changes (stretching of the neck, experimentally or naturally, as in diving, produces apnea).

8. Ventilation of the lungs can be impaired by restricting movement of the sternum because the sternum must have downward and forward movement to assist body volume increase. This is an important consideration during bird restraint.

9. Air sac infections can seriously impair ventilation, particularly if exudate plugs entry from air sacs to lungs (common in aspergillosis).

10. Hyperventilation caused by heat stress reduces the PCO_2 and bicarbonate concentration. The loss of bicarbonate causes egg shells to be thinner, and greater breakage occurs.

STUDY AIDS—RESPIRATION

Structure and Function of the Respiratory System

1. How are the nostrils of the horse adapted to the need for greater air intake?
2. What functions are served by the conchae?
3. Where is the olfactory epithelium located?
4. List the openings to the pharynx.
5. What is the function of the pharynx and syrinx?
6. What is the function of tracheal rings? Why are they incomplete dorsally?
7. What are the subdivisions of the trachea (in order from largest to smallest)?
8. Where does most of the diffusion of gas between air and blood occur?
9. Describe the pleura and mediastinal space.
10. What structures lie within the mediastinal space?

11. What happens to mediastinal pressure when intrapleural pressure decreases?

Factors Affecting Respiration and Ventilation

1. What are the mechanical activities associated with inspiration? What are some conditions for active expiration?
2. Differentiate between abdominal and costal breathing. When is either accentuated?
3. What are some commonly referred to states of breathing?
4. Know the subdivisions of lung volume. What is the difference between a lung volume subdivision and a lung capacity subdivision?
5. When expansion of the lungs is restricted, how is adequate ventilation maintained?
6. Define partial pressure.
7. What are the gases of the atmosphere and what is the approximate percentage composition of each? How would you determine the PO_2 of dry atmospheric air?
8. Why does the composition of atmospheric air differ from that of alveolar air?
9. What comprises dead space ventilation? Is physiologic dead space volume less than anatomic dead space volume? Less than tidal volume? What functions are served by dead space ventilation?
10. How do intrapulmonic and intrapleural pressures change during a respiratory cycle? Study Figure 7.32 (laboratory model of the thorax).
11. How could a condition of pneumothorax be corrected?

Diffusion of Respiratory Gases

1. Which one of the respiratory gases, O_2 or CO_2, diffuses more readily through cell membranes?

2. Read the text to understand Table 8.2 and Figure 8.12.
3. What volume of oxygen is normally transported in 100 ml of arterial blood?
4. Why does O_2 diffuse from alveoli to hemoglobin? Why does O_2 diffuse from hemoglobin to tissue cells (see Fig. 8.13)?
5. What is the relationship of CO_2 transport to the hydration reaction?
6. Why is venous blood more acidic than arterial blood?
7. What is the most plentiful compound available for buffering H^+ formed during the hydration reaction?
8. What is a carbamino compound?
9. Where is the respiratory center for the regulation of ventilation located?
10. What are the Hering-Breuer reflexes? Give three additional examples of neural mechanisms that modify the basic rhythm of respiration.
11. What are the three factors of the body fluids that influence ventilation?
12. Where are the receptors located for the detection of O_2 lack?
13. Why is there no increase in ventilation when there is O_2 lack caused by carbon monoxide poisoning?
14. How are the upper airways and alveoli kept clean from deposited particles?
15. What function is served by panting?
16. How do cats purr?
17. Define hypoxia, hypercapnia, cyanosis, and asphyxia.
18. What is pulmonary surfactant?

Avian Respiration

1. What respiratory structures account for ventilation of the avian lungs that are fixed in position?
2. Describe the relationship of the bronchi to the lungs and air sacs.
3. Where are the air sacs located? What are the two major groups?
4. Could smoke enter a broken wing-bone (humerus) and exit the trachea?

5. What are the parabronchi? Name their extensions which comprise the parabronchial mantle.
6. Where does gas exchange occur in the avian lung?
7. Is there significant gas exchange in air sacs?
8. Where would blood perfusion be more abundant, in the air sacs or air capillaries?
9. Is diaphragm contraction a factor in avian inspiration?
10. Describe how body volume changes influence inspiration and expiration.
11. Has air that enters the caudal and cranial air sacs been through a parabronchial mantle?
12. Does air that leaves the caudal air sacs go through parabronchial mantles?
13. Does air that leaves the cranial air sacs go through parabronchial mantles?
14. Study Figure 8.27 and understand how blood leaving the lung can have a lower P_{CO_2} and a higher O_2 than gas that leaves the parabronchi. Can blood leaving the mammalian lung have a lower P_{CO_2} and a higher P_{O_2} than alveolar gas?
15. Compare the hemoglobin saturation of arterial and venous blood between birds and mammals.
16. How can blowing-off excess CO_2 during heat stress lower bicarbonate concentration (think hydration reaction)?
17. What is meant by a statement that notes the utilization coefficient for most birds is about ½ versus ¼ for mammals?

SELF-EVALUATION—RESPIRATION

1. The P_{O_2} of dry atmospheric air approximates:
   a. 40 mm Hg
   b. 100 mm Hg
   ➥c. 160 mm Hg
   d. 760 mm Hg

2. Which respiratory structures serve to warm and humidify inhaled air and also to cool blood going to the brain?
   a. larynx
   b. nares
   c. conchae
   d. syrinx

3. Diffusion of gases between air and blood occurs mostly in the:
   a. respiratory bronchioles
   b. alveoli
   c. conchae
   d. heart

4. The aorta, venae cavae, esophagus, and large lymph vessels occupy a space within the thorax known as the:
   a. intrapleural space
   b. mediastinal space
   c. intrapulmonic space
   d. outer space

5. During inspiration the pressure within the mediastinal space:
   a. increases
   b. decreases
   c. remains the same

6. During expiration the intrapulmonic pressure:
   a. increases
   b. decreases
   c. goes bonkers

7. A condition of pleuritis would accentuate:
   a. abdominal breathing
   b. costal breathing

8. Return of blood to the right atrium is assisted when:
   a. the thorax is expanded (intrapleural pressure decreased from normal) during inspiration
   b. the thorax is contracted (intrapleural pressure returned to normal) during expiration

9. Alveolar P_{CO_2} is measured to be 45 mm Hg. Considering this value, one would expect atmospheric P_{CO_2} to be _____ than 45 mm Hg and venous blood P_{CO_2} to be _____ than 45 mm Hg. Select the respective words from the sets below which complete the above blanks.
   a. greater; less
   b. less; less
   c. less; greater
   d. greater; greater

10. The PO_2 of arterial blood during the development of carbon monoxide poisoning is:
    a. normal
    b. greater than normal
    c. less than normal

11. Which one of the following causes increased ventilation of the lungs?
    a. decreased CO_2 concentration in the blood
    b. increased CO_2 concentration in the blood
    c. increased PO_2 of arterial blood
    d. increased pH of the blood (decreased H^+ concentration)

12. Where is the respiratory center for the regulation of ventilation located?
    a. brain stem
    b. lungs
    c. cerebral cortex
    d. hypothalamus

13. Vagus nerve (a cranial nerve containing parasympathetic neurons) stimulation would increase all activities of the heart.
    a. true
    b. false

14. During inspiration:
    a. intrapleural and intrapulmonic pressures are decreased
    b. intrapleural and intrapulmonic pressures are increased
    c. intrapleural pressure is decreased and intrapulmonic pressure is increased
    d. intrapleural pressure is increased and intrapulmonic pressure is decreased

15. The PO_2 of blood in the pulmonary arteries is higher than the PO_2 of blood in the pulmonary veins.
    a. true
    b. false

16. The PCO_2 in the interstitial fluid compartment is higher than the PCO_2 of blood in the venules and veins.
    a. true
    b. false

17. When the lungs are expanded during inspiration:
    a. the pressure inside the venae cavae is increased
    b. the pressure inside the venae cavae is decreased
    c. there is no change in the pressure inside the venae cavae

18. Receptors for the detection of changes in arterial blood PO_2 are located in the:
    a. lungs
    b. brainstem respiratory center
    c. carotid and aortic bodies
    d. heart

19. Which one of the ventilation subdivisions is normally increased during panting?
    a. alveolar ventilation
    b. dead-space ventilation

20. The chemical form that accounts for the greatest amount of carbon dioxide transport is:
    a. CO_2 associated with amino groups of hemoglobin
    b. CO_2 in solution (dissolved)
    c. HCO_3^- (bicarbonate)

21. A difficult, labored state of breathing is termed:
    a. eupnea
    b. dyspnea
    c. hyperpnea
    d. polypnea

22. The amount of air breathed in or out during a respiratory cycle is known as the:
    a. vital capacity
    b. residual volume
    c. tidal volume
    d. functional residual capacity

23. When cats purr, which one of the following is FALSE?
    a. the muscles of the larynx that close the vocal cords and the diaphragm contract simultaneously during inspiration
    b. sound is produced by the vocal cords while they are opening
    c. the vocal cords open and close 25 times each second to produce the purring sound

24. The functional residual capacity in an animal is composed of:
    a. the inspiratory reserve volume and the tidal volume
    b. the expiratory reserve volume and the tidal volume
    c. the residual volume and the expiratory reserve volume
    d. the residual volume only

25. During the development of carbon monoxide poisoning or as observed in anemic (nonexerted) animals:
    a. ventilation of the lungs is not increased because the PO_2 of arterial blood remains normal
    b. ventilation of the lungs is increased because of hypoxemia
    c. carbon monoxide does not interfere with oxygen transport and their is no deficiency of hemoglobin, respectively

26. The bronchi that correspond to parabronchi are the:
    a. primary
    b. secondary
    c. tertiary

27. The air capillaries are immediate extensions of:
    a. parabronchi
    b. air sacs
    c. infundibuli
    d. atria

28. Compression of air sacs is associated with:
    a. inspiration
    b. expiration

29. Ventilation of the lungs occurs during:
    a. inspiration
    b. expiration
    c. both inspiration and expiration
30. Gas exchange occurs between the interface of:
    a. air capillaries and blood capillaries
    b. air sacs and blood capillaries
    c. both a and b
31. Both cranial and caudal air sacs ventilate the parabronchial mantles during expiration.
    a. true
    b. false
32. Because of cross-current ventilation, it is possible to have a lower PCO$_2$ and a higher PO$_2$ in arterial blood than in gas leaving the parabronchial mantles.
    a. true
    b. false

Suggested Readings

Comroe JH, Jr. Physiology of respiration. 2nd ed. Chicago: Year Book Medical Publishers, 1974.

Davenport HW. The ABC of acid-base chemistry. 6th ed. Chicago: University of Chicago Press, 1974.

Dellman H-D. Textbook of veterinary histology. 4th ed. Philadelphia: Lea & Febiger, 1993.

Dyce KM, Sack WO, Wensing CJG. Textbook of veterinary anatomy. Philadelphia: WB Saunders, 1987.

Fedde MR. Respiration in birds. In: Swenson MJ, Reece WO, eds. Dukes' physiology of domestic animals. 11th ed. Ithaca, NY: Cornell University Press, 1993:294–302.

Frandson RD, Spurgeon TL. Anatomy and physiology of farm animals. 5th ed. Philadelphia: Lea & Febiger, 1992.

Ganong WF. Review of medical physiology. 17th ed. East Norwalk, CT: Appleton & Lange, 1995.

Hare WCD. Ruminant respiratory system. In: Getty R, ed. Sisson and Grossman's anatomy of the domestic animals, Vol. 1. 5th ed. Philadelphia: WB Saunders, 1975:916–936.

McNaught AB, Callander R. Illustrated physiology. 3rd ed. Edinburgh: Churchill Livingstone, 1975.

Morrow PE. Some physical and physiological factors controlling the fate of inhaled substances. Health Physics 1960;2:372.

Reece WO. Respiration in mammals. In: Swenson MJ, Reece WO, eds. Dukes' physiology of domestic animals. 11th ed. Ithaca, NY: Cornell University Press, 1993:263–293.

Remmers JE, Gautier H. Neural and mechanical mechanisms of feline purring. Respir Physiol 1972;16:351.

Schmidt-Nielsen K. Animal physiology: adaptation and environment. New York: Cambridge University Press, 1975.

Schmidt-Nielsen K, Bretz WL, Taylor CR. Panting in dogs—unidirectional air flow over evaporative surfaces. Science 1970; 169:1102.

Sturgess JM. The mucous lining of major bronchi in the rabbit lung. Am Rev Respir Dis 1977;115:819.

Thews G. Pulmonary respiration. In: Schmidt RF, Thews G, eds. Human physiology. 2nd ed. Berlin: Springer-Verlag, 1989:456–488.

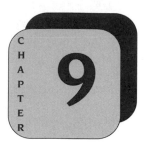

The Kidneys

The kidneys are usually thought to have the excretion of metabolic waste products as their only function. Another function, which is at least equally important, is the regulation of the volume and composition of the body's internal environment, the extracellular fluid. It has been said that the composition of the body fluids is determined not by what the mouth takes in, but by what the kidney keeps. Both functions—excretion of metabolic waste products and regulation of volume and composition of extracellular fluid—are performed by the kidneys because of their perfusion with blood, resulting in the formation of urine, a fluid of varying composition.

STRUCTURE AND FUNCTION OF THE KIDNEYS

The kidneys are paired organs suspended from the dorsal abdominal wall by a peritoneal fold and the blood vessels that serve them. They are located slightly cranial to the midlumbar region (Fig. 9.1). Because they are separated from the abdominal cavity by their envelopment of peritoneum, they are called retroperitoneal structures. Blood is carried to each kidney by a renal artery, and venous blood is conveyed away from each kidney by a renal vein. The renal artery arises directly from the aorta, and the renal vein empties directly into the caudal vena cava (Fig. 9.2).

Structure

Gross Features

The kidney is described as a bean-shaped structure for most domestic animals. In the horse, however, it is described as heart-shaped, and in cattle it is lobulated (Fig. 9.3). If a midsagittal cut is made through the kidney (Fig. 9.4), an outer cortex and an inner medulla are visible. The striations of the medulla are formed by the anatomic arrangement of the major parts that occupy the medulla, the loop of Henle of long-looped nephrons and the medullary portion of the collecting tubules (see later section on microstructure). The medullary portions of the collecting tubules are known as collecting ducts. The renal hilus

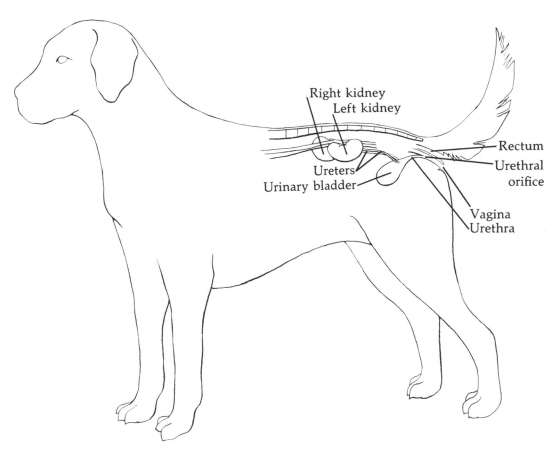

Figure 9.1. Side view of female dog showing general location of kidneys, ureters, urinary bladder, urethra, urethral orifice, and vagina.

is the indented area on the concave edge of the kidney through which the ureter, blood vessels, nerves, and lymphatics enter or leave. The renal pelvis (Fig. 9.4) is the expanded origin of the ureter within the kidney. The final discharge of urine from the many collecting ducts is received by the renal pelvis. The principal nerve supply to the kidneys is sympathetic in origin, and the fibers terminate mostly on glomerular arterioles. The ureter is a muscular (smooth muscle) tube that conveys urine from the renal pelvis to the urinary bladder. The ureter enters the bladder at an oblique angle (ureterovesicular junction), thus forming a functional valve to prevent backflow when the bladder is filling (Fig. 9.5). The urinary bladder is a hollow, muscular (smooth muscle) organ that varies in size depending on the amount of urine it contains at any one time. The smooth muscle of the urinary bladder is known as the detrusor muscle. The epithelial cell lining of the bladder accommodates for the change in size and is known as transitional epithelium. When the bladder is empty the cells appear to be piled on one another, giving it a stratified (layered) appearance. A transition occurs on filling so that the piled-up appearance gives way to a thinner epithelial stratification.

The neck of the bladder is the caudal continuation of the bladder leading to the

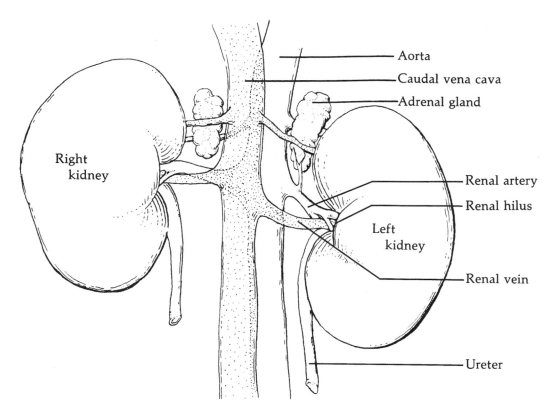

Figure 9.2. Ventral view of canine kidneys showing renal arteries, veins, and ureters and their positions relative to the aorta, vena cava, and adrenal glands.

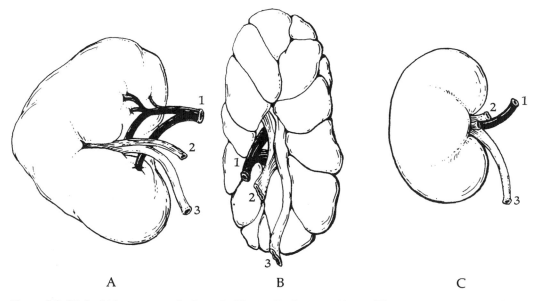

A   B   C

Figure 9.3. Right kidney, ventral view. **A.** Horse. **B.** Cow. **C.** Sheep. These represent heart-shaped, lobulated, and bean-shaped kidneys, respectively. 1, Renal artery; 2, renal vein; 3, ureter.

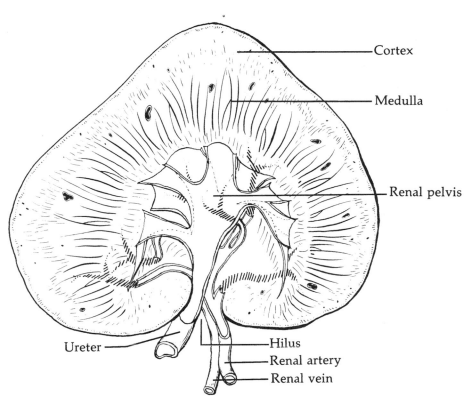

Figure 9.4. Midsagittal section of horse kidney showing cortex, medulla, pelvis, hilus, ureter, and renal artery.

urethra. The smooth muscle in the neck is mixed with a considerable amount of elastic tissue and functions as an internal sphincter.

The urethra is the caudal continuation of the neck of the bladder. It conveys the urine from the bladder to the exterior (Fig. 9.6). The external sphincter lies beyond the neck; it is composed of skeletal muscle that encircles the urethra at this point. The functional boundary between the bladder and urethra is represented by this sphincter.

Prevention of urine escape while the bladder is filling is provided for by contraction of the external sphincter and by tension passively exerted by the elastic elements in the neck of the bladder. When urine is expelled from the bladder, the external sphincter relaxes and the bladder muscles contract. The bladder muscle con-

traction opens its neck into a funnel shape. The contraction not only forces urine into the urethra but, because of the muscle fiber arrangement, the beginning of the urethra is widened.

Microstructure

The functional unit of the kidney is the nephron. An understanding of nephron function is essential for understanding kidney function. Nephron numbers vary considerably among species, and approximate numbers for several species are given in Table 9.1. Within a species the nephron numbers are relatively constant. Considering the differences in size among various breeds of dogs, it might be thought that the kidneys of large-breed dogs would contain more nephrons than the kidneys of small-breed dogs. This is not the case, however, and the larger kidney size in large dogs is compensated for by their having larger nephrons rather than more nephrons.

The mammalian kidney has two principal types of nephrons identified by (1) the location of their glomeruli and (2) the depth of penetration of the loops of Henle into the medulla. Those nephrons with glomeruli in the outer and middle cortices are called cortical or corticomedullary nephrons. They are associated with a loop of Henle that extends to the junction of the cortex and medulla or into the outer zone of the medulla. Those nephrons with glomeruli in the cortex close to the medulla are known as juxtamedullary nephrons. Juxtamedullary nephrons are associated with loops of Henle that

extend more deeply into the medulla; some extend as deep as the renal pelvis. The relationship of each nephron type to the cortex and medulla is shown in Figures 9.7 and 9.8. The juxtamedullary nephrons are those that develop and maintain the osmotic gradient from low to high in the outer medulla to the inner medulla, respectively. The percentage of nephrons having long loops of Henle (juxtamedullary nephrons) varies among animal species and ranges from 3% in the pig to 100% in the cat. In humans, the percentage of long-looped nephrons is about 14%.

A typical nephron and its component parts are shown in Fig. 9.9. The glomerulus is the tuft of capillaries through which filtration is accomplished. The afferent arteriole conducts blood to the glomerulus, and

Figure 9.5. Ureterovesicular junction (oblique entrance of ureter into the urinary bladder). **A.** Urine is conveyed to the urinary bladder from the renal pelvis by peristalsis and enters at the ureterovesicular junction. **B.** During micturition (emptying of the urinary bladder), urine is directed through the neck of the bladder to the urethra. Urine does not reenter the ureter because the ureterovesicular junction is closed by the hydrostatic pressure of urine associated with contraction of the detrusor muscle of the bladder wall.

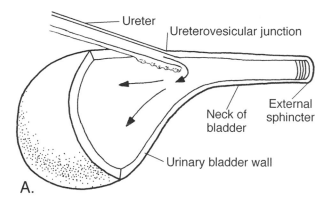

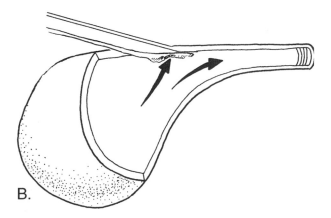

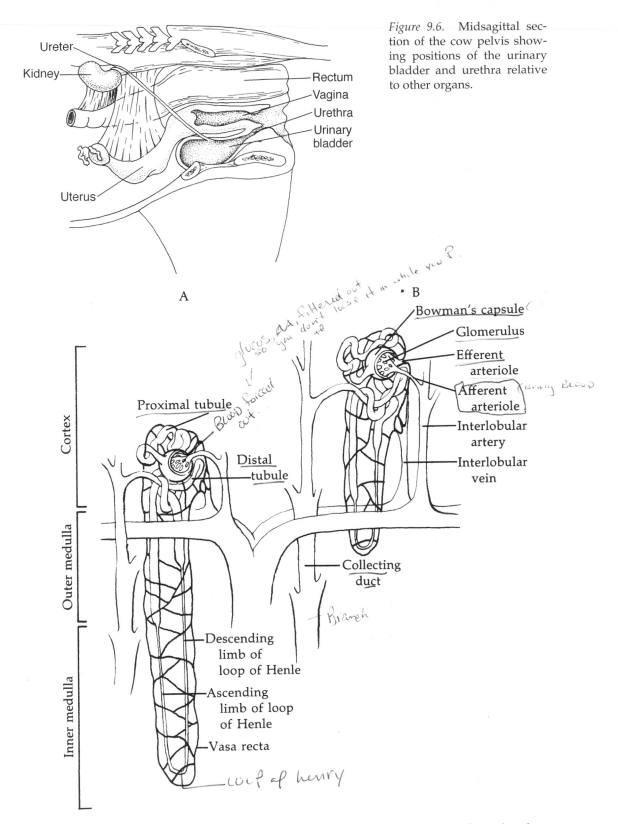

Figure 9.6. Midsagittal section of the cow pelvis showing positions of the urinary bladder and urethra relative to other organs.

Ureter

Kidney

Rectum
Vagina
Urethra
Urinary bladder

Uterus

A

B

Bowman's capsule
Glomerulus
Efferent arteriole
Afferent arteriole
Interlobular artery
Interlobular vein

Proximal tubule

Distal tubule

Collecting duct

Cortex

Outer medulla

Inner medulla

Descending limb of loop of Henle

Ascending limb of loop of Henle

Vasa recta

Figure 9.7. Types of mammalian nephrons. **A.** Juxtamedullary (long-looped) nephron. **B.** Cortical nephron.

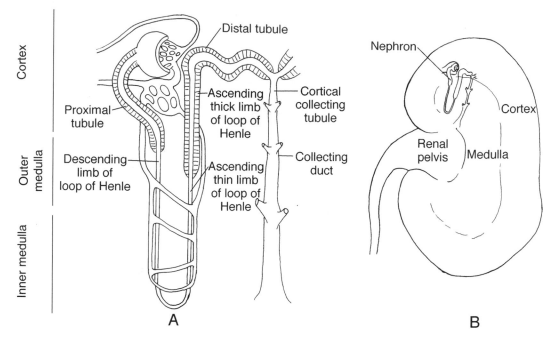

Figure 9.8. **A**. Component parts of a juxtamedullary nephron (mammalian) relative to their locations in the cortex and medulla. **B**. Midsagittal section of the kidney showing the location of a juxtamedullary nephron (exaggerated size) relative to the cortex, medulla, and renal pelvis.

the efferent arteriole conducts blood away from the glomerulus. Blood leaving through the efferent arterioles is redistributed into another capillary bed known as the peritubular capillaries; these perfuse the nephron tubules. The vasa recta are capillary branches from the peritubular capillaries associated with the long-looped nephrons. After perfusion of the kidneys, blood is returned to the caudal vena cava by the renal veins.

Filtrate from the glomerulus is collected by Bowman's capsule and is subsequently directed through the proximal tubule, loop of Henle, and distal tubule. The distal tubule empties into a cortical collecting tubule. A cortical collecting tubule is not unique to a single nephron because it receives tubular fluid from the convoluted portion of several distal tubules. When the collecting tubule turns away from the cortex and passes down into the medulla, it is known as a collecting duct. Successive generations of collecting ducts coalesce to form

TABLE 9.1. Approximate Number of Nephrons in each Kidney for Several Domestic Animals and Humans

Species	Nephrons/kidney
Cattle	4,000,000
Pig	1,250,000
Dog	415,000
Cat	190,000
Human	1,000,000

progressively larger collecting ducts. The tubular fluid is finally discharged from the larger collecting ducts into the pelvis of the kidney, and it is conveyed from there by the ureters to the urinary bladder for storage until discharge through the urethra. A summary of nephron component parts encountered by glomerular filtrate as it becomes tubular fluid and finally urine with final discharge through the urethra is shown in Figure 9.10.

The loop of Henle is composed of three segments—the thin descending limb, the thin ascending limb, and the thick ascend-

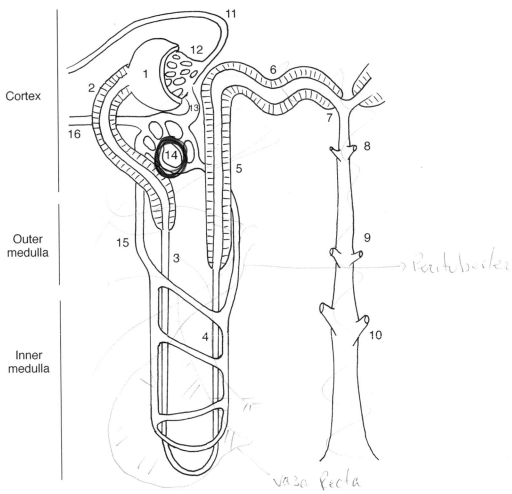

Figure 9.9. The functional nephron with blood supply. 1, Bowman's capsule, 2, proximal tubule; 3, descending limb of loop of Henle; 4, thin ascending limb of loop of Henle; 5, thick ascending limb of loop of Henle; 6, distal tubule; 7, connecting tubule; 8, cortical collecting tubule; 9, outer medullary collecting duct; 10, inner medullary collecting duct; 11, afferent arteriole; 12, glomerulus; 13, efferent arteriole; 14, peritubular capillaries; 15, vasa recta; 16, to renal vein.

ing limb. Their relative thicknesses are a result of differences in the epithelial cells and do not refer to changes in lumen diameter. The thin segment for each loop is continuous with the thin segment of the other at the hairpin curve. The descending limbs of loops of Henle of cortical nephrons only go as deep as the inner aspect of the outer medulla. The juxtamedullary nephrons have descending limbs of loops of Henle that can extend to the renal pelvis. The thin segment of the descending limb is a straight tubule continuous from the proxi-

mal tubule and is followed after its hairpin turn by the thin ascending limb. The thick segment of the ascending limb is a straight tubule continuous from the thin ascending limb. The thick segment of the ascending limb of the loop of Henle returns in its ascent to its glomerulus of origin, passes between the afferent and efferent arteriole, and proceeds from there as the distal tubule to its cortical collecting tubule. The junction of the distal tubule and glomerulus is known as the juxtaglomerular apparatus (Fig. 9.11). There are characteristic cell

240 The Kidneys

types at this location. In the tubule, the cells are collectively known as the macula densa; in the afferent and efferent arterioles they are called the juxtaglomerular cells. The juxtaglomerular apparatus is associated with regulating the amount of blood flowing to the kidney, the amount of filtration, and the secretion of renin, an enzyme involved in the formation of angiotensin II (a vasoconstrictor).

Formation of Urine

The three processes involving the nephrons and their blood supply in urine formation are 1) glomerular filtration, 2) tubular reabsorption, and 3) tubular secretion. As a result of glomerular filtration, an ultrafiltrate of plasma known as glomerular filtrate appears in Bowman's capsule. Glomerular filtrate becomes tubular fluid when it enters the nephron tubules because of the compositional changes that begin to occur immediately as a result of reabsorption from the tubular lumen and secretion into the tubular lumen (Fig. 9.12). Tubular reabsorption and tubular secretion continue throughout the length of the nephron and collecting duct, so that tubular fluid does not become urine until it enters the

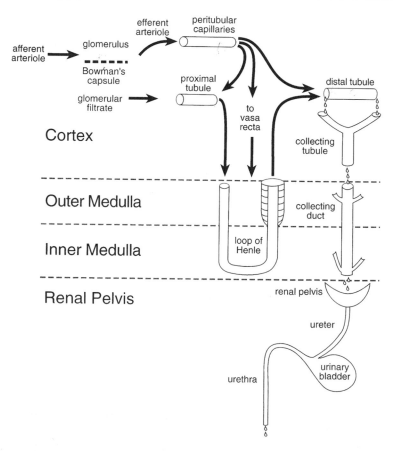

Figure 9.10. Summary of kidney blood flow and tubular fluid flow as it applies to the nephron. After removal of the filtration fraction of plasma at the glomerulus, the remaining blood that enters the efferent arteriole is distributed to the nephron as shown. The fraction of plasma filtered at the glomerulus enters Bowman's capsule as glomerular filtrate. It continues through the nephron tubules and ducts as tubular fluid. The tubular fluid is subjected to reabsorption and secretion and enters the renal pelvis as urine. Urine is finally evacuated from the urinary bladder by micturition.

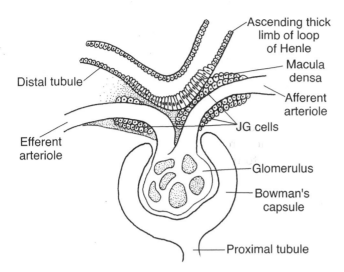

Figure 9.11. The juxtaglomerular (JG) apparatus. The JG apparatus is located at the junction of the distal tubule and its glomerulus of origin. It is associated with regulation of blood flow and filtration fraction for the nephron and with the secretion of renin, an enzyme involved in the formation of angiotensin II.

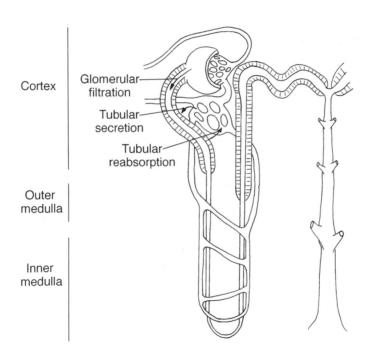

Figure 9.12. Functional nephron and processes involved in urine formation. The arrows indicate the origins and destinations of the three processes associated with the formation of urine. Following glomerular filtration, glomerular filtrate enters the proximal tubule and becomes tubular fluid. Tubular secretion is directed from the peritubular capillaries into the tubules and tubular reabsorption is directed from the tubules into the peritubular capillaries. Tubular reabsorption and tubular secretion occur throughout the length of the nephron.

renal pelvis. With the possible exception of mucus addition in the horse, there are no compositional changes in urine beyond the collecting ducts.

Distribution of Blood at the Glomerulus

The renal blood flow (RBF) refers to the rate at which blood flows to the kidneys (in ml/min). Inasmuch as plasma is the fluid part of the blood, from which the glomerular filtrate is formed, renal plasma flow (RPF) refers to that part of the RBF that is plasma. As long as there continues to be a renal blood flow, a glomerular filtrate will be formed from the plasma at the glomerulus. The rate at which it is formed is known as the glomerular filtration rate (GFR) and is measured in ml/min. Renal blood flow and RPF are also measured in ml/min, and the ratio of GFR to RPF (GFR:RPF) is referred to as the filtration fraction (FF). The FF is the fraction (or percentage) of plasma flowing through the glomerulus that becomes glomerular filtrate. The blood that continues into the efferent arterioles has an increased value for PCV and protein concentration because a fraction of the plasma has been filtered and has entered the tubules. The protein concentration is higher because, as a result of its molecular size, it is virtually prevented from being filtered with the other plasma components.

An example for the relationships of RBF, RPF, GFR, and FF, and the percentage of urine formed relative to the amount of filtrate formed in 24 hours is shown in Table 9.2.

Glomerular Filtration

The kidneys have the functional counterpart of two capillary beds, represented by the glomeruli and the peritubular capillaries. The glomeruli are considered to be a high-pressure system (high hydrostatic pressure favoring filtration), and the peritubular capillaries, which are perfused

TABLE 9.2. Approximate Values for Several Kidney Function Variables in a 11.35 kg (25 lb) Dog in a Normal State of Hydration

Variable	Value
Cardiac output (ml/min)	1500
Blood flow to kidneys (% of cardiac output)	20
Renal blood flow (ml/min)	300
Renal plasma flow (ml/min)	180
Glomerular filtration rate (ml/min)	45
Filtration fraction (decimal equivalent)	0.25
Urine volume in 24h[†] (ml)	681
Glomerular filtrate volume in 24h (ml)	64800
Volume of urine as percent of filtrate	1.05
Filtrate reabsorbed (%)	98.95

*Based upon plasma portion of hematocrit being approximately 60%.

[†]Calculated from average rate for dogs being 60 ml/kg/24h.

with blood coming from the glomerular capillary bed, are considered to be a low-pressure system (low hydrostatic pressure favoring reabsorption). As such, the glomeruli are similar to the arterial end of a typical muscle capillary, and the peritubular capillaries are similar to the venous end (see Fig. 7.34). It appears that the capillary endothelium of the glomerulus is slightly more porous than muscle capillary endothelium and larger molecules are filtered more readily. Protein molecules are relatively restricted from filtration (similar to their restriction in muscle capillaries) because of their large molecular size, but they might not be excluded altogether.

The dynamics of filtration through the glomerular membrane are illustrated in Figure 9.13. No colloidal osmotic pressure is shown on the Bowman capsule side. Although some filtration of protein (a potential source of colloidal osmotic pressure) occurs (as in muscle capillaries), the filtrate does not accumulate as it does in muscle because the hydrostatic pressure in Bowman's capsule causes the filtrate to flow away from the capsule and through

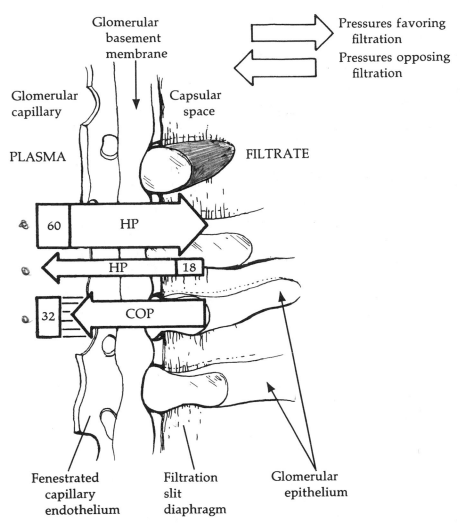

Figure 9.13. Dynamics of glomerular filtration in mammals. Bowman's capsule is separated from the glomerulus by a glomerular membrane, through which filtration occurs. The extent of filtration is determined by the difference between the pressures favoring filtration and those opposing filtration. In this illustration, filtration occurs because 60 − (32 + 18) = 10 mm Hg. Values greater than or less than 10 mm Hg would correlate with more or less filtration, respectively. Pressure values (60, 32, 18) are in mm Hg. HP, hydrostatic pressure; COP, colloidal osmotic pressure.

the nephron tubules. Therefore, the colloidal osmotic pressure in Bowman's capsule urinary space is negligible.

The GFR can be varied by changing the diameter of the afferent or efferent arterioles. Dilatation of the afferent arteriole increases the blood flow to the glomerulus, which in turn increases the hydrostatic pressure and potential for filtration. Constriction of the efferent arteriole increases the glomerular hydrostatic pressure, just as blockage of a vein increases the hydrostatic pressure in capillaries behind it. Even though RBF to the glomerulus is reduced because of the decreased outflow caused by efferent arteriole constriction, the GFR is maintained (because of the greater hydrostatic pressure), and this allows for a continued FF. These two mechanisms of maintaining the GFR are associated with the autoregulation of the GFR and RBF. Autoregulation means that GFR and RBF are maintained at rather constant values because of intrinsic mechanisms within the kidney, independent of outside nerve supply. It is believed that cells in the macula densa that are sensitive to changes in ionic concentration (Na^+ and Cl^-) can detect lowered concentrations in the tubular fluid (decreased tubular flow, thus more time for reabsorption) and signal the afferent arteriole to dilate (resulting in increased blood flow and hydrostatic pressure). At the same time, the juxtaglomerular cells secrete renin, which initiates the formation of angiotensin II. Angiotensin II is responsible for efferent arteriolar constriction (greater sensitivity of efferent arteriole to angiotensin II than of afferent arteriole), which increases a lowered hydrostatic pressure in the glomerulus. Even though systemic blood pressure might be low (the cause of renin secretion), kidney function continues because the GFR is being maintained (see upcoming section). The kidneys assist the return of the blood pressure back toward normal by reabsorbing more water from the tubular fluid, thus increasing blood volume (this occurs at the same time as the angiotensin II is having its effect). The increasing blood volume causes an increase in blood pressure. The increase in water reabsorption occurs because, while increasing the FF by efferent arteriolar constriction, efferent arteriolar blood has a higher colloidal osmotic pressure and a lower hydrostatic pressure. Both these factors favor reabsorption at the level of the peritubular capillaries. In addition, angiotensin II promotes the reabsorption of Na^+, and this also favors reabsorption of water.

Tubular Reabsorption and Secretion

For reabsorption to occur, a substance must pass from the tubular lumen, through the tubular epithelial cells, diffuse through the interstitial fluid, and enter the capillary. A substance to be secreted must leave the capillary, diffuse through the interstitial fluid, and pass through the tubular epithelial cell into the tubular lumen. A longitudinal section of tubular epithelium and its relationship to the tubular lumen and peritubular capillary is shown in Figure 9.14.

Substances important to body function, such as glucose and amino acids, enter tubular fluid by filtration at the glomerulus. Because of their relatively small molecular size, they pass easily through the glomerular membrane and their concentration in the glomerular filtrate is equal to their concentration in plasma. Unless these substances are returned to the blood, they are excreted in the urine and lost from the body. In the epithelial cells of the proximal convoluted tubules, glucose and amino acids are transferred from the tubular lumen to the interstitial fluid, from which they diffuse into the peritubular capillaries. Their transport from the tubular lumen into the tubular epithelial cell is coupled with the transport of Na^+. For example, Na^+ and glucose (or an amino acid) are coupled to the same protein carrier when moving through the brush border of the epithelial cell from the lumen to the cytoplasm of the cell (Fig. 9.15). The energy for transport is associated with the active transport of Na^+ through the basal and lateral membranes of the tubular epithelial cells. The active transport of Na^+ out of the cell at the basal and lateral borders creates a chemical gradient (lumen concentration higher) for diffusion of Na^+ from the tubular lumen into the cell cytoplasm. The transport of glucose and amino acids does not require additional energy because of their trans-

Re Proximal or Loop of Henly

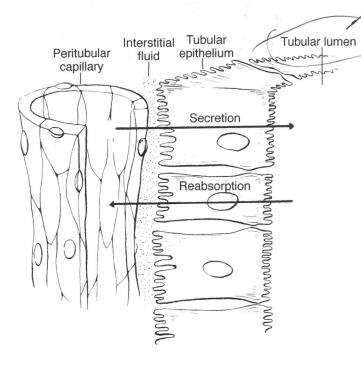

Figure 9.14. Functional nephron and processes involved in urine formation. The arrows indicate the origins and destinations of the three processes associated with the formation of urine. Following glomerular filtration, glomerular filtrate enters the proximal tubule and becomes tubular fluid. Tubular secretion is directed from the peritubular capillaries into the tubules and tubular reabsorption is directed from the tubules into the peritubular capillaries. Tubular reabsorption and tubular secretion occur throughout the length of the nephron.

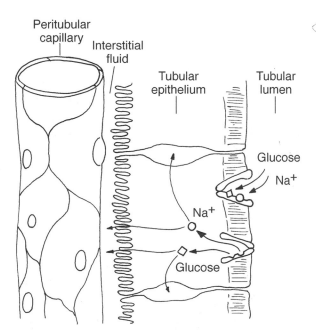

Figure 9.15. Transport of Na^+ from tubular lumen into the tubular epithelial cell and its cotransport with glucose. The protein carrier conformation permits reception of Na^+ and glucose from the lumen. Carrier conformational change permits Na^+ and glucose release into the epithelial cytoplasm. Once released the carrier returns to its original conformation for the reception of more Na^+ and glucose. The Na^+ released into the tubular epithelial cytoplasm is actively transported through the basal and lateral borders of the cells into the interstitial fluid and diffuses from there into the capillaries. Glucose follows the same pathways except that it is not actively transported. Amino acids are also cotransported with Na^+ similar to that of glucose.

port with Na^+. Once glucose and amino acids are inside the cell, and are uncoupled from their carrier, they diffuse through the basal and lateral borders into the interstitial fluid and from there into the capillaries. The protein carrier on which they were transported from the lumen into the cell with Na^+ returns to its previous conformation to transport more glucose, amino acids, and Na^+.

Because Na^+ is transported actively from the tubular epithelial cells to the interstitial fluid, an electrical gradient is established between the peritubular space and the tubular lumen (lumen negative). Because Cl^- diffuses through membranes easily, however, its diffusion from the lumen follows the transport of Na^+ so that electrical neutrality is maintained. Consequently, the lumen has a low negativity in the proximal tubule, where much of the Na^+ is reabsorbed.

The removal of Na^+, glucose, amino acids, and other substances from the lumen into the interstitial fluid and capillaries increases the concentration of water within the lumen, and water is reabsorbed by osmosis into the interstitial fluid and capillaries. Reabsorption of water into the peritubular capillaries from the interstitial fluid is favored because of the relatively low hydrostatic pressure and because of the increased colloidal osmotic pressure (loss of water, but not protein, at the glomerulus) in the peritubular capillaries. This situation is similar to that at the venous end of a muscle capillary (see Fig. 7.34).

The removal of water from the tubular lumen increases the concentration of diffusible substances (particularly urea), and they move from the lumen to the interstitial fluid and capillaries by simple diffusion. The proximal tubules reabsorb about 65% of H_2O, Na^+, Cl^-, and HCO_3^- and 100% of the glucose and amino acids that were previously filtered at the glomerulus.

Tubular secretion—the transfer of substances from the capillaries into the interstitial fluid and hence to the tubular lumen—occurs for several substances. The secretion of H^+ occurs throughout the length of the nephron tubules (except in thin limb of loops of Henle) and is coupled with the reabsorption of HCO^-. The secretion of K^+ occurs in the distal convoluted tubule and collecting tubules and ducts and is coupled with the reabsorption of Na^+. Ammonia is secreted by the nephron tubules. Its rate of secretion varies, depending on the acid-base equilibrium of the body fluids (see later text). Several organic molecules are also secreted by the tubular epithelial cells into the tubular lumen. A substance similar to penicillin is lost from the body fluids because of tubular secretion. Penicillin-like substances have been developed that persist in the body fluids for longer periods of time because their rate of secretion has been slowed.

Transport Maximum

Substances such as glucose that are associated with a carrier or that have active transport mechanisms for their reabsorption have a maximum rate at which they can be reabsorbed, known as the tubular transport maximum (T_M). When the T_M for the substance is exceeded, the substance will appear in the urine. In the disease known as diabetes mellitus, insulin is lacking, and the movement of glucose from the plasma into body cells is impaired. Glucose concentration in the plasma therefore increases, causing the plasma and tubular loads of glucose to increase. The increased tubular load exceeds the availability of carrier molecules for its transport and reabsorption, and excess glucose continues its flow through the tubules into the urine. Because it is retained within the tubules, it contributes to the effective osmotic pressure of the tubular fluid, and water is also retained. In diabetes mellitus, glucose is detected in the urine and a greater volume of urine is formed. Greater amounts of water are lost from the body in the urine, so the afflicted animal drinks more water to compensate for the urine loss. Increased urine formation is known as diuresis; when it is caused by retention of water because of greater effective osmotic pressure in the tubular lumen, it is known as osmotic diuresis.

Not all of the hundreds of thousands of nephrons have the same T_M. The first appearance of glucose in the urine does not represent the T_M for the kidney, it represents the renal threshold (the plasma concentration of a substance when it first appears in the urine). The T_M for the kidney is reached when all nephrons are reabsorbing to their maximum ability. For glucose, the renal threshold (its plasma concentration when glucose first appears in urine) is about 180 mg/dl and the T_M (its plasma concentration when further increments of glucose increase in the plasma result in similar increments of glucose increase in the urine) is about 260 mg/dl.

Countercurrent Mechanism

The countercurrent mechanism is a tubular phenomenon, associated with the loop of Henle of the long-looped nephrons, that increases the solute (principally NaCl and urea) concentration in the interstitial fluid of the kidney medulla. There is a concentration gradient of low to high from the outer medulla to the innermost aspects of the medulla. The transport of NaCl occurs from the lumen of the thick ascending limb of the loop of Henle to the interstitial fluid by an active transport (cotransport) process for Na^+ coupled with Cl^-. While the Na^+ and Cl^- are leaving the lumen, H_2O is retained because the membrane is not permeable for water. Consequently, the tubular fluid becomes quite dilute as it continues into the distal tubule. The Na^+ and Cl^- that have been transported into the interstitial fluid diffuse readily into the descending limb and out of the ascending limb of the vasa recta (capillary extensions from

the peritubular capillaries). As a result of the diffusion ease, perfusion of the medulla with blood is accomplished without removing the high solute concentration that was established.

A schematic representation of the countercurrent mechanism is shown in Figure 9.16; the nephron parts are identified by circled numbers.

The tubular fluid entering the descending limb of the loop of Henle (Fig. 9.16, 1) from the proximal tubule has an osmolality of 300 mOsm, 280 contributed from NaCl and minor electrolytes and 20 from urea (280, 20). There is a high permeability for H_2O and no permeability for Na^+, Cl^-, and urea. Water diffuses outward (osmosis) and solutes remain within. The tubular fluid at the hairpin turn has an osmolality of 1200 (1120, 80).

The thin segment of the ascending limb of the loop of Henle (Fig. 9.16, 2) is not permeable to H_2O, highly permeable to NaCl, and moderately permeable to urea. The tubule retains H_2O while NaCl diffuses outward and urea diffuses inward. A gradient for the outward diffusion of NaCl was established because the osmolality in the interstitial fluid needed for the outward diffusion of H_2O in the descending limb (and consequent increasing concentration of NaCl within) received a contribution from urea (thus, high NaCl concentration not needed). The tubular fluid osmolality when it reaches the thick segment is 500 mOsm (400, 100).

The thick segment of the ascending limb of the loop of Henle (Fig. 9.16, 3) is involved with active transport of NaCl from the lumen to the interstitial fluid and a low permeability for the diffusion of H_2O and urea. The average osmolality of fluid in the lumen that is leaving the thick ascending limb and entering the distal tubule is about 200 mOsm (100, 100), which is decidedly hypotonic.

There is continued active transport of NaCl and low permeability for H_2O and

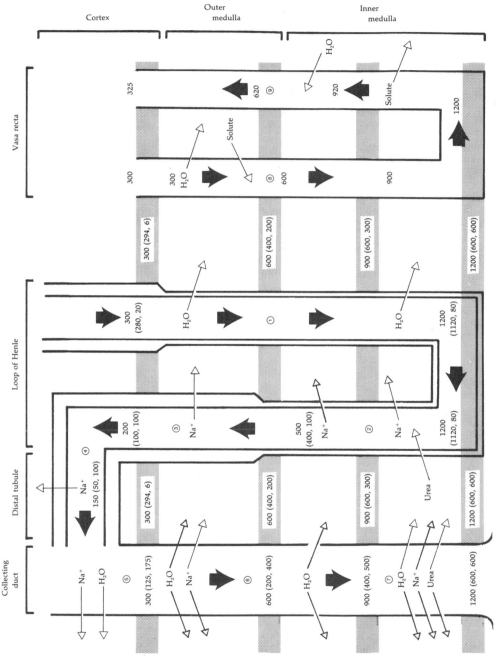

Figure 9.16. Functional aspects of the countercurrent mechanism in humans. Values shown approximate those for humans and the osmolality of tubular fluid entering the renal pelvis reflects maximum ADH secretion. The movement of Na^+ from the tubule implies a similar movement of Cl^-. 1, Descending limb of the loop of Henle; 2, thin segment of ascending limb of loop of Henle; 3, thick segment of ascending limb of loop of Henle; 4, distal tubule; 5, cortical collecting tubule; 6, outer medullary collecting duct; 7, inner medullary collecting duct; 8, descending limb of vasa recta; 9, ascending limb of vasa recta. The values of the tubular fluid osmolality are shown for each part (in mOsm); the numbers in parentheses represent the contribution to the osmolality from NaCl and minor electrolytes and from urea, respectively. For example, at the end of the cortical collecting tubule (5), the osmolality is 300 mOsm (125, 175), with 125 mOsm contributed from NaCl and minor electrolytes and 175 mOsm contributed from urea. See text for further explanation.

urea in the distal tubule (Fig. 9.16, *4*). At the end of the distal tubule, and before entering the collecting tubule, the osmolality is about 150 mOsm (50, 100).

In the cortical collecting tubule, outer medullary collecting duct, and inner medullary collecting duct (Fig. 9.16, *5, 6, and 7*), sodium reabsorption is stimulated by aldosterone, H_2O reabsorption is influenced by antidiuretic hormone (ADH), and urea reabsorption (inner medullary only) is influenced by ADH.

With maximum ADH (as shown in Fig. 9.16) there is increased permeability for H_2O and urea. At the end of the cortical collecting tubule the osmolality is 300 mOsm (125, 175), at the end of the outer medulla it is 600 mOsm (200, 400), and before it empties into the renal pelvis it is 1200 mOsm (600, 600).

With no ADH there would be no H_2O reabsorption and no urea reabsorption, but there could be continued NaCl reabsorption under the influence of aldosterone. In this situation, the osmolality of urine formed would be 130 mOsm (30, 100).

Both the descending and ascending limbs of the vasa recta (Fig. 9.16, *8* and *9*) are permeable to H_2O and solutes. Because there is an increasing osmolality in the interstitial fluid from the cortex through the inner medulla, there is osmosis of H_2O outward from the descending limb and diffusion of solutes inward. After the hairpin turn, the plasma is exposed to decreasing concentrations of solute in the interstitial fluid as it proceeds upward, the solute that was gained while going down is lost by diffusion as it ascends, and water diffuses by osmosis into the tubule. The osmolality of the plasma as it reaches the cortex is only slightly higher (325 mOsm) than it was when it entered the vasa recta.

Maximum osmolality is maintained in the interstitial fluid in the region of the hairpin turns of the loops of Henle and vasa rectae. It varies among animal species and indicates the maximum urine concentration that can exist under conditions of maximum antidiuresis (low urine output). The previous example (1200 mOsm) is representative for humans.

In addition to NaCl, urea also contributes to the high solute concentration in the interstitial medulla of the kidney. This is accomplished by a recirculation mechanism for urea between the collecting ducts and the loop of Henle. Recirculation means that urea diffuses from the inner medullary collecting ducts (as influenced by ADH) into the interstitial fluid, and from there diffuses into the lumen of the thin segment of the ascending limbs of the loops of Henle. Diffusion occurs because of the permeability of these nephron parts for urea and because of concentration differences (high to low concentration). After the entrance of urea into the loops of Henle, it is retained there because of membrane impermeability until it again arrives at the inner medullary collecting ducts, which have a variable permeability depending on the amount of ADH (see following section). The recirculation mechanism and high concentration of urea in the medulla not only assist the countercurrent mechanism but also ensure excretion of urea when urine output is low. For example, if urine is formed at the rate of 2 ml/min and it has a urea concentration of 2 mg/ml, then 4 mg of urea would be excreted each minute. If, however, urine formation is reduced to 1 ml/min (greater reabsorption of water), the concentration of urea is increased to 4 mg/ml and excretion is maintained at 4 mg/min. The concentration of urea remains high in the collecting ducts because the concentration is also high in the interstitial fluid (diffusion from the collecting duct limited by concentration difference).

HORMONES AND KIDNEY FUNCTION

Antidiuretic Hormone

Concentration of the Urine

Tubular fluid entering the distal tubules has an osmolality lower than that of plasma because of the removal of Na^+ and Cl^- that occurred in the ascending limb of the loops of Henle along with the simultaneous retention of water. The osmolality of plasma is about 300 mOsm. The epithelial cells of the collecting tubules and collecting ducts have a variable permeability for water, depending on the amount of antidiuretic hormone (ADH) that has been secreted from the posterior pituitary gland. ADH increases the permeability of the cells for water. Significant changes seem to occur in the rate of ADH secretion when there are deviations in the plasma osmolality of as little as 2% in either direction.

The degree of dehydration of the extracellular fluid is detected by osmoreceptor cells in the hypothalamus. When the cells detect dehydration they stimulate the posterior pituitary to secrete more ADH and, when overhydration is detected, the rate of ADH release is decreased. The secreted ADH is circulated by the blood to the kidney tubules, where the water permeability changes take place. Hypotonic tubular fluid entering the collecting tubules and ducts could be excreted as urine if water were not

reabsorbed. This happens in diabetes insipidus, in which there is either an absence of ADH or severely decreased amounts of ADH. Usually, when tubular fluid enters the collecting tubules and ducts, water is reabsorbed as it proceeds to the renal pelvis because it is exposed to effective osmotic pressures of increasing magnitudes in the interstitial fluid of the kidney medulla, as established by the countercurrent mechanism. It would be possible for the osmolality of the tubular fluid, and hence that of the urine, to approach the osmolality of the interstitial fluid in the innermost region of the medulla.

In the dog this would approach 2400 mOsm and the urine-to-plasma osmolal ratio (2400:300) would be approximately 8:1. The urine would have a concentration 8 times that of plasma. Some desert rodents attain a urine-to-plasma osmolal ratio of about 16:1. This ratio represents an extreme adaptation for body water conservation. Environmental water is not available for desert animals (water gain mostly metabolic water) and water losses are minimized for survival. Table 9.3 compares the

TABLE 9.3. Relationship of Structure to Concentrating Capacity in Mammalian Kidneys

Animal	Kidney size* (mm)	Long-looped nephrons (%)	Relative medullary thickness[†]	Maximum freezing point depression in urine (°C)
Beaver	36	0	1.3	0.96
Pig	66	3	1.6	2
Human	64	14	3	2.6
Dog[‡]	40	100	4.3	4.85
Cat	24	100	4.8	5.8
Rat	14	28	5.8	4.85
Kangaroo rat	5.9	27	8.5	10.4
Jerboa	4.5	33	9.3	12
Psammomys	13	100	10.7	9.2

*Kidney size = cube root of the product of the dimensions of the kidney

[†]Relative medullary thickness = medullary thickness in millimeters $\times$ 10/kidney size.

[‡]Beeuwkes and Bonventre have shown (1975) that the dog kidney does contain short-looped or cortimedullary nephrons; therefore, long-looped nephrons comprise fewer than 100% of the nephrons.

From Schmidt-Nielsen, O'Dell, eds. Structure and concentrating mechanism in the mammalian kidney. Am J Physiol 1961;200:1119–1124.

percentage of long-looped nephrons (loops of Henle extending deeply into the medulla) and relative medullary thickness of different animals. The relative medullary thickness is derived from measurements of the depth of the medulla from the corticomedullary junction to its innermost depth, which protrudes into the renal pelvis. Relative medullary thickness is believed to be a better predictor of urine concentrating ability than percentage of long-looped nephrons. As judged by freezing point depression (solute particles lower

the freezing point of solutions), the kangaroo rat has the greatest concentrating capacity for urine. As compared to humans, it appears that its innermost medullary osmolality would be about 4 times that of humans, or about 4800 mOsm. The hypothalamic-pituitary-renal association is shown in Figure 9.17.

Other Factors Affecting ADH Release

ADH release from the posterior pituitary is influenced by other factors in addition to hydration of the extracellular fluids.

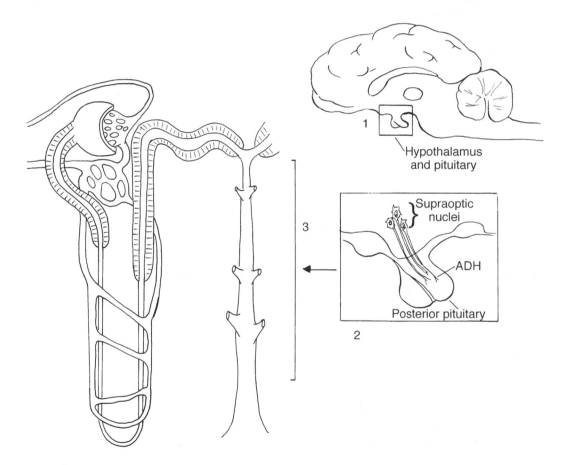

Figure 9.17. Relationships among the hypothalamus, posterior pituitary, and kidneys in the regulation of extracellular hydration. 1, Extracellular dehydration detected by osmoreceptors in the hypothalamus. Boxed area in 1 shows location in the brain of the boxed area in 2. 2, ADH (neurosecretion of supraoptic nuclei in hypothalamus) secreted into blood in response to dehydration. 3, Cortical collecting tubules and medullary collecting ducts are targets of ADH, causing increased reabsorption of H_2O.

Another aspect of water reabsorption is compensation for loss of blood volume and resultant low blood pressure. There are "volume receptors" in the walls of many large blood vessels that monitor the degree of filling of the cardiovascular system. When blood volume decreases, the receptors stimulate increased ADH secretion, and when blood volume increases, the receptors stimulate decreased ADH secretion. In both cases, blood volume is adjusted to normal by increasing or decreasing water reabsorption, respectively.

Cold environments inhibit ADH release, so urine production and water intake increase. The need for water intake results from thirst induced by water loss from diuresis. The need for water availability in cold weather is apparent.

Ethyl alcohol inhibits ADH secretion and dehydration is a consequence of alcohol consumption.

When water loss exceeds water intake, the extracellular fluid (ECF) is concentrated, resulting in hyperosmolality. A water deficit requires water intake for correction. The ECF hyperosmolality not only stimulates greater secretion of ADH so that water excretion is suppressed but also stimulates thirst so that the animal seeks water for ingestion. The osmoreceptors of the hypothalamus (see previous text) respond to effective osmotic pressure; hence the osmolality increase must be caused by substances restricted from diffusion into the osmoreceptor cells. For this reason, the osmoreceptor cells are often considered to be Na^+ receptors because Na^+ is the non-diffusible cation with the greatest concentration in the ECF. Osmolality increase as a result of urea (freely diffusible) does not stimulate the receptors.

Angiotensin II

ADH has been described relative to its role in regulating the osmolality of body fluids. Angiotensin II, another hormone, ensures a continuous GFR by increasing the FF when the RBF decreases (see previous text). Because of the increased FF, reabsorption of water occurs more readily into the peritubular capillaries, so that decreasing blood volume can be stopped. In addition, angiotensin II causes peripheral vasoconstriction, which improves a failing blood volume by reducing the total volume of the cardiovascular system. Angiotensin II also causes secretion of aldosterone, a hormone of the adrenal cortex.

Aldosterone

Aldosterone is more particularly involved with the regulation of K^+ concentration in the extracellular fluids and accordingly promotes the secretion of K^+ ions. The mechanism of K^+ secretion, however, involves the reabsorption of Na^+. Therefore, the secretion of aldosterone in response to angiotensin II has as its function the reabsorption of Na^+. This would be followed by reabsorption of water, which assists in the reestablishment of a decreasing blood volume.

Aldosterone regulates the K^+ concentration of the extracellular fluid by its activity in the cortical collecting tubules and in medullary collecting ducts. Aldosterone is secreted in response to elevated K^+ concentrations in the extracellular fluid. Even though Na^+ reabsorption is coupled with K^+ secretion (not a 1:1 exchange), aldosterone is not involved with the regulation of Na^+ concentration.

Parathyroid Hormone

Parathyroid hormone, secreted by the parathyroid glands, acts on the kidney tubules to increase reabsorption of Ca^{2+}, while at the same time promoting the excretion of phosphorus. Parathyroid hormone is secreted in response to low concentrations of Ca^{2+} in the extracellular fluid. Another role of the kidney in response to a declining Ca^{2+} concentration in the extracellular fluid involves the formation of the

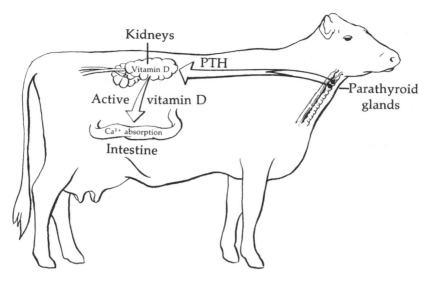

Figure 9.18. Relationship of parathyroid hormone (PTH), the kidneys, and calcium ion homeostasis in the cow. PTH from the parathyroid gland activates vitamin D in the kidney; activated vitamin D promotes absorption of Ca^{2+} from the intestine.

active form of vitamin D (1,25-dehydroc-holecalciferol), also known as calcitriol (Fig. 9.18). Active vitamin D promotes Ca^{2+} absorption from the intestine. Parathyroid hormone controls the formation of active vitamin D by the kidney.

MICTURITION

Transfer of Urine to the Urinary Bladder

During the formation of urine, the tubular fluid flows through the tubules because of a hydrostatic pressure difference that exists between Bowman's capsule and the renal pelvis. The hydrostatic pressure in Bowman's capsule is about 15–20 mm Hg and there is almost no hydrostatic pressure in the renal pelvis. Urine is transported from the renal pelvis to the urinary bladder by peristalsis in the ureters. The ureters enter the urinary bladder at an oblique angle to form a functional valve, called the ureterovesicular valve (see Fig. 9.5). Once urine has entered

the bladder, its backflow into the ureters is prevented as the bladder fills.

Micturition Reflexes

Micturition is the physiologic term for emptying of the bladder. The bladder is allowed to fill before emptying because of reflexes having control centers in the sacral spinal cord and brain stem. Receptors in the bladder wall are stretched during filling and have the reflex ability (activation of sacral spinal cord reflex center) of allowing urine to be evacuated through the neck of the bladder and external sphincter. The brain stem reflex center, however, prevents contraction of the bladder and relaxation of the external sphincter that would otherwise occur. Normal filling occurs and the cerebral cortex is aroused when sufficiently full. Voluntary control intervenes and micturition is permitted, when appropriate. Once micturition proceeds, complete emptying is ensured because of another reflex that involves flow receptors in the urethra. As long as urine is flowing, bladder contraction continues until there is no further flow (the bladder is empty).

The parasympathetics are the sole motor nerve supply to the detrusor muscle of the bladder. The sympathetics have no effect on micturition but appear to constrict the neck of the bladder during ejaculation, thus directing the ejaculate through the penile urethra rather than having backflow into the bladder.

Characteristics of Mammalian Urine

COMPOSITION. Urine is formed to keep the composition of the extracellular fluids constant, and, generally, most substances that are present in extracellular fluid are also present in urine. Also, the composition of urine varies depending on whether substances are being conserved or excreted.

COLOR. Urine is usually yellow in color. The yellow color is derived from bilirubin that was excreted into the intestine and reabsorbed as urobilinogen. Much of the urobilinogen is reexcreted by the liver into the intestine, but urobilinogen that bypasses the liver can be excreted by the kidneys into the urine. The various bilinogens are colorless but are spontaneously oxidized on exposure to oxygen. Thus urobilinogen, when partially oxidized, is known as urobilin, and it is largely responsible for the yellow color of urine.

ODOR. The odor of urine is characteristic for a species and is probably influenced by diet. For example, the characteristic odor imparted to human urine after the ingestion of asparagus is caused by the formation of asparagine (the amide form of the amino acid, aspartic acid).

CONSISTENCY. Urine has a watery consistency in most species. Horse urine is somewhat thick and syrupy, however, because of the secretion of mucus from glands in the pelvis of the kidneys and the upper part of the ureters. The urine of the horse has high concentrations of carbonates and phosphates, which seem to precipitate on standing. The secretion of mucus probably provides a carrier for the precipitated carbonates and phosphates and prevents their collection in the renal pelvis.

NITROGENOUS COMPONENT. The principal nitrogenous constituent of mammalian urine is urea. Urea is formed by the liver from ammonia, which is produced during amino acid metabolism. The body expends considerable energy in producing urea so that the toxicity of ammonia can be avoided. As compared to ammonia, urea is relatively nontoxic at normal concentrations.

OUTPUT. The output of urine varies; certain terms are used for its description. Polyuria means increased urine output, oliguria means decreased output, and anuria describes the condition of no urine output.

Continence is the normal condition of storing urine in the bladder while it fills. Continence is maintained by continuous tone of the muscle of the external sphincter and by closure of the posterior urethra (contraction of the bladder wall muscle opens the posterior urethra), which is augmented by elastic tissue. An incontinent animal dribbles urine at frequent intervals instead of permitting the bladder to fill. Spinal injuries above the sacrum are frequently the cause; in such injuries, the brain stem reflexes, which are initiated by the sacral reflexes as the bladder fills, are not effective in preventing emptying. Dysuria is a term used for describing difficult or painful urination.

RENAL CLEARANCE

Renal clearance is a measurement of the kidney's ability to remove substances from the plasma. It can be determined by the formula:

$$C_x = (U_x \dot{V})/P_x$$
(Eq. 9.1)

where C_x = clearance of substance x (ml/min), U_x = concentration of x in urine

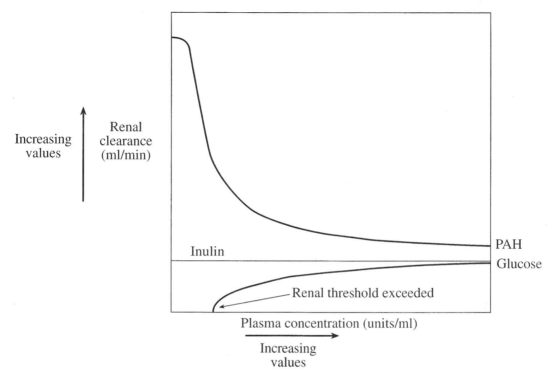

Figure 9.19. Effect of tubular reabsorption and tubular secretion on renal clearance. Glucose represents a substance that is reabsorbed from the tubules, *p*-aminohippuric acid (PAH) represents a substance that is secreted into the tubule but not reabsorbed, and inulin represents a substance that is neither reabsorbed nor secreted by the renal tubules. All of these substances are freely filtered at the glomerulus and enter the tubules. The decrease for renal clearance of PAH and the increase of renal clearance for glucose indicates a point at which their renal clearance is changed as their plasma concentration increases. See text for details.

(mg/ml), $\dot{V}$ = rate of urine formation (ml/min), and P_x = concentration of x in plasma (mg/ml). Thus, if U_x = 130 mg/ml, $\dot{V}$ = 1 ml/min, and P_x = 2 mg/ml, then C_x = (130 × 1)/2 = 65 ml/min.

$U_x \dot{V}$ (130 mg/ml × 1 ml/min = 130 mg/min) is the rate at which substance x is excreted. Accordingly, dividing the excretion rate by the concentration of the substance in plasma (130 mg/min divided by 2 mg/ml = 65 ml/min) gives the amount of plasma that would be needed each minute to provide the quantity that is excreted. Only a few substances are removed completely from the blood as it circulates through the kidney, so the renal clearance measurement does not actually describe an event, but only provides values for comparison. For example, a renal clearance value for urea of 50 ml/min does not mean that 50 ml of the RPF is completely cleared of urea and that the remainder continues through the kidney, with none extracted. Rather, it means that each ml of the RPF contributes urea to that which is excreted, but the amount excreted in the urine each minute would require all the urea in 50 ml of the RPF.

A substance such as inulin in the plasma is filtered freely at the glomerulus. It is not reabsorbed from the tubular fluid, nor is it secreted into the tubular fluid from the peritubular capillaries. All that is filtered is excreted. Because it is freely filtered, any increase in plasma concentration results in a similar excretion rate. Plasma clearance does not change (Fig. 9.19). A substance such as glucose is filtered freely at the glomerulus and, as long as the renal threshold is not reached, all that is filtered is reabsorbed and the renal clearance is zero. If the plasma concentration is increased to the point where the renal threshold is surpassed, however, part of the filtered glucose is excreted and renal clearance values begin to rise. These values can never equal the renal clearance values for inulin because some of the glucose filtered will always be reabsorbed (Fig. 9.19). A plasma substance such as *p*-aminohippuric acid (PAH), which is freely filtered and is not reabsorbed from the tubules, but is secreted into the tubules (increases the tubular load), will always have a renal clearance value greater than that of inulin because a greater proportion of the plasma load is excreted (Fig. 9.19).

Thus, information can be obtained about how different substances are handled by the kidney. Also, the health status of the kidneys can be assessed by these measurements. A diseased kidney has a lower renal clearance value for inulin than a normal kidney because the excretion rate is diminished as a result of reduced filtration (fewer functional nephrons) and the plasma concentration would be correspondingly higher. Renal clearance measurements are also used pharmacologically to determine how certain drugs alter kidney function and how they are handled by the kidney.

MAINTENANCE OF ACID-BASE BALANCE

Relationship of pH to H+ Concentration

In their role of regulating the composition of the extracellular fluid, the kidneys are important in maintaining a constant hydrogen ion concentration. The pH (negative log of H+ concentration) of the extracellular fluids seldom varies from the normal value of about 7.4. A pH change of 0.3 units doubles or halves the H+ concentration. For example, a pH of 7.4 represents a H+ concentration of 40 nEq/L. A pH of 7.1 and 7.7 represent H+ concentrations of 80 and 20 nEq/L, respectively. In these examples, the H+ has doubled or halved from the normal pH of 7.4. A pH of 7.1 represents severe acidosis and a pH of 7.7 represents severe alkalosis.

Mechanism of H+ Secretion by the Kidneys

The epithelial cells throughout the length of the nephron (except thin segment of the loop of Henle) secrete H+, but about 85% are secreted by the proximal tubule. The mechanism associated with H+ secretion is shown in Figure 9.20. The hydration reaction, $CO_2 + H_2O \leftrightarrow H_2CO_3 \leftrightarrow H^+ + HCO_3^-$ (see Equation 8.1), occurs in the cytoplasm of the tubular epithelial cell and is accelerated by the presence of carbonic anhydrase (an enzyme) within the cytoplasm. CO_2 in the extracellular fluid freely diffuses into the cells. Increased amounts of CO_2 promote more hydration and decreased amounts reduce hydration. After hydration, the H+ formed is secreted into the tubular lumen in exchange for a Na+ (countertransport). The H+ that is secreted combines with the bicarbonate tubular buffer to form H_2CO_3, which is further dehydrated to the CO_2 and H_2O that become a part of urine. Dehydration at this location is facilitated by carbonic anhydrase located on the brush border. The HCO_3^- formed from hydration within the cell diffuses into the extracellular fluid, accompanied by the Na+ exchanged for the H+. The extracellular fluid loses a H+ and gains a HCO_3^-. The gain of HCO_3^- (into the extracellular fluid) and the loss of HCO_3^- (from the tubular fluid) just about balance each other, so that pH equilibrium is maintained. When excess hydrogen ions are produced, another tubular buffer, the phosphates, are used for the exchange with H+ (Fig. 9.21). If

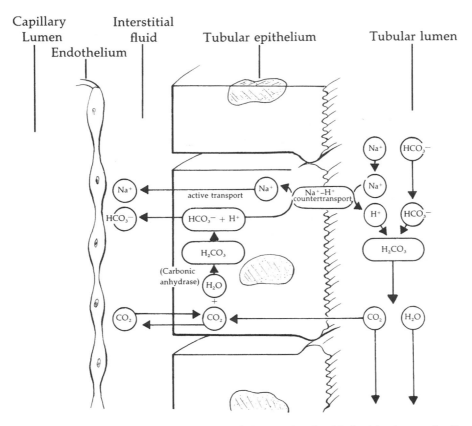

Figure 9.20. Mechanism for the renal secretion of H+ associated with the bicarbonate buffer system in the tubular fluid.

acidosis persists, the formation and secretion of ammonia by the tubular epithelial cells (Fig. 9.22) increases so that the H+ can continue to be secreted without lowering the pH of the tubular fluids.

An increase in intracellular pH of the tubular epithelial cells, as might be caused by acidosis not related to increased CO_2, is also a stimulus for increased secretion of H+ by the tubular epithelial cells.

Role of Respiratory System

Equally important in maintaining acid-base equilibrium in the extracellular fluids is the respiratory system. During transport from the body cells to the lungs, CO_2 diffuses into the erythrocytes and is hydrated under the influence of carbonic anhydrase. The H+ that is formed is buffered, and HCO_3^- diffuses into the plasma. When blood passes through the pulmonary capillaries, the diffusion of CO_2 to the alveoli is favored and the hydration reaction (see previous text, and Equation 8.1) is reversed quickly, so that H+ is lost from the extracellular fluid. Increases in unbuffered H+ cause ventilation of the lungs to increase. Accordingly, the gradient for loss of CO_2 into the pulmonary alveoli increases and hydrogen ions are lost at an increased rate. Furthermore, increases in CO_2 also increase ventilation so that extra hydrogen ions from increased hydration are lost at the lungs. The role of pulmonary ventilation in regulating H+ concentration can thus clearly be seen.

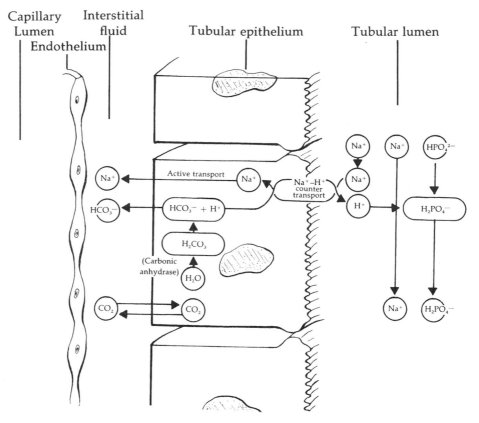

Figure 9.21. Mechanism for the renal secretion of H$^+$ associated with the phosphate buffer system in the tubular fluid.

Chemical Buffer Systems

Chemical buffer systems constitute the first line of defense in maintaining constant pH of the extracellular fluids. The principal chemical buffer systems are the bicarbonate, phosphate, and protein systems.

Mechanisms of Action

The bicarbonate system is represented by $NaHCO_3$ and H_2CO_3; they react with acid and base as follows:

$$HCl + NaHCO_3 \rightarrow H_2CO_3 + NaCl$$
(Eq. 9.2)

$$NaOH + H_2CO_3 \rightarrow NaHCO_3 + H_2O$$
(Eq. 9.3)

In Equation 9.2, the basic component of the system reacts with an acid to form a weaker acid and a salt. In Equation 9.3, the weak acid component reacts with a base to form a weaker base and H_2O.

The phosphate buffer system is represented by NaH_2PO_4 and Na_2HPO_4. They react similarly to acid and base, respectively:

$$HCl + Na_2HPO_4 \rightarrow NaH_2PO_4 + NaCl$$
(Eq. 9.4)

$$NaOH + NaH_2PO_4 \rightarrow Na_2HPO_4 + H_2O$$
(Eq. 9.5)

Proteins act as buffers because their molecules contain a large number of acidic and basic groups. The basic groups (R-NH$_2$) act as buffers by taking up H$^+$ and forming cations (R-NH$_3^+$). The acidic groups (R-COOH) act

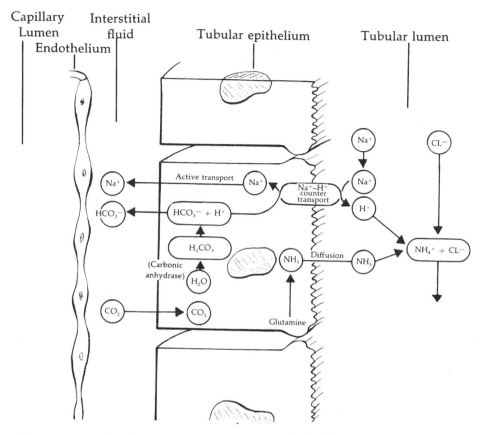

Figure 9.22. Mechanism for the secretion of H⁺ associated with the secretion of ammonia by the tubular epithelial cells.

as buffers by losing H^+ and forming anions ($R\text{-}COO^-$).

Relative Merits of Buffer Systems

The bicarbonate buffer system is rather weak because (1) the pH of the body fluids is about 7.4 and the pK (negative logarithm of the dissociation constant) of the system is 6.1 (buffering power greatest when pH = pK), and (2) the concentration of the buffering elements is not high. The bicarbonate system is unique, however, because it can be adjusted by the respiratory system and the kidneys (i.e., the components are elements of the hydration reaction).

The concentrations of the phosphate buffer components are relatively low in the extracellular fluids, but are higher in the intracellular fluids. Accordingly, the phosphate buffer system is more important as an intracellular buffer, not only because of concentration, but also because its pK (6.8) is closer to intracellular pH. Phosphate buffer is also important as a buffer in the kidney tubular fluids when H^+ is secreted.

Because of their abundance, the proteins of the body cells, plasma, and hemoglobin (protein of red blood cells) are important chemical buffers. Anemic animals (low hemoglobin concentration) quickly become acidic when they are exerted. Hemoglobin is normally the most plentiful chemical buffer in the body.

The various buffer systems are not isolated from each other in the body.

According to the isohydric principal, any condition causing H+ change results in a balance of all the buffer systems, so they change at the same time (the buffers buffer the buffers).

AVIAN RENAL PHYSIOLOGY

There are many similarities between birds and mammals in urine formation and elimination. Also, there are many differences. Similarities include the three phenomena of urine formation: glomerular filtration, tubular reabsorption, and tubular secretion. Also, they are able to modify the concentration of ureteral urine so that it may have an osmolality that is above or below that of plasma. Differences between mammals and birds include in birds the presence of two major nephron types, the presence of a renal portal system, formation of uric acid instead of urea as the major end product of nitrogen metabolism, and postrenal modification of ureteral urine.

Anatomical Features

Avian kidneys are paired retroperitoneal structures that are fitted closely to the bony depressions on the dorsal wall of the fused pelvis. Each kidney has cranial, middle, and caudal lobes. Ureters transport urine from the kidneys to the cloaca (mammalian urinary bladder not present). The cloaca is a common collection site not only for the urinary organs but also for the digestive and reproductive organs (Fig. 9.23). Each lobe has lobules (Fig. 9.24) and a lobule gives the appearance of a mushroom, with its cortex corresponding to the cap of the mushroom and the medulla corresponding to the stem.

Avian kidneys are characterized by having two nephron types, reptilian and mammalian (Fig. 9.25). The reptilian types lack loops of Henle and are located in the cortex. They are not capable of concentrating urine. Mammalian-type nephrons have well-defined loops of Henle that are grouped into a medullary cone (Fig. 9.24), the part of the lobule that corresponds to the stem of a mushroom. Other structures in the medullary cone are those that would be found in the medulla of a mammalian kidney, the collecting ducts and vasa recta. The medullary structures enter at the wider cortical end of the cone. The extent of the vasa recta is shown in Figure 9.26. Osmolality of the medullary interstitial fluid increases from its beginning near the cortex to the tip of the cone. The osmotic gradient is established by the loops of Henle and is maintained by the vasa recta as in mammalian kidneys and permits the excretion of urine that has an osmolality greater than plasma. All tubular fluid, whether from nephrons of the reptilian or the mammalian-type, is exposed to the osmotic gradient because of the exit of the collecting tubules and ducts through the cone to join the common ureteral branch (Fig. 9.24).

Avian kidneys can alternate between the use of reptilian-type and mammalian-type nephrons, depending on the need for water conservation. Greater use of mammalian-type nephrons would promote greater water conservation. When both nephron types are functional, 25% of the filtrate comes from mammalian-type nephrons and 75% comes from reptilian-type nephrons.

Renal Portal System

A unique feature of the avian kidney is its renal portal system for part of the blood supply that perfuses the tubules. The renal portal blood is venous blood that comes to the kidney from the hind limbs via the external iliac and sciatic veins (Fig. 9.27). This venous blood enters the kidney from its periphery, supplying afferent blood to the peritubular capillaries. Within the peritubular capillaries, it is mixed with effer-

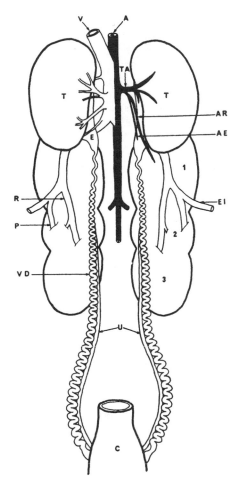

Figure 9.23. Ventral view of organs and associated structures of the dorsal abdominal cavity of a rooster (male chicken). A, abdominal aorta; AE, epididymal artery; AR, cranial renal artery; C, cloaca; E, epididymis; EI, external iliac vein; P, caudal renal portal vein; R, renal vein; T, testis; TA, testicular artery; U, ureters; V, caudal vena cava; VD, ductus deferens; 1, 2, and 3, cranial, middle, and caudal lobes of the left kidney, respectively. From Hodges R. The histology of the fowl. New York: Academic Press, 1974.

ent arteriolar blood coming from the glomeruli (Fig. 9.28). The mixture perfuses the tubules and proceeds to the central vein of the lobule. The renal portal system supplies one-half to two-thirds of the blood to the kidneys. There is a valve, known as a renal portal valve, located at the juncture of the right and left renal veins and their associated iliac veins (Fig. 9.27). Closure of the valve would have the potential of diverting more blood to the renal portal system, and they may be controlled by factors that regulate blood flow to the kidneys.

Uric Acid Formation and Excretion

The metabolism of proteins and amino acids results in the production of nitrogenous end products. Among each of the many different kinds of animals, either ammonia, urea, or uric acid accounts for two-thirds or more of the total nitrogen excreted. Accordingly, animals are divided into three groups depending on whether their main nitrogenous excretory product is ammonia, urea, or uric acid. Because ammonia is a very toxic substance, it must either be excreted rapidly or converted to a substance that is less toxic, such as urea or uric acid. Ammonia excretion is encountered only in animals that are entirely aquatic wherein it can be quickly discharged into their aquatic environment. The urea excreting group is found among mammals and amphibians.

In reptiles and birds, uric acid is formed instead of urea because these animals develop in egg shells that are impervious to water. The excretion of urea obligates water excretion (because of its effective osmotic pressure) and, because there is only limited water in eggs, it must be conserved. Uric acid reaches a certain concentration and it precipitates. As a precipitate (no effective osmotic pressure), there is no water obligated in its excretion. If urea were excreted, it would be necessary to eliminate the liquid urine formed and this is not possible within eggs.

Just as urea is formed in the liver of mammals from ammonia, so is uric acid formed in the liver of birds from ammonia. The kidneys of birds are also a site for the formation of uric acid. Uric acid precipitates in the tubules because the extra blood from the renal portal system that perfuses the tubules leads to greater tubular secre-

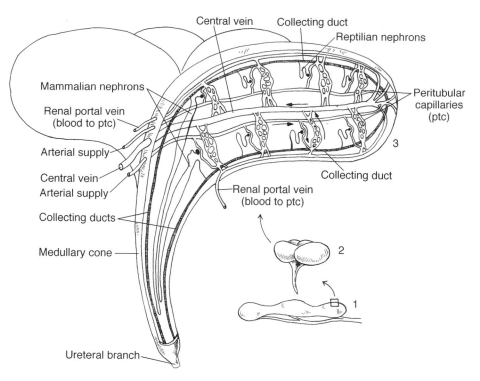

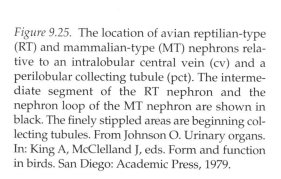

Figure 9.24. Arrangement of reptilian and mammalian nephrons within a lobule. 1, an avian kidney with its three lobes. 2, a lobule from a lobe. 3, the inner structure of a lobule. Reptilian nephrons do not have loops of Henle. Mammalian nephrons are located near the medullary cone and extend their loops of Henle into the cone. The tubular fluid from both nephron types are received by common collecting ducts that also extend into the medullary cone where it is exposed to interstitial fluid concentration gradients similar to mammalian kidneys. All urine from a lobule leaves by a common ureteral branch. Modified from Braun EJ, Dantzler WH. Function of mammalian type and reptilian type nephrons in kidney of desert quail. Am J Physiol 1972;222:617.

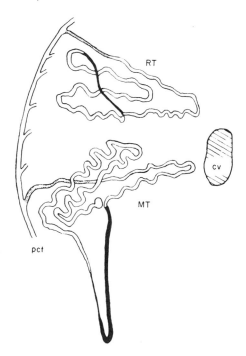

Figure 9.25. The location of avian reptilian-type (RT) and mammalian-type (MT) nephrons relative to an intralobular central vein (cv) and a perilobular collecting tubule (pct). The intermediate segment of the RT nephron and the nephron loop of the MT nephron are shown in black. The finely stippled areas are beginning collecting tubules. From Johnson O. Urinary organs. In: King A, McClelland J, eds. Form and function in birds. San Diego: Academic Press, 1979.

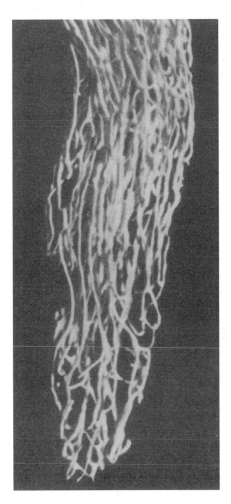

Figure 9.26. The vasa recta and associated capillary plexus from an avian kidney medullary cone. "Microfil" injection via ischiadic artery. From Johnson O. Urinary organs. In: King A, McClelland J, eds. Form and function in birds. San Diego: Academic Press, 1979.

tion and, consequently, greater tubular concentration. The greater amounts in the tubules exceed uric acid solubility, and it precipitates. Uric acid continues in the tubules in its precipitated form and appears in the urine as a white coagulum. Because uric acid is no longer in solution, it does not contribute to the effective osmotic pressure of the tubular fluid, and obligatory water loss is avoided.

Modification of Ureteral Urine

After presentation of ureteral urine to the cloaca, there may be retrograde flow into the colon. In the colon, Na^+ is reabsorbed and water is reabsorbed by osmosis. The same phenomenon could occur in the ceca if retrograde flow occurred to that level. There is no water reabsorbed from the cloaca even though there may be some Na^+ reabsorption.

Concentration of Avian Urine. The permeability of the collecting tubules and collecting ducts responds to ADH as in mammals. Accordingly, with a need for water conservation, the tubular fluid reaches osmotic equilibrium with the interstitial fluid surrounding the tubules, and it becomes hyperosmotic to plasma as collecting tubules and ducts pass through the medullary cone. The hypertonicity of the interstitial fluid of the medullary cone is created by NaCl transport from ascending limbs of the loops of Henle. The maximum concentration of urine that is attainable in birds is much less than for mammals and is about 540 mOsm/kg H_2O, which is the concentration of the interstitial fluid at the tips of the medullary cones. A maximum urine to plasma osmolal ratio would be about 1.58:1.

Urine Characteristics and Flow

Bird urine is cream colored and contains thick mucus. The precipitated uric acid is mixed with the mucus, whereby the mucus secretion facilitates transport of the precipitate similar to the mucus in equine urine that facilitates the transport of the carbonates and phosphates that precipitate. Urine flow for hydrated chickens is reported to be about 18 ml/kg/hr and for hydrated turkeys it is about 30 ml/kg/hr.

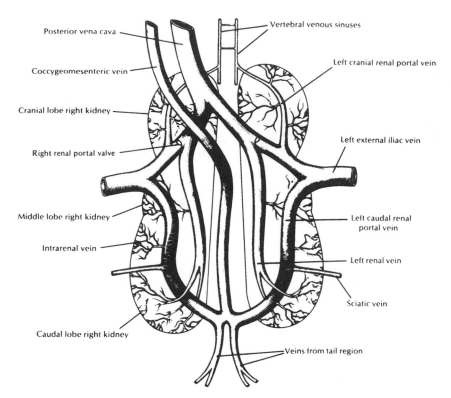

Figure 9.27. The veins associated with the renal portal system of birds. Blood arrives from the hind limbs via the external iliac and sciatic veins. Also shown is a renal portal valve. Its closure has potential for diverting more blood to the renal portal system. From Sturkie PD. Avian physiology. 4th ed. New York: Springer-Verlag, 1986.

Figure 9.28. Intralobular blood flow. Intralobular artery (ia) blood supplies afferent arterioles (aa) going to glomeruli (g). Blood leaving the glomeruli via efferent arterioles (ea) enters the peritubular capillaries and mixes with blood from branches of the renal portal (RP) veins. Peritubular blood enters the central vein (CV) of each lobule. Arrows indicate direction of blood flow. From Johnson O. Urinary organs. In: King A, McClelland J, eds. Form and function in birds. San Diego: Academic Press, 1979.

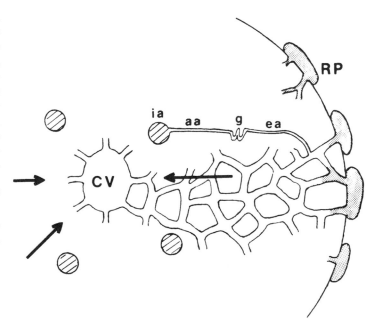

STUDY AIDS—THE KIDNEYS

Structure and Function of the Kidneys

1. Study the shape of kidneys from different species.
2. What is the location of the kidney cortex and medulla? What is the renal hilus and renal pelvis?
3. What is the difference between the ureter and the urethra?
4. What is the relationship between the ureterovesicular junction and prevention of backflow of urine from the bladder to the kidney?
5. Do large breed dogs have significantly greater numbers of nephrons in their kidneys than small breed dogs?
6. What is the difference between a cortical nephron and a juxtamedullary nephron?
7. What is the difference between plasma, glomerular filtrate, tubular fluid, and urine?
8. Be able to follow fluid from plasma in the afferent arteriole through the several components of the nephron to its final discharge from the urethra.
9. Define RBF, RPF, GFR, and FF. Which variable (RBF, RPF, or GFR) represents the largest volume? What is an approximate value for the percentage of glomerular filtrate that is excreted as urine?
10. What are the two capillary beds that perfuse the nephrons? Which one resembles the arterial end of a muscle capillary and which one resembles the venous end?
11. Study the capillary dynamics associated with filtration at the glomerulus (Fig. 9.12).
12. What are the three processes associated with urine formation (Fig. 9.11)?
13. What nephron part accounts for the greatest amount of reabsorption?
14. What is meant by transport maximum and how does it differ from renal threshold?
15. What is the function of the countercurrent mechanism?
16. What is the tone of tubular fluid as it enters the distal tubule?
17. Where is the degree of dehydration of the extracellular fluid detected?
18. Where does ADH exert its influence?
19. What is the direction of water diffusion (i.e., collecting duct to medullary interstitial fluid or vice-versa) when ADH secretion is increased?
20. What blood vessels collect water reabsorbed into the interstitial space of the medulla?
21. What is the approximate urine-to-plasma osmolal ratio in the dog? How does this compare to that of humans? Would greater urine concentration be possible where the ratio is increased?
22. Review the role of angiotensin II in maintaining an appropriate FF in the face of lowered blood pressure. Also, what is its role in adjusting blood pressure back to normal?
23. What is the function of aldosterone? How does aldosterone secretion assist in restoring blood volume?
24. What is the relationship of parathyroid hormone, the kidneys, and calcium ion homeostasis?

Micturition

1. What is meant by micturition?
2. Where are the reflex control centers located for micturition?
3. Talk through the events involved in filling of the urinary bladder and micturition.
4. Which division of the autonomics is involved in micturition?
5. Make a statement about the composition, color, odor, consistency, nitrogenous component, and output of mammalian urine.

Renal Clearance

1. What is meant by renal clearance?
2. Can renal clearance be an index about kidney function?
3. With normal kidney function there is total reabsorption of glucose. What would the renal clearance be for glucose with normal kidney function?

Maintenance of Acid-Base Balance

1. Study the secretion of H^+ by the kidney.
2. Does the secretion of H^+ result in reclaiming bicarbonate for the extracellular fluid?
3. Would greater H^+ production and secretion involve greater "reabsorption" of HCO_3^-?
4. Is pulmonary ventilation increased when the PCO_2 of extracellular fluids increase? Does this result in the greater elimination of H^+?
5. Is hemoglobin a chemical buffer of the body?

Avian Renal Physiology

1. Understand the division of the kidneys of birds into lobes and lobules and the structural detail of a lobule.
2. What are the two nephron types associated with avian kidneys?
3. What is the location of each nephron type within a lobule?
4. What is lacking in the reptilian nephron that makes it incapable of concentrating urine?
5. Where are the loops of Henle of the mammalian nephrons located within a lobule?
6. What structures are located in the medullary cone?
7. Would the tubular fluid from reptilian nephrons be exposed to the osmotic gradient in the medullary cone on its exit from the kidney?
8. What is the exit route for ureteral urine?
9. What is the cloaca?

10. Avian kidneys can alternate between reptilian and mammalian nephron types. Which nephron type would promote greater water conservation?
11. Describe the renal portal system.
12. Where does renal portal blood enter the vascular supply that perfuses the renal tubules?
13. What is the value of two sources of blood perfusing the tubules?
14. What is the value of having uric acid precipitated in the tubules?
15. What is the principal nitrogenous component of avian urine?
16. What organs in birds are sites for the conversion of ammonia to uric acid?
17. What is the principal site for the postrenal modification of ureteral urine?
18. What is the extent of urine concentration in birds (osmolality maximum)?
19. What color is bird urine and what is the function of its being mixed with mucus?
20. How much urine could be produced by a 3-kg hen in a 24-hour period?

SELF-EVALUATION—THE KIDNEYS

1. Which one of the following nephron parts is first encountered by blood entering from the afferent arteriole?
   a. Bowman's capsule
   b. glomerulus
   c. proximal convoluted tubule
   d. loop of Henle
2. Where would one expect to find the lowest hydrostatic pressure?
   a. glomerulus
   b. peritubular capillaries
   c. renal vein
   d. renal artery
3. The composition of glomerular filtrate is the same as tubular fluid.
   a. true
   b. false

4. Which one of the following is not associated with diabetes mellitus?
   a. increased urine formation
   b. renal threshold for glucose is exceeded
   c. increased thirst
   d. lack of antidiuretic hormone (ADH)

5. The principal nitrogenous constituent of mammalian urine is:
   a. amino acids
   b. uric acid
   c. urea
   d. ammonia

6. The kidneys and lungs have no role in the maintenance of body acid-base balance.
   a. true
   b. false

7. Which one of the following measurements would be the lowest at any one time?
   a. renal plasma flow
   b. renal blood flow
   c. glomerular filtration rate

8. Which one of the following nephron parts is associated with the establishment of a high salt concentration in the medulla of the kidney?
   a. Bowman's capsule
   b. proximal tubule
   c. loop of Henle
   d. distal tubule

9. When antidiuretic hormone from the posterior pituitary is released in greater amounts, what will happen to the fluid in the collecting ducts of the kidney?
   a. it will become more dilute
   b. it will remain the same
   c. it will become more concentrated

10. Which one of the following nephron parts accounts for the largest amount of water, glucose, amino acid, and vitamin reabsorption?
   a. glomerulus
   b. distal tubule
   c. proximal tubule
   d. collecting tubule

11. Tubular fluid is transported from Bowman's capsule to the renal pelvis by:
   a. action of cilia
   b. peristalsis
   c. hydrostatic pressure gradient
   d. bucket brigade

12. Which one of the following hormones promotes the tubular reabsorption of Na^+ and the tubular secretion of K^+?
   a. antidiuretic hormone
   b. secretin
   c. aldosterone
   d. oxytocin

13. If excess glucose fails to be reabsorbed (renal threshold exceeded), the effective osmotic pressure in the tubular lumen:
   a. increases
   b. decreases
   c. becomes ineffective

14. Loss of solute (Na^+, Cl^-) and retention of H_2O that occurs in the ascending limb of the loop of Henle causes the tubular fluid to be _____ as compared to plasma.
   a. hypotonic
   b. hypertonic
   c. isotonic

15. What prevents the backflow of urine from the bladder into the ureters?
   a. angle of ureter entrance at the ureterovesicular junction
   b. a discrete muscular sphincter
   c. constant peristaltic waves toward the bladder
   d. there is nothing to prevent it

16. The physiologic term for emptying the bladder is:
   a. parturition
   b. micturition
   c. defecation
   d. ammunition

17. A renal clearance value for urea of 50 ml/min means that:
    a. 50 ml of the RPF are completely cleared of their urea and the remainder continue through the kidney with none extracted
    b. 50 ml of filtrate are formed each minute and all of the urea is excreted
    c. each ml of the RPF contributes urea to that which is excreted but the amount excreted in the urine each minute would require all of the urea in 50 ml of the RPF

18. What hormone acts upon the kidney to activate vitamin D which in turn increases Ca^{2+} absorption from the intestine?
    a. calcitonin
    b. thyroxine
    c. aldosterone
    d. parathyroid hormone

19. Increases in P_{CO_2} from poor ventilation would increase the secretion of H^+s by the kidney.
    a. true
    b. false

20. Increased $[H^+]$ caused by poor kidney function and consequent reduced H^+ secretion would stimulate ventilation and increase CO_2 loss, which would assist in lowering $[H^+]$.
    a. true
    b. false

21. Which one of the following nephron components is lacking in reptilian nephrons?
    a. proximal tubule
    b. loop of Henle
    c. distal tubule
    d. collecting tubule

22. Renal portal system blood is:
    a. venous blood
    b. arterial blood

23. Reptilian nephron tubular fluid goes directly to the ureters and escapes the medullary cones where it could become concentrated.
    a. true
    b. false

24. The avian nephron type that provides for water conservation is the:
    a. reptilian nephron
    b. mammalian nephron

25. Renal portal blood enters the vascular supply perfusing the renal tubules at the level of the:
    a. glomerulus
    b. peritubular capillaries
    c. vasa recta
    d. vena cava

26. The principal nitrogenous component of avian urine is:
    a. ammonia
    b. urea
    c. uric acid

27. Uric acid precipitates in the renal tubules in order to:
    a. avoid ammonia toxicity
    b. avoid obligation of water excretion
    c. make it more slippery
    d. have a better mix with feces

28. Ammonia is converted to uric acid in birds:
    a. in the liver
    b. in the kidneys
    c. in the liver and kidneys

29. Water reabsorption from urine deposited in the cloaca may occur in the:
    a. cloaca
    b. colon
    c. colon and cecum

30. A urine to plasma osmolal ratio of 3:1 is common in birds.
    a. true
    b. false

Suggested Readings

Cormack DH. Ham's histology. 9th ed. Philadelphia: JB Lippincott, 1987.

Johnson OW. Urinary organs. In: King AS, McClelland J, eds. Form and function in birds, Vol. 1. New York: Academic Press, 1979:183–235.

Laiken ND, Fanestil DD. Body fluids and renal function. In: West JB, ed. Best & Taylor's physiological basis of medical practice, Sect. 4. 12th ed. Baltimore: Williams & Wilkins, 1990:438–544.

Reece WO. The kidneys. In: Swenson MJ, Reece WO, eds. Dukes' physiology of domestic animals. 11th ed. Ithaca, NY: Cornell University Press, 1993:573—603.

Schmidt-Nielsen B, O'Dell R. Structure and concentrating mechanism in the mammalian kidney. Am J Physiol 1961;200:1120.

Straffen RA. The urinary tract. In: Brobeck JR, ed. Best & Taylor's physiological basis of medical practice. 10th ed. Baltimore: Williams & Wilkins, 1979:5-95–5-102.

Sturkie PD. Kidneys, extrarenal salt excretion, and urine. In: Sturkie PD, ed. Avian physiology. 4th ed. New York: Springer-Verlag, 1986:359–382.

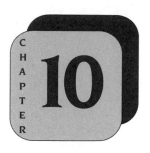

Digestion and Absorption

The maintenance of life requires that animals obtain nutrients essential for the body processes from food. Animals can live for a period of time without food; in such a situation, the body stores of energy and finally the tissues themselves are broken down and metabolized through biochemical conversion. During prolonged and continued deprivation of food, however, death finally ensues as a result of starvation.

It is generally believed that food is in the body after its acquisition and ingestion, but the digestive tract is a hollow, tubelike structure that extends from the mouth to the anus, so materials within its lumen are still, strictly speaking, outside the body. Therefore, the acquisition of food must be followed by processes that divide food into smaller parts through both physical and chemical means, so that the structural units or other simple chemical compounds can finally enter the body by crossing the intestinal barrier. The process associated with this division (or, as often stated, degradation of food to more basic units) is called digestion, and the process of crossing the intestinal epithelium and entering

the blood is called absorption. The reactions and conversions necessary to provide energy, build tissues, and synthesize secretions constitute intermediary metabolism. The continuance of intermediary metabolism in the body depends on digestion and absorption.

THE DIGESTIVE TRACT

Animals are classified, according to the diet in their natural state, as carnivorous, omnivorous, or herbivorous. The extremes are represented by the carnivorous, or flesh-eating, animals and by the herbivorous, or plant-eating animals. Those subsisting on both flesh and plants are omnivorous animals. Because of the diversity of diet, various parts of the digestive system developed in different ways. Whereas the dog, a carnivorous animal, has an inconspicuous cecum, the horse, a herbivorous animal, has a voluminous cecum. The cecum of the horse facilitates the digestion of coarse plant materials by microbial fermentation. Only minimal fermentation is

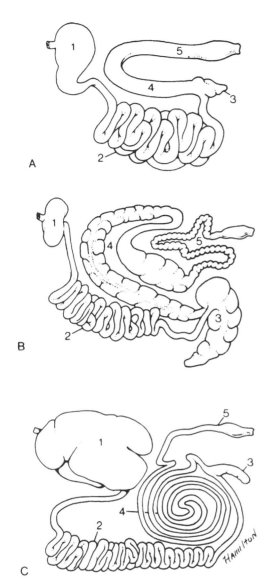

not only has a relatively long small intestine for digesting and absorbing foodstuffs not requiring fermentation, but it also has an expanded part of its colon in which fermentation of the fibrous parts of its diet takes place. A comparison of the gastrointestinal tracts of the dog, horse, and cattle (a ruminant) is shown in Figure 10.1.

The principal parts of the digestive tract as it courses through the body are the mouth, teeth, tongue, pharynx, esophagus, stomach, small intestine, and large intestine. The salivary glands, liver, and pancreas serve as accessory organs of the digestive tract. Generally, the digestive tract among the various animal species has the same parts, but the size and function of the parts for any one species differ according to the characteristics of the natural diet.

Mouth

The mouth is the most cranial part of the digestive tract and is often referred to as the oral cavity. It is where food is first received and where reduction in the size of food particles begins. Associated with reduction in size, the food particles are mixed with saliva, so that subsequent swallowing of the food mass (bolus) is facilitated. The teeth and tongue are structures within the mouth that assist digestion.

Teeth

The teeth mechanically reduce the size of ingested food particles by grinding, and at the same time increase the surface area of the food for chemical and microbiologic degradation. Teeth are also used for cutting; in this way food can first be presented to the mouth. In some species, the teeth serve a protective function when used to inflict wounds and a food-gathering function when used to capture and kill other animals.

The four types of teeth are described according to their location and function. The incisors are the most forward teeth in the mouth and are used principally for cut-

Figure 10.1. Comparisons of gastrointestinal tracts of the dog (**A**), of the horse (**B**), and of cattle (**C**). *1,* Stomach; *2,* small intestine; *3,* cecum; *4,* ascending colon in dog; large colon in horse; coiled colon (ansa spiralis) in cattle; *5,* descending colon. From Dyce KM, Sack WO, Wensing CJG. Textbook of veterinary anatomy. 2nd ed. Philadelphia: WB Saunders, 1996.

necessary in the dog, so its cecum is minimally developed. Whatever fermentation is required in the dog occurs mainly in the colon. The pig is an omnivorous animal. It

TABLE 10.1. Dental Formulas and Eruption Times for Permanent Teeth

Teeth	Horse	Cow	Sheep	Pig	Dog
	PERMANENT FORMULA				
	3 1 3 or 4 3	0 0 3 3	0 0 3 3	3 1 4 3	3 1 4 2
	2(I–C–P—M–)	2(I–C–P–M–)	2(I–C–P–M–)	2(I–C–P–M–)	2(I–C–P–M–)
	3 1 3 3	4 0 3 3	4 0 3 3	3 1 4 3	3 1 4 3
	PERMANENT ERUPTION				
Incisors					
I1	2½ yr	1½–2 yr	1–1½ yr	1 yr	3–5 mo
I2	3½ yr	2–2½ yr	1½–2 yr	16–20 mo	3–5 mo
I3	4½ yr	3 yr	2½– 3 yr	8–10 mo	4–5 mo
I4		3½–4 yr	3½–4 yr		
Canines					
C	4–5 yr			9–10 mo	4–6 mo
Premolars					
P1	5–6 mo	2–2½ yr	1½–2 yr	12–15 mo	4–5 mo
P2	2½ yr	1½ -2½ yr	1½–2 yr	12–15 mo	5–6 mo
P3	3 yr	2½–3 yr	1½–2 yr	12–15 mo	5–6 mo
P4	4 yr			12–15 mo	5–6 mo
Molars					
M1	9–12 mo	5–6 mo	43–5 mo	4–6 mo	5–6 mo
M2	2 yr	1½ yr	9–12 mo	8–12 mo	6–7 mo
M3	3½–4 yr	2–2½ yr	1½–2 yr	18–20 mo	6–7 mo

I, incisors; C, canines; P, premolars; M, molars; wk, week; mo, month; yr, year.

From Frandson RD, Spurgeon TL. Anatomy and physiology of farm animals. 5th ed. Philadelphia: Lea and Febiger, 1992.

ting; they are sometimes called "nippers." Next to the incisors are the canine teeth, also known as fangs, eye teeth, and tusks. The shape of the canines permits their use for tearing and separation of a food mass. The premolars are located posterior to the canines, and their shape and size is more suitable for grinding. This function is also carried out by larger teeth located caudal to them, the molars. The molars and premolars are collectively called cheek teeth.

A dental formula indicates the numbers of incisors (I), canines (C), premolars (P), and molars (M) on one side of the mouth. For the permanent teeth of the cow, the dental formula is I 0/4 C 0/0 P 3/3 M 3/3. The numerator of the fraction represents the teeth in the upper jaw and the denominator represents the teeth in the lower jaw. The formula represents the number of teeth on one side of the mouth, so the total number is twice that shown. For the cow

the total number of teeth is 32. The cow has a firm dental pad in place of the upper incisors, which provides for the compression necessary to shear forage against the lower incisors. Dental formulas and eruption times for various species are listed in Table 10.1.

Several terms are used to describe the exposed surfaces of a tooth. The grinding (table) surface makes contact with a tooth from the opposite jaw and is the principal wearing surface. The side of the tooth next to the tongue is called the lingual surface. The outer surface is labial if next to the lips and buccal if next to the cheek. The contact surface is next to a neighboring tooth of the same arcade (row). The upper arcades of cheek teeth (molars and premolars) are slightly wider apart than the lower arcades of cheek teeth. Also, the upper cheek teeth have a wider table surface than the lower cheek teeth. The rotation of the jaw associ-

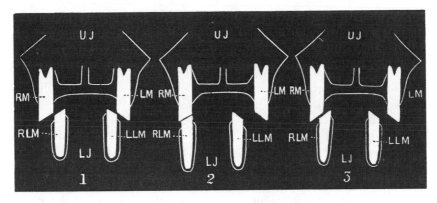

Figure 10.2. Schematic transverse section of the upper and lower jaws of the horse at the level of the fourth molars showing the position of the tables of the teeth during rest and mastication. *1.* Position of the teeth during rest. The outside edge of the lower row is in apposition with the inside edge of the upper. *2.* Jaws fully crossed, masticating from left to right (lower jaw movement). The tables of both upper and lower molars now rest on each other. *3.* Position halfway through mastication. The outer half of the lower teeth wears against the inner half of the upper. Note the potential for developing "points" on the cheek side of the uppers and on the tongue side of the lowers (*UJ,* upper jaw; *LJ,* lower jaw; *RM,* right molar; *LM,* left molar, *RLM,* right lower molar; *LLM,* left lower molar). From Smith F. Manual of veterinary physiology. 5th ed. Chicago: Alexander Eger, 1921.

ated with chewing usually provides for even wear of the table surfaces, but uneven wear can develop, particularly in horses, in which points are formed that inflict injury to the buccal or lingual membranes (Fig. 10.2). Eating becomes painful and the points must be filed off with a dental rasp. The procedure of removing the points is referred to as floating the teeth.

The age of horses can be approximated by examining the lower incisors, determining whether the permanent incisors have erupted, and examining for characteristics associated with wear. The three pairs are the central (I1), intermediate (I2), and corner (I3) incisors, respectively, according to their location from the midline to the outside. A rule of thumb for their eruption is 2½, 3½, and 4½ years for I1, I2, and I3, respectively. A horse is said to have a full mouth when all three pairs of permanent incisors have erupted.

Wear characteristics are related to tooth structure (Fig. 10.3A,B). The progression of wear is shown in Figure 10.3C. A mouth is said to be in wear when two complete enamel rings are present on the table surface of each incisor. Approximate ages for each pair to be in wear are 6, 7, and 8 years for I1, I2, and I3, respectively. Finally, a judgment is made about disappearance of the infundibulum (which eliminates the inner enamel ring) and appearance of the pulp cavity (dental star). The loss of the inner enamel ring and appearance of the dental star occur at about 11, 12, and 13 years of age for each pair of I1, I2, and I3, respectively; a horse has a smooth mouth when these occur in all three pairs of incisors. A rough approximation of age in a horse as determined by the incisors is 5, 10, and 15 years for full mouth, in wear, and smooth mouth. Much variation occurs naturally, depending on diet and associated wear. The practice of aging horses by "mouthing" was more common when dealers abounded in the draft horse market. Similar practices occur in cattle and sheep husbandry and are related more to eruption than to wear characteristics.

Tongue

The tongue is a muscular organ used to maneuver the food mass within the mouth. The tongue can be differentiated microscopically from other muscle tissues because it has fibers oriented in three directions. The multidirectional orientation attests to its extreme mobility. The tongue not only moves food to the table surfaces of the cheek teeth, but also serves as a plunger to move food into the esophagus. It assists some animals in seizing food and bringing it to the mouth.

The rough surface of the tongue is provided for by numerous projections, known as papillae. These provide traction for moving the food within the mouth of the animal and help in grooming their own or their offspring's hair surface (Fig. 10.4).

The digestive process is assisted by the discriminatory taste buds located on the tongue surface within the vallate and fungiform papillae (see Chapter 2). Discrimination is a more significant factor when food is obtained in its native

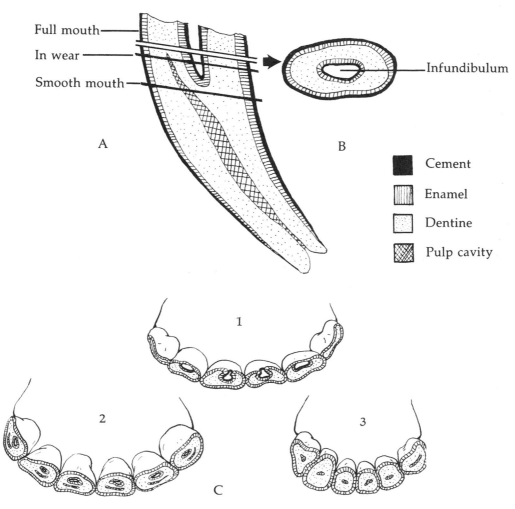

Figure 10.3. Incisors of the horse showing wear characteristics. **A.** Longitudinal section. **B.** Transverse section. **C.** Table surfaces illustrating full mouth (*1*), in wear (*2*), and smooth mouth (*3*).

(unprocessed) state. Distinction can then be made between harmful and proper foods.

Pharynx

The pharynx is the common passageway for food and air and is located posterior to the mouth (Fig. 10.5). The pharynx opens into the mouth and into the nasal cavities, eustachian tubes, larynx, and esophagus. During its passage through the pharynx, food is prevented from entering the larynx and nasal cavities because of reflex and

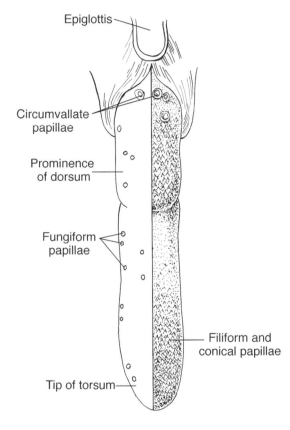

Figure 10.4 A view of the dorsal surface (dorsum linquae) of a bovine tongue with special emphasis on its roughness provided by the papillae. In front of the prominence are large and horny filiform and conical papillae with sharp points directed backward. These papillae impart to the tip especially, its rasp-like roughness making it very efficient in the prehension of food. One-half of tongue not shown with fungiform and conical papillae for contrast.

mechanical factors associated with swallowing. The eustachian tubes are air passages leading from the pharynx to the middle ear that provide for air pressure within the middle ear to be equalized to atmospheric pressure. Distortions of the tympanic membrane (eardrum) that might otherwise occur are thereby prevented.

Esophagus

The esophagus is a muscular tube extending from the pharynx to the stomach. During its course to the stomach, the esophagus traverses the thorax within the mediastinal space, in which it is subjected to pressure changes associated with that space. The esophagus finally passes through its opening in the diaphragm and enters the stomach within the abdominal cavity. Food and water are moved from the pharynx to the stomach by contraction waves in the muscular wall. The esophagus is normally closed at the pharyngeal end by tonic activity of the cranio-esophageal sphincter. It remains closed at the opening to the stomach (the cardia), not because of an anatomic sphincter, but because of a closure that is physiologic in nature. The lumen of the esophagus is normally closed, which produces folds in its inner surface. During passage of a bolus the folds are extended, so that a minimum of stretch is necessary. Unusually large objects extend the folds and stretch the mucosal and submucosal layers, and they can also become lodged at points of constriction (e.g., the thoracic inlet).

The pharyngeal opening to the esophagus lies just above the glottis, the opening to the larynx. On its way to the stomach, the esophagus courses along the left side of the trachea. Bolus transport can be observed by watching the left side of the neck (this is particularly apparent in cattle).

The muscle fibers of the esophagus are arranged circularly and longitudinally. In

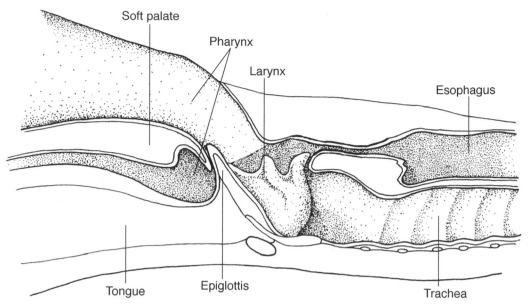

Figure 10.5 Sagittal section of the pharynx, esophagus, and trachea. The darker stippled areas relate to the route of food intake. Reflexes associated with swallowing facilitate the safe passage of food from the pharynx into the esophagus.

most animals they are striated, but in some animals a part of the caudal portion is smooth muscle. Because of the muscular nature of the esophagus, it is recovered at slaughter as an edible source of certain meat products. The esophagus is sometimes referred to as the *wiesand* (from the German for esophagus).

Stomach

Food is received by the stomach for storage (pending further digestion) and for the beginning of digestion. Because the stomach serves a storage function, it is a dilated portion of the digestive tube. As viewed from the outside, it is seen to be subdivided into parts, which are continuous with one another. The cardia (entrance area) is located nearest the esophagus and is continued by the fundus, which is the dome-shaped part of the stomach. The fundus is adjacent to the corpus (the rounded base or bottom) and together they constitute the middle portion, the one most subject to

enlargement. The antrum is the constricted part of the stomach that joins the duodenum. The inner aspect of the stomach has specific regions according to cell type: the esophageal, cardiac gland, fundic gland, and pyloric gland regions. The fundic gland region includes the entire space between the cardiac gland (nearest the cardia) and pyloric gland regions (near the pylorus); these glands are sometimes called the gastric glands. The cardiac, gastric, and pyloric glands all secrete mucus. In addition, the gastric glands secrete hydrochloric acid (HCl) and pepsinogen by their parietal and neck chief cells, respectively. The pyloric glands also secrete the hormone gastrin.

The esophageal region is the area immediately around the cardia. The epithelium of the esophageal region is continuous with the lining of the esophagus. It varies in size, depending on the species, and is nonglandular. The several regions of the stomach lining for the horse, pig, and ruminant are shown in Figure 10.6.

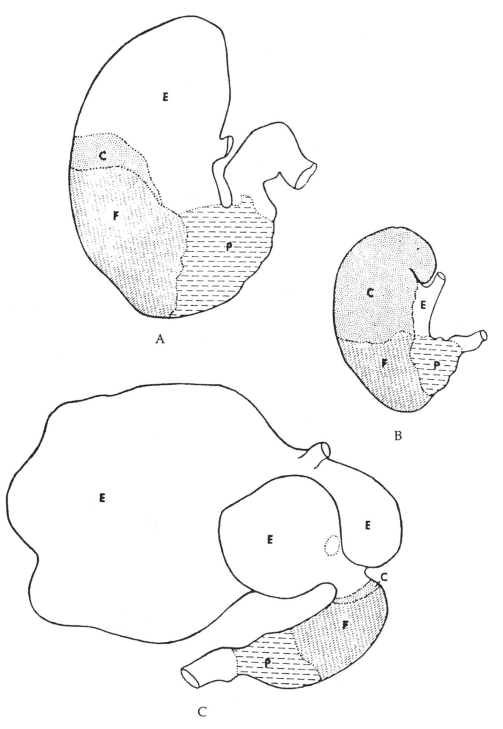

Figure 10.6. Inner regions of the stomach. **A.** Horse. **B.** Pig. **C.** Ruminant. *E*, Esophageal region; *C,* cardiac gland region; *F*, fundic gland region; *P*, pyloric gland region. From Frandson RD. Anatomy and physiology of farm animals. 5th ed. Philadelphia: Lea & Febiger, 1992.

The previously described stomach is often referred to as the nonruminant stomach, but it is also characteristic of the "true stomach" of the ruminant. The other compartments of the ruminant stomach precede the true stomach and are called forestomachs (the rumen, reticulum, and omasum); these are followed by the true stomach, or abomasum. The primary function of the forestomachs in ruminants is to allow for fermentation necessitated by their diet. Ruminant digestion is considered in more detail in the section called The Ruminant Stomach.

Small Intestine

The stomach contents enter the small intestine after their preparation in the stomach. The small intestine is comprised of three sections as it proceeds caudally from the antrum: the duodenum, jejunum, and ileum. The duodenum makes a loop as it turns to cross from the right to the left side. Closely related to the duodenum is the pancreas. The duodenum receives pancreatic secretions involved in digestion through a pancreatic duct (Fig. 10.7). The duodenum also receives bile formed in the liver through the common bile duct, which transports bile from the liver or gallbladder to the intestine. Most digestion and absorption takes place in the small intestine for those animals not requiring extensive fermentation of their ingested food.

The inner layer of the small intestine, having intimate contact with the contents of the lumen, is comprised of an epithelial cell layer known as the mucosa (Fig. 10.8). The submucosa is a connective tissue layer that provides space for blood vessels, lymph vessels, and nerve fibers. In addi-

Figure 10.7. Dorsal view of the canine stomach, duodenum, and pancreas. *1,* right lobe of pancreas; *2,* body of the pancreas; *3,* left lobe of pancreas; *4,* pancreatic ducts. The common bile duct is received into the duodenum in close association with the anterior pancreatic duct. From Adams DR. Canine anatomy: a systemic approach. Ames, IA: Iowa State University Press, 1986.

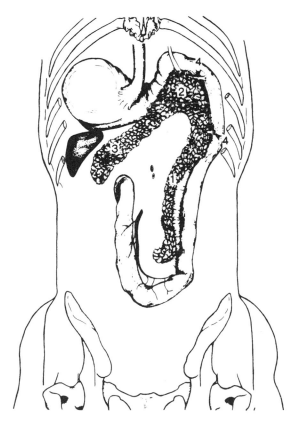

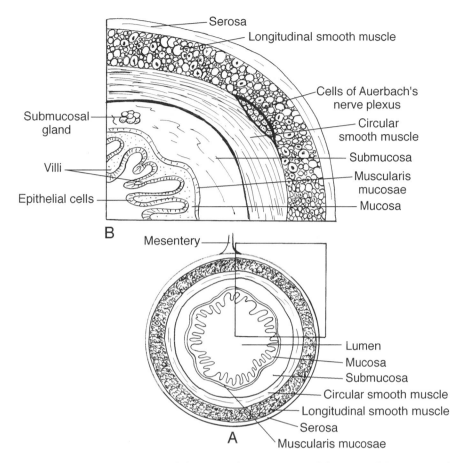

Figure 10.8. Schematic representation of the general organizational features of the mammalian gastrointestinal tract. **A**. Cross-section of small intestine with its mesenteric suspension that envelops the intestine as its serosa. **B**. Boxed section from **A** to show greater detail. The Auerbach nerve plexus controls gastrointestinal movements. Meissner's plexus (not shown) is in the submucosa and it controls secretions and blood flow. The muscularis mucosae produces folds in the mucosa for amplification of surface area.

tion, a sparse layer of smooth muscle fibers is in the submucosa, known as the muscularis mucosae. The muscularis mucosae appears to produce folds in the mucosa, thereby increasing surface area. These folds change location to bring different parts of the intestine into more intimate contact with the luminal contents. Individual fibers from the muscularis mucosae attach to villi and cause villus movement when contracting. This facilitates lymph movement and placement of the villus into new

areas of luminal fluid. Beneath the submucosa are circular and longitudinal muscle layers comprised of smooth muscle fibers. Contraction of these muscles is associated with mixing and propulsive movements of intestinal content.

A nerve network (Meissner's plexus) in the submucosa is important in controlling secretions of the epithelial cells and blood flow. This network (plexus) also serves a sensory function—it receives signals from stretch receptors and from the gut epithe-

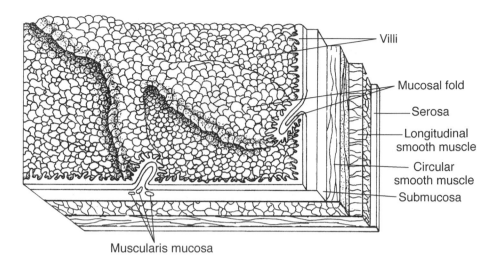

Figure 10.9. A layered section of intestine as viewed from its inner surface. The folds are produced by strategic contraction of the muscularis mucosae. The projections from the surface represent the villi, another means of surface amplification.

lium. Another nerve plexus (Auerbach's plexus), between the inner circular and outer longitudinal muscle layers, is important in controlling gastrointestinal movements. These two nerve plexuses are referred to as the enteric nervous system, and extend from the esophagus to the anus. Although the enteric nervous system has its own "pacemakers" and conduction fibers similar to those of the heart, it also has connections with the autonomic nervous system (sympathetic and parasympathetic fibers) that can alter the degree of activity of the enteric nervous system.

The outer layer of the intestine is the serosa. It covers the intestine and is continuous with the mesentery, which is the suspension for the intestine within the abdominal cavity. The mesentery in turn is continuous with the lining of the abdominal cavity, the peritoneum.

A large surface area is presented to the lumen of the small intestine (Fig. 10.9). The small intestine has considerable length; average lengths for several species are given in Table 10.2. Its length is accommodated within the abdomen by looping and coiling. Another feature is the unfolding of the intestinal surface, which can be observed when the intestine is opened for inspection. The folds, or plications, are covered with villi, and the individual epithelial cells that cover the villi have their own microvilli on the luminal surface. The microvilli provide for the greatest amplification of surface area and constitute the brush border (Fig. 10.10). The amplification just described provides the small intestine with about 600 times more surface area than that of a smooth cylinder (of comparable volume).

Figure 10.11 illustrates the epithelial surface of the small intestine in more detail. The crypts of Lieberkühn are cloistered groups of undifferentiated cells between adjacent villi. These are the only cells of the villi that undergo cell division. Renewal of cells for the villi is provided by the migration of new cells from the crypts toward the tips of the villi. The migration of new cells occurs simultaneously with the continued loss or extrusion of older cells from the villi tips. Moderate physical or functional loss of villus cells, either through attrition or disease, can be replaced by the dividing cells at the crypt.

TABLE 10.2. Lengths of Intestinal Parts for Several Species

Animal	Part of Intestine	Relative Length (%)	Average Absolute Length (m)	Ratio of Body Length to Intestine Length
Horse	Small intestine	75	22.44	1:12
	Cecum	4	1.00	
	Large colon	11	3.39	
	Small colon	10	3.08	
	Total	100	29.91	
Ox	Small intestine	81	46.00	1:20
	Cecum	2	0.88	
	Colon	17	10.18	
	Total	100	57.06	
Sheep and goat	Small intestine	80	26.20	1:27
	Cecum	1	0.36	
	Colon	19	6.17	
	Total	100	32.73	
Pig	Small intestine	78	18.29	1:14
	Cecum	1	0.23	
	Colon	21	4.99	
	Total	100	23.51	
Dog	Small intestine	85	4.14	1:6
	Cecum	2	0.08	
	Colon	13	0.60	
	Total	100	4.82	
Cat	Small intestine	83	1.72	1:4
	Large intestine	17	0.35	
	Total	100	2.07	
Rabbit	Small intestine	61	3.56	1:10
	Cecum	11	0.61	
	Colon	28	1.65	
	Total	100	5.82	

From Argenzio RA. General functions of the gastrointestinal tract and their control and integration. In: Swenson MJ, Reece WO, eds. Dukes' physiology of domestic animals. 11th ed. Ithaca, NY: Cornell University Press, 1993.

The normal villous epithelial cell replacement time (migration from crypt to tip) is faster in younger than in older animals (about 2 to 4 versus 7 to 10 days). The undifferentiated cells can become absorptive, mucus-producing, or endocrine cells, which then perform the necessary functions of the small intestine.

The blood supply and lymphatic vessels for a villus are shown in Figure 10.12. The arrangement of capillaries and lymph vessels provides for capillary exchange of nutrients and fluids and for lymphatic removal of large molecules not accommodated by return to the capillaries. For substances to be absorbed into the blood from the epithelial cells, they must traverse the epithelial cell membrane, basement membrane, interstitial fluid, and capillary membrane. Large molecules not entering the capillaries enter the central lacteals. Blood from the veins of the intestine enters the liver through the portal vein before it returns to the right ventricle of the heart. Lymph from the central lacteals bypasses the liver and reenters the blood through the thoracic duct.

Large Intestine

Contents from the terminal part of the ileum enter the large intestine at the cecum (ileocecal junction), as in the horse, at the colon (ileocolic junction), as in the dog, or

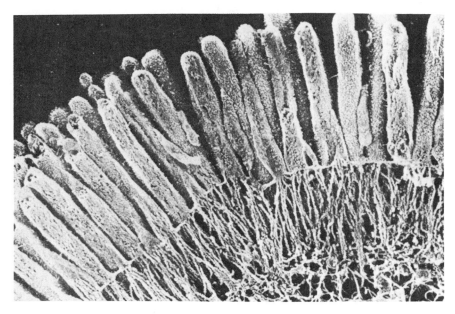

Figure 10.10. Photomicrograph of microvilli extending from a small intestine epithelial cell. The cordlike structures extending downward from the microvilli are contractile actin filaments. From Fawcett DW. Bloom & Fawcett: a textbook of histology. 11th ed. Philadelphia: WB Saunders, 1986. Courtesy of N. Hirokawa and J. Heuser.

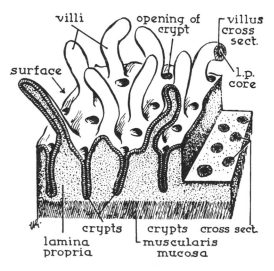

Figure 10.11. Three-dimensional representation of the small intestine lining. The villi are finger-like processes with cores of lamina propria that extend into the lumen. The crypts of Lieberkühn are depressions into the lamina propria. From Ham AW. Histology. 7th ed. Philadelphia: JB Lippincott, 1974.

at the cecum and colon (ileocecocolic junction), as in the ruminant and pig.

The large intestine consists of the cecum and colon. Development of the large intestine varies among animals according to diet. Fermentation occurs to some extent in the large intestine of all animals, but is a more widespread process in the cecum and colon of herbivorous animals. In ruminants, the forestomachs constitute the principal location for fermentation; in nonruminant herbivores (simple herbivores), the cecum and colon provide for fermentation. Enzymatic digestion occurs after fermentation in ruminants, and the bacterial and protozoan cells are themselves digested. In simple herbivores enzymatic digestion precedes fermentation, so only fermentation products and not microbes are available for digestion and absorption.

Food requiring further digestion by fermentation usually enters or is diverted into the cecum unless it is developed

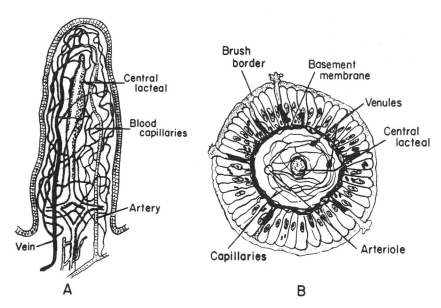

Figure 10.12. Functional organization of the villus. **A.** Longitudinal section. **B.** Cross section showing the epithelial cells and basement membrane. From Guyton AC. Textbook of medical physiology. 7th ed. Philadelphia: WB Saunders, 1991.

poorly, as in the dog. The colon continues from the cecum to its termination at the anus; it consists of ascending, transverse, and descending parts. All animals have a transverse and descending colon, but the arrangement between the cecum and transverse colon differs among species. The dog and cat have an ascending colon between the cecum and transverse colon (Fig. 10.13), but the horse, pig, and ruminant have a counterpart to the ascending colon. In the pig and ruminant this is known as the ansa spiralis (coiled colon) and in the horse the ascending colon is replaced by the large colon, which consists of a ventral colon and a dorsal colon. The ansa spiralis, which resembles a coiled bedspring, is shown in Figure 10.14 for the pig. The coil is directed downward as it leaves the cecum and returns upward, coiled inside the downward coil. The coiled colon for ruminants (Fig. 10.15) resembles a cartwheel. When the colon leaves the cecum it is coiled to the hub; it then reverses at the hub to be recoiled to

the rim, and from there proceeds to the transverse colon.

In the horse the cecum is a large, comma-shaped structure that extends from the pelvic inlet to the abdominal floor, with its tip just behind the diaphragm (Fig. 10.16). It is mainly located on the right side of the horse. The ventral colon continues craniad from the base of the cecum, which is near the pelvic inlet, to the diaphragm, where it turns caudad and returns to the pelvic inlet. Another turn is made cranially and it continues as the dorsal colon, located above the ventral colon. The ventral and dorsal colons can be described as double horseshoes because one appears to be on top of the other. A turn is made at the diaphragm and the dorsal colon continues for a short distance and joins the transverse colon, which is directed toward the left side of the horse. The descending colon in the horse is called the small colon.

The cecum and colon of the pig and horse are sacculated as a result of the presence of

Figure 10.13. Dorsal view of the dog cecum and colon (large intestine). The dog, a carnivore, has no special arrangement for its ascending colon. The rectum is the pelvic portion of the descending colon that terminates at the anus.

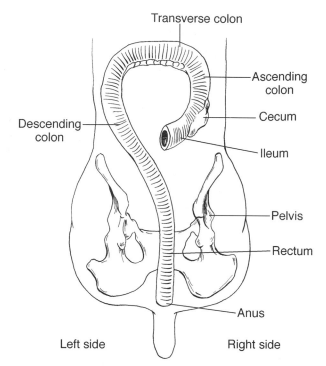

Figure 10.14. Schematic representation of the intestinal tract of the pig. *1,* rectum; *2,* cecum; *3,* ileum; *4,* ansa spiralis (coiled colon); *5,* descending colon; *6,* transverse colon; *7,* second curve of duodenum; *8,* jejunum. From Engel HH, St. Clair LE. Anatomy. In: Leman AD, et al, eds. Diseases of swine. 6th ed. Ames, IA: Iowa State University Press, 1986.

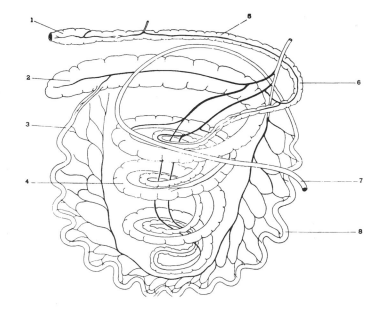

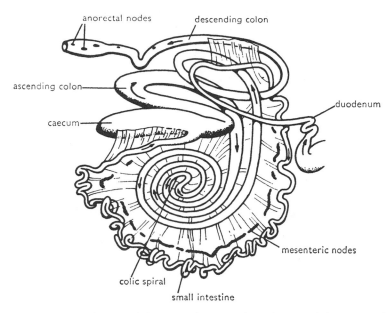

Figure 10.15. Gastrointestinal tract of the cow showing the colic spiral (ansa spiralis). From Dyce KM, Wensing CJG. Essentials of bovine anatomy. Philadelphia: Lea & Febiger, 1971.

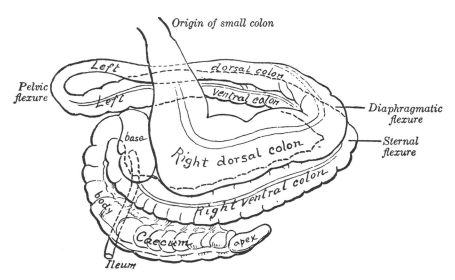

Figure 10.16. Schematic representation of the cecum and colon of the horse. From Getty R. Sisson and Grossman's The anatomy of the domestic animals. 5th Ed. Philadelphia: WB Saunders, 1975.

longitudinal bands of muscle. The sacculations, called haustra, appear to act as buckets. By accommodating extra volume they can help to prolong the retention of contents, thus allowing more time for microbial digestion (Figs. 10.14 and 10.16).

The descending colon terminates at the anus. The part of the descending colon located within the pelvis is known as the rectum. It is relatively dilatable and serves to store feces before its expulsion.

The anus is the junction of the terminal part of the digestive tract with the skin. It closes by means of a muscular sphincter comprised of smooth and striated muscle fibers.

Accessory Glands

The salivary glands, pancreas, and liver supply secretions to the digestive tract and provide for digestion within the lumen. These secretions are in addition to those supplied by the many glands of the stomach and intestine and include electrolytes, water, digestive enzymes, and bile salts. This combination of secretions causes dietary substances to be degraded within the lumen, so that the new substances can interact with the epithelial enzymes.

The salivary glands consist of three pairs of well-defined glands and of some lesser defined, scattered salivary tissue. The larger glands are known as the parotid, mandibular, and sublingual salivary glands. These are connected to the oral cavity by one or more excretory ducts that have openings through the cheeks or tongue. The general location of the salivary glands is shown in Figure 10.17 for the dog.

Salivary glands are serous, mucous, or mixed, depending on their secretion. A serous secretion is a watery, clear fluid as compared to mucus, which is a viscid, tenacious material that acts as a protective covering throughout the digestive tract. A mixed gland secretes both serous and

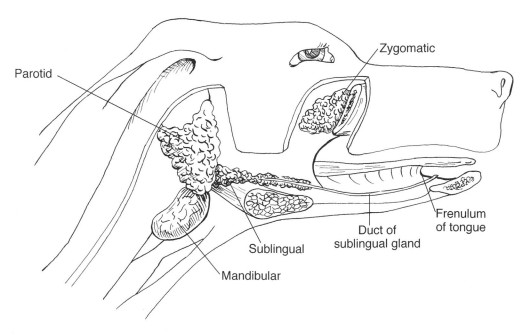

Figure 10.17. Location of salivary glands in the dog. They are paired glands, and only those on the right side are shown. The right mandible has been removed to show the sublingual salivary gland and its duct. The duct empties on a small papilla located near the anterior end of the frenulum (midventral fold of the tongue).

mucous fluids. Blood vessels and nerves enter each gland where the ducts exit. Innervation is provided by the sympathetic and parasympathetic divisions of the autonomic nervous system.

The pancreatic gland has both endocrine and exocrine functions—it produces hormones (endocrine) and digestive secretions (exocrine). The pancreas is always located near the first part of the duodenum and appears as an elongated gland of loosely connected aggregated nodules. The main pancreatic duct enters the first part of the duodenum close to the common bile duct, which comes from the liver (Fig. 10.7). In sheep and goats, the pancreatic duct empties directly into the common bile duct, so that a mixture of bile and pancreatic juice enters the duodenum. The accessory duct, if present, opens a short distance from the main duct. The endocrine portions of the pancreas (islets of Langerhans) are isolated groups of cells scattered throughout the gland. The beta cells produce insulin and the alpha cells produce glucagon. Secretions from the alpha and beta cells are made directly into the blood (ductless secretions). Islet cells are clearly visible with the use of a microscope (Fig. 10.18).

The liver is a multipurpose organ; its production of bile and bile salts is only one of its many important functions. The epithelial cells of liver lobules are metabolically active in synthesis, storage, and metabolic conversions. The location of the liver varies among species, but it is always located immediately behind the diaphragm. In ruminants it tends to be on the right side. The lobules of the liver are clearly demarcated; in the pig they are surrounded by visible connective tissue septa. Other animals have fewer connective tissue divisions and accordingly cannot be seen. The liver and its location in a pig is shown in Figure 10.19.

The liver receives arterial blood for its many cells from the hepatic artery and venous blood through the portal vein from the stomach, spleen, pancreas, and intestines. Blood from both sources is circulated through the sinusoids (second capillary bed of the hepatic portal system). Here it is detoxified and modified before re-entering the central vein (second venous drainage of hepatic portal system) for return to the hepatic veins; and from there it proceeds to the heart through the caudal vena cava. The arrangement of a liver lobule with its triad of vessels and ducts (branches of portal vein, hepatic artery, and bile duct) is shown in Figure 10.20. Bile flows opposite to the direction of blood flow in the hepatic artery and portal vein branch.

The largest part of the macrophage system is present in the liver and is represented by the fixed macrophages, the Küpffer cells. Küpffer cells are highly phagocytic and remove foreign materials entering the blood from the stomach and intestines. They also remove tissue debris, such as old and fragile erythrocytes.

Composition of Foodstuffs

The six basic foodstuffs are classified chemically as carbohydrates, proteins, fats, water, inorganic salts, and vitamins. These are found in varying amounts in the foods that are ingested; a balanced diet must contain some proportion of each. Herbivorous animals can have a diet consisting of roughages and concentrates. Roughages are foods that contain a high percentage of cellulose; they generally have a low digestibility. Concentrates are comprised of seeds from plants and most of their by-products, and are more digestible than roughages. Feeding practices help dictate whether animals receive a high-roughage or high-concentrate diet.

Carbohydrates

Carbohydrates are classified as monosaccharides, disaccharides, or polysaccharides, depending on the number of five (pentose) or six (hexose) carbon units they

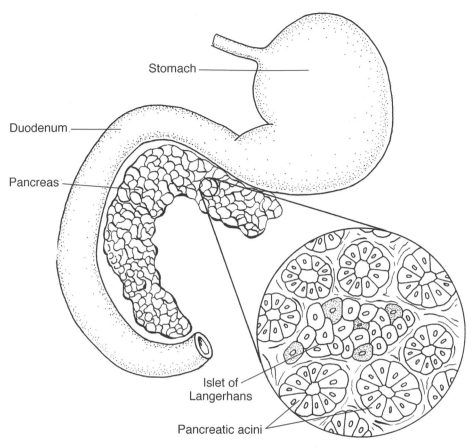

Figure 10.18. Location of the pancreas and its general appearance. The pancreas is always located near the first part of the duodenum and appears as an elongated gland of loosely connected aggregated nodules. The inset from the pancreas shows an islet of Langerhans (endocrine) situated among a number of pancreatic acini, the exocrine (digestive secretions) portion.

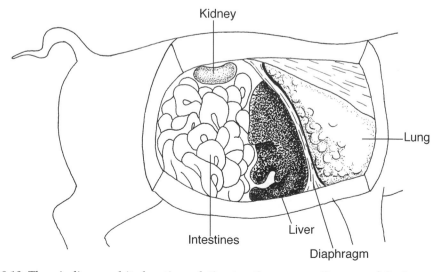

Figure 10.19. The pig liver and its location relative to other organs. Because of the large amount of interlobular connective tissue, the lobules are mapped out sharply. For this reason, the liver is much less friable (easily broken) than that of other animals.

contain. The monosaccharides include ribose (a five-carbon sugar), glucose, fructose, and galactose (Fig. 10.21). The disaccharides are chemical combinations of two molecules of monosaccharides and include sucrose, maltose, and lactose (Fig. 10.22). Disaccharides are degraded (broken down) to monosaccharides through the process of hydrolysis (splitting with water). The hydrolysis of sucrose yields one molecule each of glucose and fructose; the hydrolysis of maltose yields two molecules of glucose; and the hydrolysis of lactose yields one molecule each of glucose and galactose. The polysaccharides are molecules that contain multiple (more than two) numbers of simple sugars, most of which are hexoses. Polysaccharides important to animals

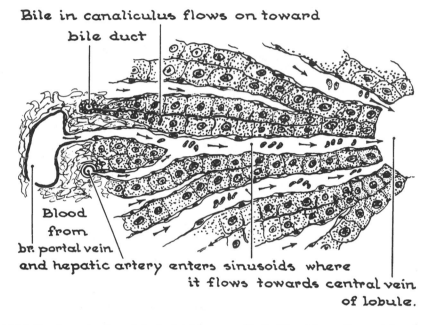

Bile in canaliculus flows on toward bile duct

Blood from br. portal vein and hepatic artery enters sinusoids where it flows towards central vein of lobule.

Figure 10.20. Portion of a liver lobule (highly magnified). Blood from the portal vein and hepatic artery flows into sinusoids (lined with Küpffer cells) and empties into the central vein. Bile travels in the opposite direction in canaliculi to empty into bile ducts in the triad areas. From Ham AW. Histology. 7th ed. Philadelphia: JB Lippincott, 1974.

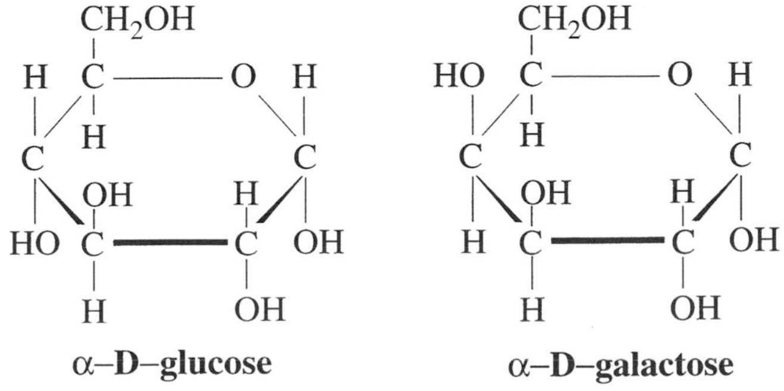

α–D–glucose   α–D–galactose

Figure 10.21. Chemical structure of monosaccharides are represented by glucose and galactose.

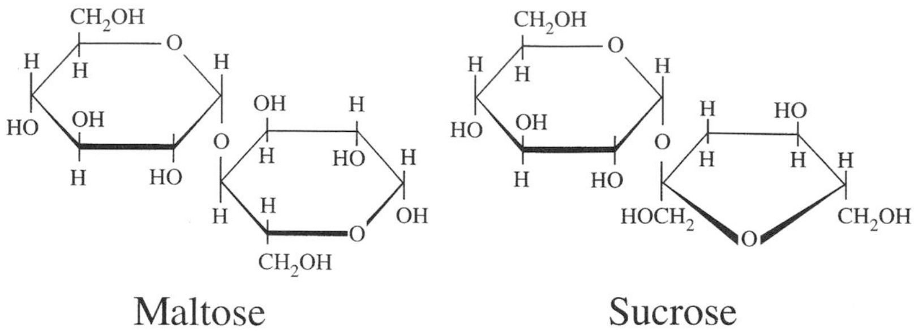

CH₂OH ... O ... H ... H ... H ... HO ... OH ... OH ... H ... H ... HO ... O ... H ... HO ... H ... H ... H ... OH ... CH₂OH

CH₂OH ... O ... H ... H ... H ... HO ... OH ... H ... HO ... H ... H ... H ... HO ... H ... H ... HOCH₂ ... O ... CH₂OH

Maltose   Sucrose

Figure 10.22. Chemical structure of disaccharides as represented by maltose and sucrose.

Figure 10.23. Schematic representation of the highly branched glycogen molecule. Each bead of the chain represents a glucose molecule. From Conn EE, Stumpf PK. Outlines of biochemistry. New York: John Wiley & Sons, Inc. © 1963 John Wiley & Sons, Inc.

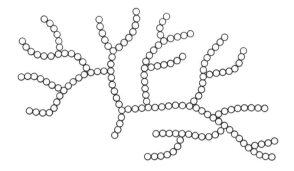

are starch, glycogen, and cellulose. Starch is a food reserve of most plants; when eaten it serves as an excellent source of energy. Starch is degraded through hydrolysis to maltose, a disaccharide, and finally to glucose, a monosaccharide, so it can be absorbed. Glycogen represents the principal carbohydrate reserve in animals; it is stored in the liver and in muscles. It is a highly branched molecule of glucose units (Fig. 10.23) and can be degraded as needed to glucose, and thereby used for energy. Cellulose is the structural component of plants. It can be digested only by enzymes of cellulose-splitting microorganisms that function mainly in herbivorous animals (forestomachs of ruminants, cecum and colon of simple herbivores). Cellulose is similarly hydrolyzed to glucose.

Proteins

Proteins are complex, high-molecular-weight, large, colloidal molecules that con-tain a high percentage of amino acids. In addition to carbon, hydrogen, and oxygen, proteins also contain nitrogen. Hydrolysis of proteins yields amino acids, the building blocks of protein. The coupling of amino acids to form proteins occurs at the carboxyl group of one amino acid with the amino group of another, accompanied by the loss of a water molecule. The degradation of proteins involves the addition of water and the reforming of the amino acids (hydrolysis).

The linkage of amino acids (called the peptide bond) to form a protein is shown in Figure 10.24. Dipeptides consist of 2 amino acids. Oligopeptides consist of more than 2, but not more than 10, amino acids. Polypeptides consist of more than 10, but not more than 100, amino acids. Polypeptides are classified as proteins when they contain more than 100 amino acids. The essential amino acids are those that cannot be synthesized at all or rapidly

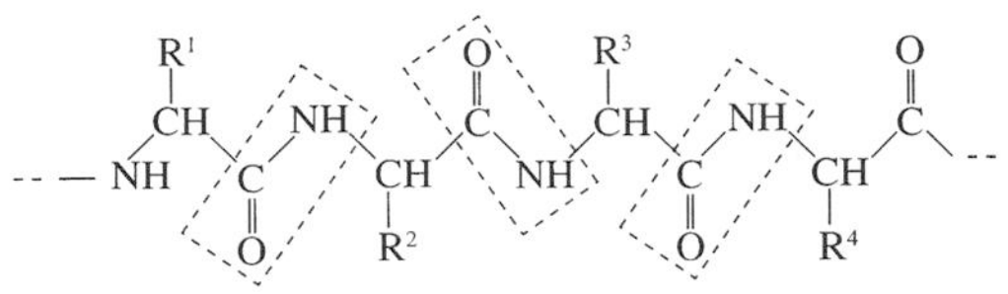

Figure 10.24. A polypeptide chain, the basic primary structure of a protein. The peptide bonds are shown by the areas boxed by dashed lines.

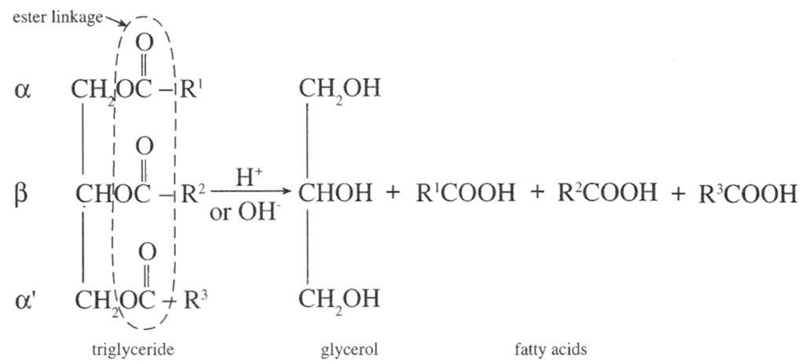

Figure. 10.25. Hydrolysis of a simple lipid. Three molecules of long-chain fatty acids and one molecule of glycerol are released when a triglyceride molecule is hydrolyzed. The great majority of lipids are triglycerides. Lipids are esters of glycerol and fatty acids. The ester linkages are shown within the area circumscribed by the dashed lines.

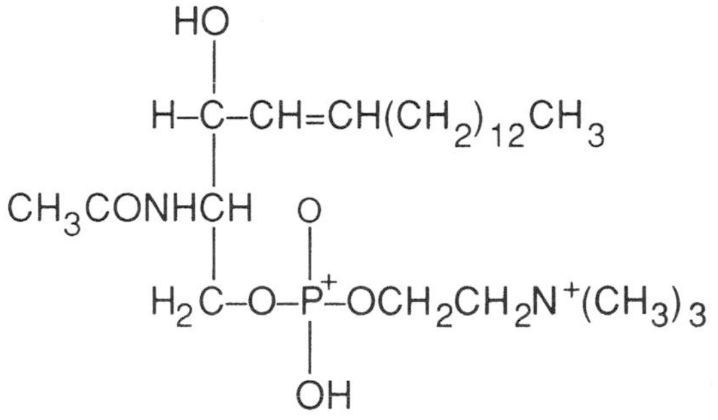

Figure 10.26. Sphingomyelin. This phospholipid is common to myelin sheaths of nerve fibers.

enough to permit normal growth; they must therefore be provided for in the diet. The nonessential amino acids are those that can be synthesized by the animal in sufficient quantities to ensure normal growth. Protein quality is important; the highest quality protein is one that provides all the essential amino acids in the exact proportions required. A lower quality protein either lacks essential amino acids or does not supply them in proper proportions. Manufacturing processes can change a high-quality protein to one of lower quality.

Lipids

The lipids include fats and related substances. Neutral fats (triglycerides) are esters (formed by the reaction between an acid and an alcohol) produced by three molecules of fatty acids combining with one molecule of glycerol (Fig. 10.25). Phospholipids are complex lipids that contain phosphate (Fig. 10.26); in addition, they usually contain glycerol, fatty acids, and a nitrogenous base. Phospholipids are important structural elements of cell membranes and of sphingomyelin (a phospholipid), which occurs in myelin sheaths of nerves. Thromboplastin, another phospholipid, is involved in blood coagulation.

Cholesterol (Fig. 10.27) is a fatty substance derived from triglycerides. It is a high-molecular-weight alcohol; its sterol nucleus is synthesized from degradation

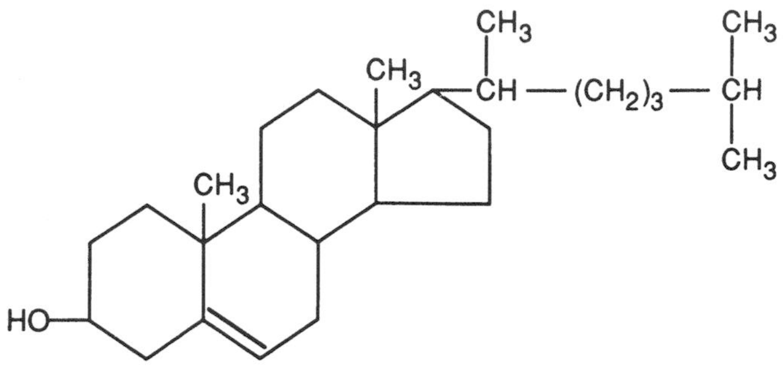

Figure 10.27. Chemical structure of cholesterol.

products of fatty acid molecules. Approximately 80% of all cholesterol formed in the body is conjugated in the liver to form bile salts, which are then transported to the intestine for use in digestion. Cholesterol is also an important structural component of cell membranes.

Accessory Foods

Minerals, vitamins, and water are considered to be accessory foods, and carbohydrates, fats, and proteins are called proper foods. The principal distinction is that proper foods supply energy, whereas accessory foods are essential for life but do not supply energy. The role of water as an accessory food has been described (Chapter 5).

Minerals are inorganic foodstuffs. The combined amount in a diet can be determined by burning; when this is done, the mineral is referred to as ash. Minerals are important for many body functions. Their presence in plasma is only a reflection of their presence in cells and other body fluids. Minerals can be actual components of body chemicals or act as catalysts for chemical reactions. Certain minerals (e.g., calcium and phosphorus) might be required for diets in substantial amounts, but others (e.g., cobalt and manganese) might be required only in minute amounts. These belong to a group known as trace minerals. Mineral functions, deficiencies, toxicities, and interrelationships are summarized in Table 10.3.

Vitamins

The vitamins are a group of chemically unrelated organic compounds. They generally function as metabolic catalysts, usually in the form of coenzymes. A summary of their functions and deficiency symptoms is presented in Table 10.4.

PHYSICAL AND MECHANICAL FACTORS

Prehension

The first factor necessary for the digestive process is prehension, the seizing and conveying of food into the mouth. The lips, teeth, and tongue are the principal prehensile structures in domestic animals. The highly mobile upper lip is a useful prehensile organ in the horse, especially when eating from a feedbox containing grain. When pasturing, the horse draws the lips back and uses the incisor teeth to sever grass.

The upper lip of cattle is rather immobile and the tongue is used as a prehensile organ. The tongue is highly mobile and can grasp grass (aided by the papillae), bringing it to the mouth between the lower incisors and upper dental pad. An upward movement of the head accomplishes shearing of the grass. Because of its use as a prehensile organ, the tongue is vulnerable to injury by sharp or pointed objects that might be in the way of the grasping movement. "Wooden tongue" in cattle is a

TABLE 10.3. Summary of Individual Mineral Functions, Deficiencies, Interrelationships, and Toxicities

Mineral	Major Functions	Specified Deficiency Symptoms	Major Interrelationships and Toxicities
Calcium (Ca)	Bone and teeth formation; blood coagulation; muscle contraction; nerve function; cell permeability; milk production; eggshell formation	Rickets (young, osteomalacia (adult); tetany; thin-shelled eggs; reduced egg production; hypocalcemia or milk fever in dairy cattle	Vit. D involved in absorption and bone deposition; excess PO_4 decreases absorption; excess Mg decreases absorption, replaces Ca in bone and increases Ca excretion; Ca: P ratio should be 1:1 to 2:1
Phosphorus (P)	Bone and teeth formation: phosphorylation; high-energy phosphate bonds; PO_4 chief anion radical of intracellular in acid-base balance	Rickets (young), osteomalacia (adult); reduced egg production	Vit. D involved in renal reabsorption and bone deposition; excess Ca and Mg causes decrease in should be 1:1 to 2:1; in ruminants, excess P can cause urinary calculi
Sodium (Na)	Major cation of extracellular fluid, where it is involved in osmotic pressure and acid-base equilibrium; preservation of normal muscle cell irritability; cell permeability	Reduced growth; eye disturbances with corneal lesions; reproduction impairment (infertility males, delayed sexual maturity in females)	Salt toxicity readily occurs in nonruminants with levels above 8% in diet; staggering gait, blindness, nervous disorders, and hypertension
Chlorine (Cl)	Major anion involved in osmotic pressure and acid-base balance (chloride shift); hydrochloric acid in digestion	Hypochloremic alkalosis (usually due to physiologic disturbance as vomiting rather than deficiency); reduced growth	Toxicity unlikely
Magnesium (Mg)	Enzyme activator primarily in glycolytic system; bone formation	Vasodilation; hyperirritability with convulsions, loss of equilibrium, and trembling; tetany	Excess upsets Ca and P metabolism; toxicity not likely
Potassium (K)	Major cation of intracellular fluid, where it is involved in osmotic pressure and acid-base balance; muscle activity	Hypokalemia; lethargic condition with high incidence of coma and death; diarrhea, distended abdomen, and untidy appearance	Excess reduces Mg absorption; Mg deficiency reduces K retention, leading to K deficiency
Sulfur (S)	Sulfur containing amino acids; SH groups function in tissue respiration; component of biotin and thiamine	Primarily reduced growth effect due to sulfur amino acid requirement for protein synthesis	Toxicity unlikely
Iron (Fe)	Cellular respiration (hemoglobin, cytochromes, myoglobin)	Hypochromic-microcytic anemia (less than normal amount of hemoglobin and fewer red cells)	Ca:P ratio influences absorption; Cu required for proper metabolism; pyridoxine deficiency decreases absorption

TABLE 10.3. Summary of Individual Mineral Functions, Deficiencies, Interrelationships, and Toxicities—*Continued*

Mineral	Major Functions	Specified Deficiency Symptoms	Major Interrelationships and Toxicities
Copper (Cu)	Cofactor in several oxidation-reduction enzyme systems; hemoglobin synthesis bone formation maintenance of myelin of nerves; hair pigmentation	Fading hair coat or lack of wool; nervous symptoms or ataxia; lameness, swelling of joints, and fragility of bones; anemia	Excess Mo, Zn inhibit its utilization and storage; toxicity occurs at levels above 250 ppm with much the same symptoms as deficiency
Zinc (Zn)	Component or cofactor of several enzyme systems, including peptidases and carbonic anhydrase; needed for bone and feather development	Poor hair or feather development and slipping of wool; rough and thickened skin or parakeratosis in swine	High Ca or Phytate ties up Zn; excess Zn interferes with Cu metabolism and can cause anemia
Manganese (Mn)	Thought to be an activator of enzyme systems involved in oxidative phosphorylation, amino acid metabolism, fatty acid synthesis, and cholesterol metabolism; bone formation (organic matrix); growth and reproduction	Poor growth; shortened long bones; impaired reproduction (testicular degeneration of males, defective ovulation of females); perosis or slipped tendon in poultry	Excess Ca and P decreases absorption; toxicity unlikely
Cobalt (Co)	Component of Vitamin B_{12} needed by rumen bacteria for growth and B_{12} synthesis	Anemia (varies from normocytic-normochromic to megaloblastic or macrocytic; deficiency in ruminants causes reduced appetite, reduced growth and body weight, and eventually death	Related to B_{12}; toxicity unlikely
Iodine (I)	Thyroxine formation	Goiter; stillbirths; hairless pigs or woolless lambs at birth	Long-term intake of high amounts of I reduces thyroid uptake of I
Selenium (Se)	Not completely known but thought to be involved in vitamin E absorption and/or retention	Mortality in poultry; if E is also deficient or suboptimal: exudative diathesis (chicks), muscle dystrophy (lambs), liver necrosis (pigs)	Chronic toxicity: blind staggers—10–20 ppm; alkali disease—5–10 ppm; acute toxicity: 20 ppm and above—sudden death; SO_4 protector against toxicity
Molybdenum (Mo)	Purine metabolism; stimulates microbial activity in rumen	Lack of conversion of xanthine to uric acid, but not likely to be deficient in natural diet	Excess interferes with Cu activation of enzymes; causes anemia and diarrhea; SO_4 protects against toxicity
Fluorine (F)	Traces protect against teeth decay	Excesses of F are of more concern than deficiencies in livestock production	Levels above 5–10 ppm block vital oxidative enzymes by interfering with Mn; causes bone deformities, enamel defects, and organ degeneration; Ca and Al salts protect against toxicity; F is a cumulative poison—thus, toxicity may not be noted until after some time

From Jurgens MH. Animal feeding and nutrition. 7th ed,. Dubuque, IA:Kendall/Hunt, 1993. Reprinted with permission.

TABLE 10.4. Vitamins: Summary of Their Functions, Deficiency Symptoms, and Selected Comments

Vitamin	Main Functions	Deficiency Symptoms	Comments
A	Bone formation (mucopolysaccharide release); vision (rhodopsin); epithelial tissue maintenance; glucose synthesis (adrenocortical hormones); growth	Xerophthalmia; night blindness; hyperkeratosis; skeletal lesions and bone remodeling; poor growth reproductive failures; reduced egg production and hatchability	Hypervitaminosis can cause hyperostosis, hyperkeratosis; most of the same symptoms that occur with deficiency; both carotene and vitamin A are readily destroyed by oxidation
D	Bone formation (Ca absorption, P absorption from renal tubules, osteoblast formation and calcification); CHO metabolism (phosphorylation); growth (related to bone formation)	Rickets (growing period), osteomalacia (adults); soft eggshells and reduced egg production and hatchability	Hypervitaminosis can cause decalcification of skeleton and calcification of soft tissue; most mammals can use either D_2 or D_3, but poultry require D_3
E	Antioxidant; muscle structure (muscle dystrophy); reproduction (seminiferous epithelium)	Muscle dystrophy; encephalomalacia; exudative diathesis; reproductive failures; steatitis	Relatively nontoxic; utilization dependent on adequate Se
K	Prothrombin formation and blood clotting	Spontaneous hemorrhages and increased blood clotting time, with lowered prothrombin levels	Relatively nontoxic; antagonists of K include dicoumarol and warfarin
Thiamine	Coenzyme, thiamine pyrophosphate	Polyneuritis and convulsions (head retraction in chickens); cardiovascular disturbances; beriberi (humans); anorexia and emaciation	Relatively nontoxic; seldom deficient in livestock; antagonist of thiamine is an enzyme called thiaminase, found in some fish feeds
Riboflavin	Coenzyme, FMN and FAD dehydrogenase (hydrogen acceptance); important in CHO and protein metabolism	Ectodermal lesions; dermatitis and hair loss; curled toe paralysis in birds; moon blindness in horses; leg troubles in pigs	Nontoxic; common swine or poultry rations will be low or deficient
Pantothenic acid	Coenzyme A; acyl transferase	Dermatitis, loss of hair, and greying of hair; spastic gait goose stepping or posterior incoordination and paralysis; enteritis; poor growth and reproduction	Relatively nontoxic; low content in cereal grains; commonly deficient for swine or poultry
Niacin	Coenzyme, DPN and TPN; hydrogen transport	3Ds: dermatitis, diarrhea, and dementia; pellagra in humans; irritability inflammation and ulceration of mouth, tongue, and digestive tract (black tongue in dog)	Vasodilation with itching and burning of skin; fatty liver; not available from grains to the pig; can be synthesized in body tissue from surplus tryptophan
Pyridoxine	Coenzyme, pyridoxal phosphate; amino acid decarboxylation, transamination, and removal of sulhydryl groups: red blood cell formation	Convulsions, neuritis, and hyperirritability; hypochromic-microcytic anemia; increased excretion xanthurenic acid	Convulsion and death occur in hypervitaminosis; normally adequate in livestock rations

TABLE 10.4. Vitamins: Summary of Their Functions, Deficiency Symptoms, and Selected Comments—*Continued*

Vitamin	Main Functions	Deficiency Symptoms	Comments
Biotin	Coenzyme, carboxylase; carboxylation; β-decarboxylation; CO_2 fixation	Dermaitis and loss of hair (spectacle eye in rats and mice); reduced growth; perosis in chicks	Nontoxic; rendered unavailable by raw eggwhite; normally adequate from diet or intestinal synthesis
Folacin (folic acid)	One carbon carrier; related to B_{12} metabolism	Macrocytic anemia and leukopenia; cervical paralysis in turkeys; poor growth	Nontoxic; unlikely to be deficient for livestock
Choline	Methyl donor; lipotropic substance; constituent of acetylcholine and phospholipids (nerve impulses)	Fatty liver and kidney degeneration; poor reproduction and lactation in swine; perosis in chicks	Persistent diarrhea occurs with hypervitaminosis; choline can be synthesized in body, especially with a high-protein diet
B_{12}	Labile methyl group metabolism. Isomerization reactions; closely linked with folacin	Macrocytic anemia with megaloblastic marrow; from neurologic disturbances; hatching problems in chicks; reduced growth	Nontoxic; not available plant sources; usually deficient in swine diets
Inositol andPara-aminobenzoic acid	Not clearly established	None demonstrated in livestock	Unlikely to be deficient for livestock
Vitamin C	Collagen formation; hydrogen transport (activation of folic acid)	Scurvy-slow wound healing, spongy gums, swollen joints, hemorrhaging, and anemia	Nontoxic; synthesized in body tissue of farm livestock

From Jurgens MH. Animal feeding and nutrition. 7th ed. Dubuque, IA:Kendall/Hunt, 1993. Reprinted with permission.

chronic inflammation caused by an organism introduced through an eating-associated injury.

The tongue is also an active prehensile organ in sheep. The cleft upper lip of sheep facilitates grazing close to the ground. Close shearing is particularly useful when grass is in short supply.

The heavy snout and pointed lower jaw of pigs are adaptations for rooting. Characteristic head movements of rooting are retained by pigs when grain is eaten from a feeder.

Dogs and cats convey liquids to the mouth with the tongue, whereby the free end is contracted to form a ladle. Other domestic animals drink water by suction. Most birds fill the beak with water by dipping and then lifting the head to allow the water to enter the esophagus by gravity. The pigeon, however, drinks by suction.

Mastication

Mastication refers to the mechanical breakdown of food in the mouth. It is commonly called chewing and is carried out to varying degrees by different animals. The fibrous nature of the diet of herbivores requires more chewing than the meat diet of carnivores. In the latter, chewing is of short duration; the teeth are used mostly for tearing and for gnawing on bones in a more leisurely fashion. The table surfaces of the cheek teeth of herbivores wear unevenly, which facilitates more efficient mastication of their diet.

A bolus of food (rounded or oblong) is formed by the mastication process. The bolus might be imperfectly formed by animals that gulp their food. The food material of the bolus is mixed with saliva. The mucous secretion of saliva provides a certain adhesiveness and, coupled with its serous secretion, lubricates the food mass for easier transport through the esophagus.

Deglutition

Deglutition is the act of swallowing or conveying the food mass from the mouth to the stomach. This complex process involves a number of reflexes that are coordinated by a swallowing center in the brain. There are three stages of swallowing: (1) through the mouth (voluntary), (2) through the pharynx (reflex), and (3) through the esophagus (reflex). Swallowing begins as a voluntary activity and is followed by reflex activity. Some degree of consciousness is required for swallowing because of the voluntary stage. Unconscious animals can inhale vomitus because of lack of the voluntary state and because the reflex centers are depressed and do not respond to receptor stimulation in the mouth and pharynx. The reflexes move the food and close the glottis and nasal cavity, thereby preventing food from entering these parts. The sequence of reflexes is as follows:

1. Respiration is inhibited and the danger of inhaling food is minimized.
2. The glottis (opening to the larynx) is closed.
3. The larynx is pulled upward and forward.
4. The base of the tongue can now fold the epiglottis (forward projection from the glottis) over the glottis as the tongue plunges the bolus from the mouth into the pharynx.
5. The soft palate is elevated, which closes the nasal cavity from the pharynx.
6. The pharynx contracts to direct food into the esophagus.
7. A reflex peristaltic wave in the esophagus is initiated, which transports the bolus into the stomach.

A representation of food about to be forced into the esophagus and the associated displacement of the soft palate, epiglottis, pharynx, and tongue is shown in Figure 10.28.

Smooth Muscle Activity

Once food reaches the stomach, its movement is controlled by the activity of the smooth muscle in the wall of the stomach and intestine. Muscle activity is spontaneous (myogenic) and is modulated by the autonomic nervous system. Smooth muscle is an excitable tissue, and the resting membrane potential of about -50 mV is subject to fluctuation. The fluctuations are represented by slow waves characterized by slow, transient, undulating changes of the resting membrane potential that are propagated for varying distances. When the peak (toward positive) of a slow wave reaches threshold, a spike potential (true action potential) is observed, and muscle contraction follows. With greater encroachment of the peaks of slow-wave potentials upon the threshold potentials, the greater the frequency of the spike potentials, and gastrointestinal muscle contraction is sustained for a longer period.

The duration of spike potentials is longer in gastrointestinal smooth muscle than in nerve fibers because, in addition to the inflow of Na^+ associated with depolarization, there is also an inflow of Ca^{2+}; the "channels" that permit Ca^{2+} to enter are slower to open and close than the Na^+-only channels of nerve fibers. In addition, the calcium ions that enter are associated with the actin and myosin interaction of contraction. A representation of spikes superimposed on slow waves is shown in Figure 10.29. Less negative values (toward positive) are associated with depolarization, and more negative values (further from threshold) are associated with hyperpolarization. The rhythmical frequencies of the slow waves represent the maximum frequency for contraction and act as pacemakers. Parasympathetic stimulation causes the resting membrane potential to

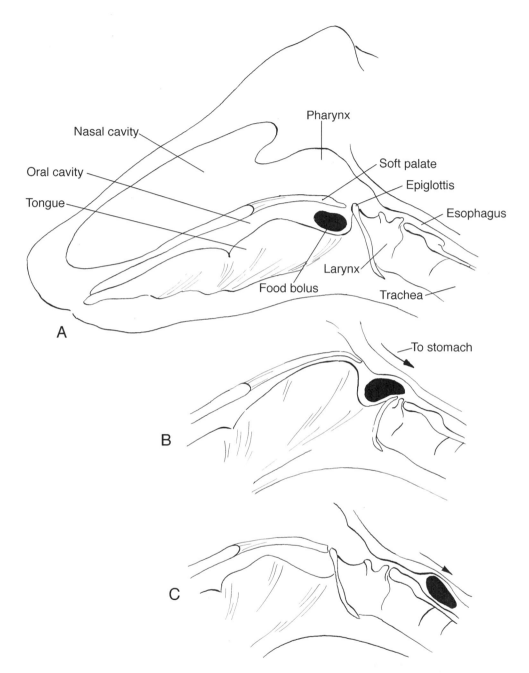

Figure 10.28. Displacement of structures associated with swallowing a food bolus. **A**. A food bolus is moved through the mouth and plunged into the pharynx near the base of the tongue during the voluntary stage of swallowing. This begins the reflex stages. **B**. Pharyngeal stimulation leads to inhibition of respiration and closing of the glottis (opening to the larynx and trachea). The posterior direction of the base of the tongue elevates the soft palate, closing off the nasal cavity, and the epiglottis, closing off the glottis. Pharyngeal contraction forces food bolus into esophagus. **C**. A peristaltic reflex is initiated by presence of food bolus in the esophagus; bolus is transported to stomach by peristalsis; pharyngeal structures return to normal position.

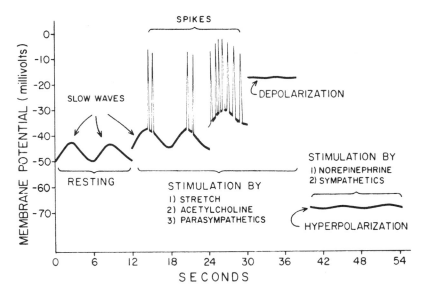

Figure 10.29. Membrane potentials in mammalian intestinal smooth muscle. Note the slow waves, spike potentials, and directions of depolarization and hyperpolarization. From Guyton AC. Textbook of medical physiology. 8th ed. Philadelphia: WB Saunders, 1991.

approach threshold, resulting in depolarization, and increases spiking that results in more vigorous gastrointestinal activity, whereas sympathetic stimulation hyperpolarizes and reduces spiking that results in decreased gastrointestinal activity.

Segmentation and Peristalsis

Segmentation is represented by contractile waves that travel short distances, and peristalsis is represented by contractile waves that travel longer distances. The peristaltic waves are usually conducted in an aboral direction (toward the anus), because the pacemaker for the intestine is located in the longitudinal muscle of the duodenum, near the entrance of the bile duct, and the pacemaker for the stomach is located near the greater curvature. An important intrinsic reflex for the small intestine is the peristaltic reflex. This is initiated by distention of the bowel, which activates local reflexes and causes stimulation of activity cranial to and inhibition of activity caudal to the distention. The cranial activity creates a zone of higher pressure that drives contents into the relaxed area caudal to the distention. The moving contents propagate the reflex and provide for movement of the contents aborally (Fig. 10.30). There is also an extrinsic reflex for the small intestine that responds to peritoneal irritation, which can inhibit gastrointestinal activity. The hormones gastrin and cholecystokinin are known to stimulate gastrointestinal smooth muscle, but the hormone secretin is inhibitory. These hormones control the rate of content passage.

Physical Functions of the Stomach and Intestine

Stomach

The most important functions of the stomach are storage of ingested food, mixing of the food with secretions, and control of the emptying of its contents. The parts of the stomach mentioned above (fundus, corpus, and antrum) are suited to these functions. The fundus receives and stores contents by adapting its volume, so that excessive pres-

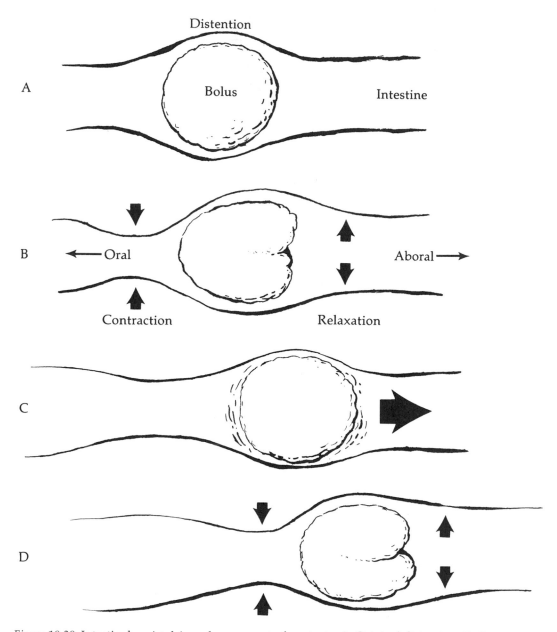

Figure 10.30. Intestinal peristalsis and movement of contents. **A.** Original distention. **B.** Contraction occurs cranial to the distention and relaxation caudal to the distention. **C.** Contraction and relaxation followed by movement of contents in an aboral direction. **D.** New distention point initiates a new locus of contraction and relaxation that continues aborally as a wave.

sure does not develop. The corpus serves as the mixing vat for saliva, food, and gastric secretions. The antrum serves as the pump by regulating the propulsion of food past the pyloric sphincter into the duodenum. The antrum contractions, together with a contracted pyloric sphincter, cause the contents to return to the corpus for additional mixing. Liquid leaves the stomach at a faster rate than solid materials, so adequate time is given for required solubilization and beginning digestion of solid materials.

The maximum number of contractions of the antrum is controlled by the slow waves. For the stomach, these occur at the rate of four or five each minute. The slow waves do not, however, necessarily result in contraction. Contraction depends on the superimposition of spikes that are created when the stomach is distended with food. Stomach distention causes receptors in the stomach wall to be activated; this in turn increases vagal tone (parasympathetic tone) so that the slow waves are closer to threshold and spike more readily. The spikes (action potentials) are followed by contraction waves.

DELAY OF GASTRIC EMPTYING. Inhibition to emptying is produced through a neural mechanism (enterogastric reflex) and an endocrine mechanism (enterogastrone reflex). The receptors for these mechanisms are present in the duodenum. The osmoreceptor, an important receptor in this regard, monitors the osmotic pressure of the material entering the duodenum. The gastric contents could be hyperosmotic and, if emptied into the duodenum, would result in fluid being withdrawn from the blood to achieve osmotic equilibrium of the contents. This does not occur in the stomach because of its lower permeability to water. The osmoreceptors detect the hypertonicity and inhibit gastric emptying via a neural mechanism so that slow emptying occurs and rapid loss of water from the blood is prevented.

Excess protein or carbohydrate is also effective in inhibiting gastric emptying. It is believed that their influence is mediated through the osmoreceptor neural mechanism. Other receptors respond to high hydrogen ion concentrations and cause delays in gastric emptying until the gastric content previously emptied into the duodenum has been neutralized by secretions from the pancreas and liver. These two reflexes are mediated by a neural mechanism. A hormonally mediated delay to gastric emptying occurs in response to lipids entering the duodenum. Cholecystokinin is released in response to the presence of lipids, and delayed emptying provides sufficient time for fat digestion. Another hormone, gastric inhibitory polypeptide (GIP), is secreted by the jejunal mucosa in response to the presence of lipids and carbohydrate, and it also delays gastric emptying.

The following list summarizes the factors that delay gastric emptying and thus permit time for adequate digestion:
1. Enterogastric reflexes (neural mechanisms)
   a. Osmoreceptors in duodenum respond to hypertonic content (hypertonicity can be caused by the presence of products of protein and carbohydrate digestion as well as electrolytes)
   b. Hydrogen ion receptors in duodenum respond to high hydrogen ion concentration
2. Enterogastrone reflexes (endocrine mechanisms)
   a. Cholecystokinin released from duodenal mucosa in response to lipids
   b. Gastric inhibitory polypeptide (GIP) released from jejunal mucosa in response to lipids and carbohydrate

EMESIS. Emesis (vomiting) is an emptying of the cranial part of the duodenum and stomach in an orad (toward the mouth) direction. A series of reflexes are involved to initiate antiperistalsis and closure of the glottis and nasal cavity. Swine, dogs, and cats vomit easily. Vomiting is a protective mechanism to help prevent absorption of noxious substances. Vomiting in ruminants occurs as an ejection of abomasal content into the forestomachs; thus, ejection from the mouth does not occur. Vomiting in the horse is rare because of the difficulty in opening the cardia from a reverse direction. Dilatation of the horse's stomach because of pressure from attempted vomiting can occur to the point of rupture. The reflexes of vomiting are controlled by a vomiting center in the brain.

Small Intestine

The small intestine provides movements that both mix the contents and propel the contents aborally as digestion proceeds. The flow of contents must be controlled for two major reasons: (1) to provide proper mixing of luminal contents with pancreatic enzymes and bile; and (2) to provide time for luminal digestion of carbohydrates, fat, and proteins and for maximum exposure of digested nutrients to the mucosa of the small intestine. One means of delaying transport is to delay transit time in the ileum. This can occur because of the greater number of segmental contractions (short-distance contractions) at that location. Segmental contractions are more effective in mixing than propelling, thus resulting in the delay. They are isolated contractions (not propagated) that cause movement of content, both orally and aborally. Segmental contractions can occur in sets so that the concentric contractions are spaced at intervals along the intestine. One set might relax and a new set occur at points midway between those in the previous set (Fig. 10.31). Small intestine activity can be increased or decreased by parasympathetic and sympathetic stimulation, respectively. Similarly, the hormone

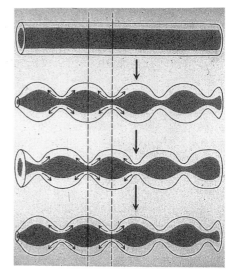

Figure 10.31. Segmentation contractions of the small intestine. This is followed by movement of the luminal contents (small arrows). The dashed, parallel, vertical lines define a segment of small intestine for successive patterns in time (large arrows). From Vander AJ, Sherman JH, Luciano DS. Human physiology: the mechanisms of body function. 4th ed. New York: McGraw-Hill, 1985.

secretin inhibits and cholecystokinin stimulates small intestine motility.

Large Intestine

The large intestine provides for microbial digestion and for reabsorption of electrolytes and water. Both these functions take longer than the digestion and absorption that occurs in the small intestine. Fermentation of the magnitude that occurs in the large intestine of the horse requires a large volume of buffered fluid to neutralize the acidic end products of microbial digestion. The motor activity of the large intestine provides for the delay time. Cecal contractions help to mix the contents and remove gas, with controlled emptying into the colon. Haustral contractions are isolated events in the colon and help to mix the contents. The stationary haustral contractions increase resistance to flow in either direction.

Peristaltic movements in the colon occur in either an oral or aboral direction. In an oral direction they produce retrograde flow, which delays movement of ingesta. Retrograde flow coupled with anatomic narrowing delays filling of various parts of the colon. Anatomic narrowing occurs at the pelvic flexure in the horse, where the ventral colon turns to become the dorsal colon. Accordingly, filling of the dorsal colon is delayed. The frequency of slow wave activity in the small intestine decreases in the aboral direction, but the frequency of slow waves in the colon decreases in the oral direction for the first half of the colon and accounts for the retrograde movement of contents (see previous text). Mass movement of ingesta in the aboral direction is accomplished by prolonged bursts of spikes migrating in the aboral direction that are independent of slow wave activity. The bursts of spikes are followed by prolonged and powerful contractions of the circular smooth muscle, which results in mass movement of the ingesta.

Much of the activity of the colon is thus directed toward the delay of transit and filling of its parts (reservoir function). Increased colonic activity is therefore associated with constipation and decreased activity is associated with diarrhea.

Intestinal Transport of Electrolytes and Water

The secretion of water and electrolytes into the digestive tract has many purposes. These secretions are derived from the extracellular fluids. They are particularly voluminous in herbivorous and omnivorous animals. An important function of the intestine is the return of water and electrolytes to the extracellular fluid before they are lost in the feces. The major reabsorption sites for these substances are the distal small intestine and the large intestine. Reabsorption of secretions is compromised in diarrhea and other conditions,

and if the problem is not corrected or the secretions replenished, an animal can soon die because of blood volume loss and circulatory collapse.

Defecation

Defecation is a complex reflex act in which feces are evacuated from the terminal colon and rectum. The frequency of defecation varies among animals but can occur 5 to 10 times daily in vigorous horses, 10 to 20 times daily in cattle, and 2 to 3 times daily in carnivores. The reflex is assisted or inhibited by certain voluntary muscles.

The time required for food to pass through the digestive tract varies among species. Studies were carried out in various species using dye stained (marked) food. The average time for food passage was determined because ingested food that is marked is mixed with food ingested at other times. The average time for pigs was found to be 48 hours, and for horses it was 24 to 48 hours. Because of the voluminous forestomach in cattle, the dilution of marked food with other food is increased and makes its initial appearance in feces in 12 to 24 hours. About 80% of the initial amount is passed by 3 to 4 days, and final evacuation is complete by 7 to 10 days.

DIGESTIVE SECRETIONS AND THEIR FUNCTIONS

Secretions

Saliva

In all animal species, salivary secretions facilitate mastication and deglutition because of the watery nature of the salivary secretions and the lubrication that is provided. The volume of the salivary secretion varies, but it is greatest in herbivorous animals. A cow can secrete from 100 to 200 L/d (25 to 50 gal/d). In addition to its lubrication function, saliva increases the potential for evaporation and cooling for panting animals. Saliva has an additional important function in ruminants, in which large volumes of buffered fluid are needed to support microbial fermentation in the rumen and to neutralize the large amounts of acids that are produced as a result of fermentation. To meet the buffering demand, ruminant saliva contains bicarbonate and phosphate buffers. Phosphates are particularly supportive of bacterial growth. In ruminants, salivary secretion is continuous, but the flow of saliva varies with activity and increases with feeding and rumination. Saliva has important antifoaming characteristics and might play a role in reducing the foaming tendency of certain diets. Consequently, increased salivary flow during eating might help to prevent dietary bloat. In cattle, about 80% of the water entering the stomach is provided by salivary flow derived from extracellular fluid. The need for reabsorption of the water from the large intestine is obvious (see previous section, Intestinal Transport of Electrolytes and Water).

The major digestive enzyme produced by the salivary glands is amylase. Among the domestic animals, amylase is most abundant in the saliva of pigs. In contrast, the amount of amylase in human saliva is 100 times that present in pigs.

In addition to the spontaneous secretion of saliva from certain glands in some species (parotid glands in ruminants), secretion is controlled by the autonomic nervous system. Parasympathetic stimulation increases salivary flow that is low in protein (more watery). Sympathetic stimulation, however, has less effect on flow rate, but increases the amount of protein and mucin and renders saliva more tenacious. The increase in flow rate is brought about by central stimulation from the salivary center and by the mechanical stimulation of receptors in the mouth and stomach. The central component is sometimes referred to as the psychic component (e.g.,

when an animal salivates in anticipation of food).

Gastric Secretions

In addition to mucus, which is usually secreted throughout the length of the digestive tract, the stomach secretes pepsinogen, HCl, and gastrin. Pepsinogen and HCl are secreted into the lumen of the stomach, and gastrin (a hormone) is secreted into the blood. Specific glandular regions are identified within the stomach; their extent varies among species (Fig. 10.6). Generally, the cardiac region secretes only mucus. The fundic gland region secretes HCl and pepsinogen (HCl by parietal cells and pepsinogen by neck chief cells) and the pyloric gland region secretes mucus and gastrin. A variable amount of surface (depending on species) around the cardia has epithelium similar to that of the skin (stratified squamous). This area serves a protective function in the same sense that mucus protects other parts of the digestive tract.

HCl and pepsinogen initiate the digestion of protein. Pepsinogen is a precursor of pepsin, a proteolytic enzyme. Conversion of the precursor to its active form in the lumen prevents proteolytic digestion of the producing cell. The conversion of pepsinogen to pepsin occurs in the lumen under the influence of HCl and begins at about pH 5. Optimal activity of pepsin occurs at pH 1.8 to 3.5 and initiates gastric protein digestion.

When H^+ is secreted into the lumen by the gastric cell, HCO_3^- is simultaneously secreted into the blood. H^+ is formed in the cell from CO_2 according to the following hydration reaction:

$$CO_2 + H_2O \leftrightarrow H_2CO_3 \leftrightarrow H^+ + HCO_3^-$$

H^+ is secreted into the stomach lumen, and HCO_3^- is secreted into the blood in exchange for Cl^-. The chloride ion is subsequently secreted into the stomach lumen with H+ (Fig. 10.32). The increase in plasma bicarbonate concentration that occurs after a meal is known as the alkaline tide, in which the blood pH increases. It is a transient situation that lasts until the pancreas becomes active in secreting HCO_3^-. An amount equivalent to the amount of HCO_3^- that entered the blood from the gastric parietal cells is returned to the duodenum by the pancreatic cells.

Because of the high H+ concentration in the stomach, a barrier exists to prevent diffusion of H+ back to the blood. The tight junction between cells is extremely effective and even prevents diffusion of H_2O through the epithelium. This is why highly hypertonic solutions can enter the duodenum—they are not diluted by the diffusion of water into the stomach.

Gastric acid secretion is stimulated by acetylcholine (ACh), gastrin, and histamine. Acetylcholine is the parasympathetic secretion; it acts directly on the parietal cells to secrete HCl and on the gastrin (G) cells to secrete gastrin. Gastrin in turn stim-

ulates HCl and pepsinogen secretion. Chemical releasers of gastrin are digested proteins and amino acids in the stomach. Histamine is an amino acid derivative present in most body tissues. It is believed that the local gastric mucosal histamine stimulates HCl secretion by potentiating the action of gastrin or by direct stimulation.

Inhibition of gastric acid secretion occurs when the pH of the gastric contents decreases to pH 2 or lower. The acid acts directly on the G cells. Inhibition to gastric acid secretion also originates from the intestine in response to acidic, fatty, and hypertonic solutions entering the duodenum from the stomach. These same substances are also effective in inhibiting gastric emptying. The inhibition is mediated by neural or hormonal mechanisms. The neural mechanism provides inhibitory neurons that synapse with the parasympathetic fibers going to the G cells. The hormones released into the blood from intestinal cells in response to acidic, fatty, and hypertonic solutions are secretin and

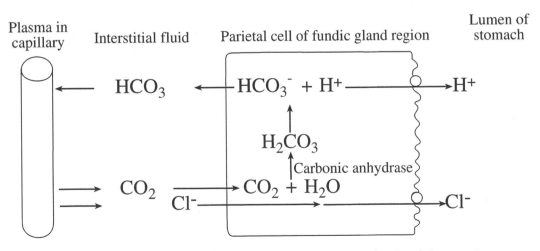

Figure 10.32. Mechanism of hydrochloric acid secretion by parietal cells of the gastric mucosa. Carbonic anhydrase facilitates the formation of H_2CO_3 from CO_2 that diffuses into the cells from the interstitial fluid. H_2CO_3 dissociates into H+ and HCO_3^-. H+ and Cl- are actively secreted by the parietal cells into the lumen of the stomach, and this causes a gradient for diffusion of Cl- from the plasma. The loss of Cl- from plasma is followed by diffusion of HCO_3^- into plasma so that electrical neutrality is maintained. Accordingly, plasma bicarbonate concentration increases after ingestion of food and is associated with the secretion of HCl into the lumen of the stomach.

cholecystokinin (CCK). When secreted, these circulate to the stomach and occupy the site on the parietal cells that gastrin would have occupied, thus preventing gastrin stimulation of HCl secretion.

The secretion of pepsinogen is stimulated by the same stimuli as those for HCl, except that secretin enhances pepsinogen secretion (but inhibits HCl secretion). It would seem that there is less need for inhibiting pepsinogen secretion inasmuch as protein digestion is to be favored.

Intrinsic factor is a mucoprotein secreted by the gastric mucosa that interacts with vitamin B_{12} to form a complex that binds to receptors in the ileum to facilitate vitamin B_{12} absorption. The secretion of intrinsic factor correlates closely with H^+ secretion, and it is also secreted by the parietal cells.

In addition to the gastric secretions mentioned above, the young ruminant secretes an enzyme called rennin. This enzyme is a milk-coagulating enzyme; in the presence of Ca^{2+} it forms a coagulum from milk. This coagulum delays the passage of milk so that more protein digestion occurs in the stomach. The offspring of other animals do not secrete rennin—it is thought that HCl accomplishes the needed coagulation. The need for rennin in ruminants might relate to their proportionately larger intake of milk at a single nursing than is observed for other animals.

The factors that regulate gastric secretions can be summarized as follows:
1. Stimulation
   a. Acetylcholine
   b. Gastrin
   c. Histamine
   d. Secretin (pepsinogen only)
2. Inhibition
   a. Within stomach: decrease of pH to 2
   b. From duodenum: presence of acidic, fatty, and hypertonic solutions
   (1) Neural mechanism—inhibitory neurons to parasympathetic fibers that stimulate G cells
   (2) Hormonal mechanism—secretion of secretin and cholecystokinin, which then occupy gastrin sites on parietal cells (HCl secretors); gastric inhibitory polypeptide (GIP) is released in response to fat or glucose and inhibits all gastric secretions

Pancreatic Secretions

Only the exocrine secretions (HCO_3^- and digestive enzymes or precursors) of the pancreas are involved in the digestive process. The secretion of HCO_3^- is needed to neutralize the HCl concentration of the stomach contents that enter the duodenum and also for neutralization of acids produced from fermentation in the large intestine. Enzymes and enzyme precursors are needed for digestion in the intestinal lumen so that the products of degradation can be absorbed. These secretions are somewhat more unique in omnivores and nonruminant herbivores. In these animals, a large volume of buffered fluid is needed for the microbial digestion that occurs in the cecum and colon. The digestive enzymes provide for small intestine digestion, and the larger volume of fluid and HCO_3^- serve a function similar to that of saliva in the ruminant. In the horse, the rate of enzyme secretion is low in comparison to that of other species. This might occur because a greater proportion of the horse's ingested food is of a type that requires microbial digestion beyond the small intestine.

There is a continuous flow of pancreatic fluid in the horse, even under basal (nonfeeding) conditions. This ensures that an adequate volume of buffered fluid (containing HCO_3^-) is present for the continuous fermentation in the cecum and colon. The rate can be increased under stimulation. In contrast, the dog might have almost no fluid flow from the pancreas under basal conditions, but high rates of flow are produced under stimulation. This pattern is appropriate because the dog eats less frequently, and because little fermentation occurs in the large intestine and a large volume of buffered fluid is not needed.

The pancreas secretes all the enzymes and enzyme precursors (proenzymes) necessary for the digestion of proteins, fats, and carbohydrates. The proteases are secreted in proenzyme form and include trypsinogen, chymotrypsinogen, elastase, and carboxypeptidases A and B. Trypsinogen is activated by enterokinase to form trypsin only after it reaches the intestinal lumen. Enterokinase is present in the intestinal epithelium and the reaction occurs at the brush border. Trypsin then becomes the activator for the other proenzymes. Digestion of the pancreas is prevented because the proteolytic enzymes are secreted as proenzymes. Spontaneous conversion of trypsinogen to trypsin is prevented in the pancreas by the presence of trypsin inhibitor.

Pancreatic lipase hydrolyzes dietary triglycerides into substances that can then be absorbed. Bile salts are needed to activate pancreatic lipase.

Pancreatic amylase is secreted in its active form. This carbohydrate enzyme hydrolyzes starch to maltose, a disaccharide. No free glucose is formed by pancreatic amylase hydrolysis.

The exocrine secretions of the pancreas are controlled by autonomic nerves as well as by the gastrointestinal hormones gastrin, CCK, and secretin. Parasympathetic stimulation increases the secretion of enzymes and proenzymes, with little secretion of electrolytes and water in most species. Increased water and electrolyte secretion, however, does accompany parasympathetic stimulation in the pig and horse (these animals need large volumes of water and HCO_3^- for large intestine fermentation). Gastrin that is secreted when the parasympathetics are stimulated can also stimulate the pancreas to release enzymes and proenzymes, so the parasympathetic effect on the pancreas is potentiated. Two hormones secreted when the stomach contents enter the intestine are secretin and CCK. Secretin release is stimulated by acid perfusion of the duodenum and causes the pancreas to secrete HCO_3^-. Secretin was the first hormone discovered (in 1902, as the result of work by Bayliss and Starling). The hormone CCK is secreted in response to the presence of protein and fat in the duodenum and causes the pancreas to secrete enzymes and proenzymes. Secretin and CCK are synergistic to each other—that is, the presence of one enhances the effect of the other.

Biliary Secretion

Bile is a greenish-yellow solution of bile salts, bilirubin, cholesterol, lecithin, and electrolytes (Na^+, K^+, Cl^-, and HCO_3^-). Bile salts are synthesized continuously by hepatic cells, but the quantity needed for digestion far exceeds the rate of production by the liver. Bile salts are, therefore, recirculated from the intestine (after being used in the intestine) to the hepatic cells, where they are resecreted (enterohepatic circulation). Because of this reuse of bile salts, an adequate amount is available for efficient digestion. Bile salts are synthesized from cholesterol and, in the process, some cholesterol, as well as bile salts, is secreted into the bile. The bile salts and lecithin form a soluble micelle (colloidal particle) with the cholesterol, thereby preventing cholesterol precipitation and gallstone formation. The solubility, however, depends on an alkaline solution, which is provided by HCO_3^-.

Bile is secreted continuously in all species and can be transported to the gallbladder and stored for later use or transported directly to the intestine. While in the gallbladder, bile can be concentrated by absorption of NaCl or of $NaHCO_3$ and water. The degree of concentration depends on the length of storage. In animals that eat once or twice a day, bile is highest in concentration, but its concentra-

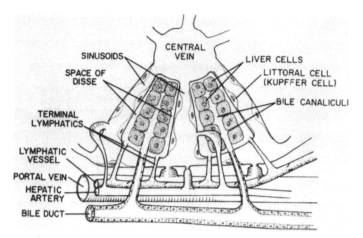

Figure 10.33. Schematic representation of the microstructure of a liver lobule and its association with bile secretion. Most of the bile salts are reabsorbed from the intestine by active transport (others lost in feces) and enter the portal vein and pass to the liver (enterohepatic circulation). They are quickly absorbed from the sinusoids into the liver cells and are then resecreted into the bile canaliculi by active transport. The bile salts then enter the bile duct from the canaliculi. Small amounts of bile salts are secreted continuously by the liver cells and this accounts for that which is lost in the feces. In addition, the secretion of bile salts by the liver is stimulated by the amount being recirculated. Therefore, the larger the amount recirculated, the higher their rate of secretion. From Guyton AC, Taylor AE, Granger HJ. Dynamics and control of the body fluids. Philadelphia: WB Saunders, 1975.

tion is low in ruminants and the pig because they eat frequently and bile is therefore discharged from the gallbladder frequently. The horse does not have a gallbladder and a large flow of hepatic bile continuously enters the duodenum; it is the only domestic animal without a gallbladder. The opening of the common bile duct into the duodenum is controlled by the sphincter of Oddi. Contraction of the gallbladder and relaxation of the sphincter are controlled by CCK, which is released in response to the presence of lipids and amino acids in the small intestine.

Bile secretion by the liver is stimulated primarily by the amount of bile salts being recirculated. On reaching the liver, the bile salts are absorbed from the hepatic sinusoids (portal circulation) into the hepatic cells and are then resecreted into the bile canaliculi by active transport (Fig. 10.33). Cations and water diffuse passively, so that the newly formed bile is iso-osmotic with plasma. Therefore, the larger the amount of

bile salts recirculated, the higher is the rate of secretion of bile. Bicarbonate and other electrolytes are secreted by the bile duct epithelium as well (biliary secretion), and their secretion is increased by CCK, secretin, and gastrin. The secretion of biliary bicarbonate is an important source of buffer for the intestine in some species. In the sheep, the rate of biliary secretion of HCO_3^- is much higher than that of the pancreatic secretion, and the liver plays a greater role than the pancreas in neutralizing the H^+ in the duodenum.

Fat in the intestine is emulsified (breakdown of fat globules into smaller globules) by the bile salts and by the lecithin present in the bile. This provides a greater surface area for digestion by the luminal lipases (lipid enzymes). Another important function of the bile salts is the removal of the products of lipid digestion (free fatty acids and monoglycerides) from the area of digestion so that digestion can continue without recombination to triglycerides. The bile salts accomplish this transport function by forming soluble micelles. In this form the digestion products are moved easily by diffusion to the intestinal epithelium for absorption.

A summary of the major gastrointestinal hormones and their association with gastric, pancreatic, and biliary secretions is presented in Figure 10.34.

Breakdown and Absorption of Carbohydrates, Proteins, and Fats

Most of the digestion and absorption of the soluble carbohydrates, proteins, and fats occurs in the small intestine (except in ruminants). Only minimal hydrolysis of starches is thought to occur in the stomach (in pigs from salivary amylase), where the digestion of protein begins through the activity of pepsin. The intestinal phases of digestion for the nonruminant are described later; these consist of those processes that occur in the lumen and on the brush border of the epithelial cells.

CARBOHYDRATES. The only carbohydrate enzyme secreted by the pancreas that is present in the lumen of the intestine is amylase. Amylase hydrolyzes starch to maltose. Further degradation of starch occurs at the brush border surface under the influence of maltase, and the resulting glucose is absorbed by active transport into the epithelial cells. Sucrose and lactose (disaccharides) do not have a luminal phase of digestion and their hydrolysis occurs at the brush border under the influence of sucrase and lactase. Glucose and fructose from sucrose, and glucose and galactose from lactose, are then absorbed, glucose and galactose by active transport and fructose by facilitated diffusion. Fructose is converted to glucose inside the epithelial cell and enters the portal vein blood in that form. Because the intracellular concentration of fructose is kept low, nearly all the fructose in the intestine can be absorbed by facilitated diffusion. Glucose and galactose require the presence of Na^+ for their active

transport (co-transport) into the cell. This is similar to the process in which glucose and amino acids are transported from the tubular lumen of the kidney nephron into the tubular epithelial cell (see Fig. 9.15).

PROTEINS. The pancreatic proteases are categorized commonly as exopeptidases (carboxypeptidases A and B) and endopeptidases (trypsin, chymotrypsin, and elastase). The exopeptidases hydrolyze proteins into smaller units and the endopeptidases hydrolyze the smaller units into oligopeptides (fewer than ten amino acids) and amino acids. Many oligopeptides must be degraded further because peptides with more than three amino acids cannot be absorbed. Further hydrolysis occurs at the brush border under the influence of oligopeptidases. The amino acids, dipeptides, and tripeptides are absorbed by active transport. Further degradation of dipeptides and tripeptides occurs within the cytoplasm of the epithelial cells.

The active transport of amino acids and peptides requires the presence of Na^+, as for glucose and galactose.

FATS. Dietary triglycerides are coarsely emulsified in the stomach as a result of stomach motility, whereby they are mixed with phospholipids and other chyme (a mixture of food with gastric secretions) components. Further emulsification occurs on entering the small intestine because of the presence of bile salts and lecithin. Further mixing with pancreatic lipase results in the formation of free fatty acids, monoglycerides, and glycerol. Micellar solutions (microemulsions) are formed with bile salts to provide for their ready transport to the brush border. Glycerol, fatty acids, and monoglycerides are absorbed by simple diffusion.

The fatty acids and monoglycerides are resynthesized to triglycerides inside the epithelial cell. The triglycerides are grouped with cholesterol and phospholipids and are given a protein covering to

Figure 10.34. The major mammalian gastrointestinal hormones and their association with gastric, pancreatic, and biliary secretions. **A.** Gastrin: *1*, stimulates secretion of HCO_3^- and H_2O from bile duct epithelium; *2*, stimulates HCl and pepsinogen secretion; *3*, stimulates secretion of pancreatic enzymes. **B.** Secretin: *4*, inhibits HCl secretion and stimulates pepsinogen secretion; *5*, stimulates secretion of HCO_3^- and H_2O from pancreas; *6*, stimulates secretion of HCO_3^- and H_2O from bile duct epithelium. **C.** Cholecystokinin: *7*, inhibits HCl secretion; *8*, stimulates secretion of pancreatic enzymes; *9*, stimulates contraction of gallbladder and relaxation of sphincter of Oddi, and stimulates secretion of HCO_3^- and H_2O by bile duct epithelium.

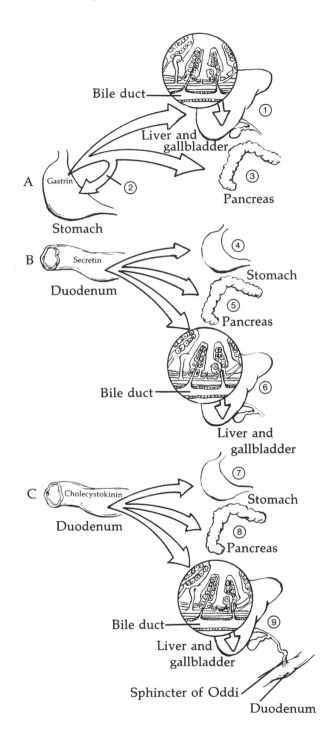

form a chylomicron. Chylomicrons are similar to micelles in that they are water-soluble and thus facilitate the transport of the water-insoluble triglycerides. The water solubility conferred by the protein coat permits exit from the cell, so that the chylomicron can enter the central lacteal (lymphatic capillary) of the villus (Fig. 10.12) for delivery to the blood.

Microbial Digestion in the Large Intestine

No enzymatic digestion occurs in the large intestine of mammals. The digestion that occurs results from microbial digestion, which is significant for the nonruminant herbivores and omnivores. The end products of digestion are volatile fatty acids (VFAs), mainly acetic, propionic, and butyric acids (Fig. 10.35). VFAs are important energy sources after absorption. The microorganisms associated with ruminant digestion are subsequently digested to provide amino acids, but the microorganisms involved with large intestine digestion in mammals are not digested and are voided with the feces. Some species, such as the rabbit, practice coprophagy (eating their feces), so that the microorganism protein is then subjected to small intestine enzymatic degradation.

An animal such as the horse obtains as much as 75% of its energy requirement from large intestinal absorption of VFAs. Even though dogs and cats have little need for microbial fermentation as a source of energy from VFAs, it is an important mechanism from a water conservation standpoint. Any nutrients that escape enzymatic degradation or absorption contribute to an effective osmotic pressure (because the nutrients would not be absorbed) and retain water. Thus, large intestine fermentation salvages otherwise lost calories in the form of VFAs and decreases the effective osmotic pressure of large intestine contents, so that water can be reabsorbed.

THE RUMINANT STOMACH

Animals that regurgitate and remasticate their food are called ruminants. There are two suborders of ruminant animals, (1) Ruminantia, which includes the deer, moose, elk, reindeer, caribou, antelope, giraffe, musk, ox, bison, cow, sheep, and goat; and (2) Tylopoda, which includes the camel, llama, alpaca, and vicuna. The principal difference between the two suborders is that Tylopoda do not have an omasum. Another difference is that Tylopoda have areas of cardiac glands that open into ventral sacculated surfaces of the reticulum and rumen. These small sacs have given rise to the myth that the camel stores water in its rumen, but no evidence has been found to support the idea that more water is present in the camel rumen than in the rumen of other ruminants.

The ruminant stomach is adapted for fermentation of ingested food by bacterial and protozoan microorganisms. Energy is obtained through fermentation that would not otherwise be made available. In their natural environment, the diet of ruminants

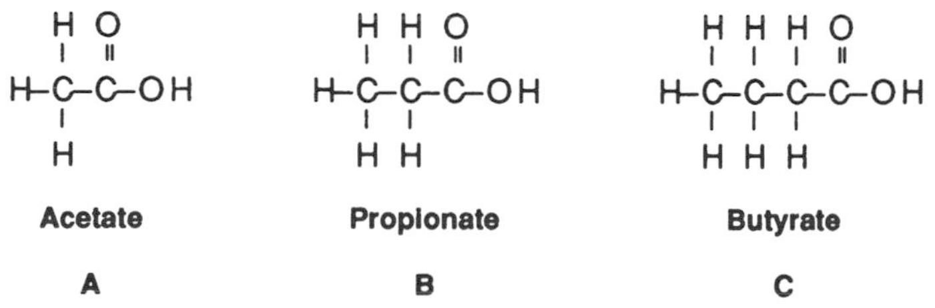

Figure 10.35. Chemical structure of principal volatile fatty acids derived from fermentation in the rumen and large intestine. **A.** Two carbon atoms. **B.** Three carbon atoms. **C.** Four carbon atoms.

includes mostly growing, mature, or dried grass, and the mammalian digestive enzymes cannot digest the cellulose in these materials. Microbial enzymes, however, can digest the plant cells through the fermentation process. Fermentation requires controlled conditions for a maximum rate of degradation; these are provided through appropriate secretions, motility, and temperature. Regurgitation and remastication (associated with rumination) assist fermentation by providing more finely divided material and thus a greater surface area for microbial digestion. Foraging ruminants often seize and swallow food over a prolonged period, with only a relatively short time given to mastication. Remastication is done during times of relative quiescence. Reinsalivation is also accomplished during remastication, and the additional saliva is also beneficial to the fermentation process.

Structure and Function

The ruminant stomach is comprised of four compartments: the (1) rumen (paunch), (2) reticulum (honeycomb), (3) omasum (many plies), and (4) abomasum (true stomach). The relationship of the compartments to each other is shown in Figures 10.36 and 10.37. The first three compartments are also known as the forestomach because they precede the so-called true stomach. The forestomach is lined with stratified squamous epithelium and constitutes the esophageal region of the stomach (see Fig. 10.6). The rumen occupies a prominent portion of the viscera on the left side of the animal; its relationship to the thoracic viscera is shown in Figure 10.36. Note the proximity of the reticulum to the heart. The viscera, as seen from the right side, is shown in Figure 10.37. The abomasum is mostly on the right side. When the

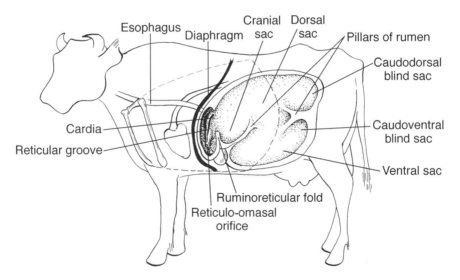

Figure 10.36. The stomach of cattle (left view). The rumen and reticulum (shown) are two of the three compartments of the forestomach that precede the true stomach (abomasum). The reticuloomasal orifice is the passageway to the third compartment known as the omasum. The rumen is divided into a number of sacs by muscular pillars. Pillar contraction is essential for movement of rumen content. The dashed line illustrates the extent of the rib cage.

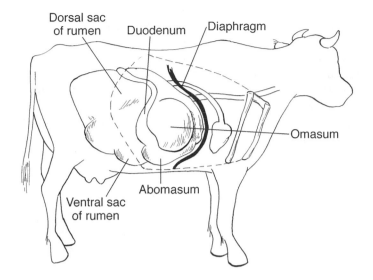

Figure 10.37. The stomach of cattle (right view). The omasum is the third compartment of the forestomach that has a short omasal canal which connects the reticulo-omasal orifice with the omasoabomasal orifice. The dashed line illustrates the extent of the rib cage.

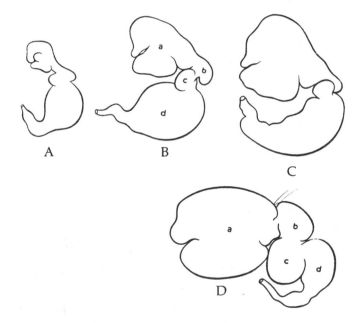

Figure 10.38. Relative sizes of the bovine stomach compartments at various ages. **A.** 3 days old. **B.** 4 weeks old. **C.** 3 months old. **D.** Adult. *a,* rumen; *b,* reticulum; *c,* omasum; *d,* abomasum. From Nickel R, Schummer A, Seiferle E. The viscera of the domestic mammals. 2nd ed. Berlin: Verlag Paul Parey, 1979.

rumen and reticulum are distended with gas (tympanites, or bloat) pressure is applied in all directions, but becomes serious when pressure on the diaphragm prevents thoracic enlargement (needed for inspiration) and pulmonary ventilation is severely impaired. Tripe, a food product, is made from the rumen and reticulum when cattle are slaughtered. The rumen and reticulum are condemned for human food if they are ulcerated. The feeding of high-concentrate rations is associated with ulceration and condemnation.

The abomasum is the largest compartment of the newborn ruminant's stomach (Fig. 10.38). Forestomach development is associated with roughage intake and is lacking in calves that are fed only milk. Young ruminants usually begin ingesting limited roughage when they are 1 to 2 weeks old, and brief periods of rumination begin soon thereafter.

In the adult ruminant, the rumen is the largest forestomach compartment. It is separated from the much smaller reticulum by the ruminoreticular fold (Fig. 10.36). Food enters the rumen through the cardiac opening of the esophagus and is deposited in the cranial sac (atrium) of the rumen (Fig. 10.36). The next contraction of the cranial sac transfers the contents into the reticulum, from which they can be "pumped" by contractions of the reticulum to the cardiac opening for regurgitation, into the omasum through the reticulo-omasal orifice for transfer to the abomasum or for further digestion and absorption by the many plies of the omasum, or to more caudal parts of the rumen. Dense metal objects are often retained in the reticulum. If they are pointed objects, reticular contractions can result in their penetrating thoracic viscera (the heart or lungs), causing inflammation. This condition is known as traumatic pericarditis (heart involvement) or, more commonly, hardware disease.

The reticular groove (Fig. 10.36) functions as a conduit for milk from the cardiac opening to the reticulo-omasal opening, from which it is conveyed to the abomasum through the omasal canal. Closure of the reticular groove (formerly called the esophageal groove) is a reflex initiated when receptors in the mouth and pharynx are stimulated. The reflex loses its responsiveness with age. Although certain chemicals have been shown to bring about closure of the reticular groove in adult ruminants, no function has been described for it in the adult.

The various pillars of the rumen (Fig. 10.36) are muscular folds, which, when contracted, can move and mix large volumes of rumen content. Two to three cycles of rumen contraction occur each minute. These can be felt when the hand is placed into the left paralumbar fossa (depression cranial to the pelvic hooks or tuber coxae,

caudal to the ribs, and ventral to the lumbar vertebrae). Assessment of rumen function is often made by this technique.

A permanent opening into the rumen at the paralumbar location is known as a rumen fistula. These surgical interventions have been used for obtaining samples and for making various physiologic measurements for many years. The fistula openings are plugged during times of nonuse. A classic example of a rumen fistula is shown in Figure 10.39.

The functions of the ruminant stomach compartments can be summarized as follows:

1. The rumen allows for soaking and fermentation of bulk fibrous food and, because of its motility, the contents are continually mixed.

2. The reticulum serves as a pump that causes liquid to flow into and out of the rumen. The flow of liquid directs ingesta into the rumen, regulates its passage from the rumen to omasum, supplies moisture to rumen contents, and floods the cardia before regurgitation.

3. The omasum provides for continued fermentation and absorption (absorption enhanced by large luminal surface

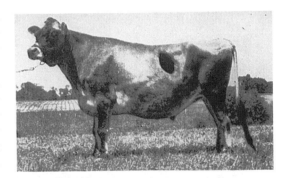

Figure 10.39. "Bill," a Jersey steer with a large rumen fistula. The animal was born in May 1942, the fistula was made in March 1943 and, after a leg injury, the steer was euthanized in January 1955. This photograph was taken in June 1954. When not in use, the fistula was kept closed with a pneumatic plug. From Dukes HH. The physiology of domestic animals. 7th ed. Ithaca, NY: Cornell University Press, 1955.

related to the plies or leaves), and regulation of onward propulsion between the reticulum and abomasum.

4. The abomasum provides true stomach functions. Digestion of degraded roughages and concentrates begins for fermentation residues that have not been already absorbed. Also, the microbes of fermentation are prepared for their own digestion. Using microbes for nutrition of their host is an advantage ruminants have over nonruminant herbivores.

Rumination

The process of bringing food material back from the ruminant stomach to the mouth for further mastication is known as rumination. Rumination is a cycle of activity composed of four phases: (1) regurgitation, (2) remastication, (3) reinsalivation, and (4) redeglutition. It is a reflex initiated by mechanical stimulation of receptors in the mucosa of the reticulum and rumen in the area of the cardia.

The rumination cycle begins with regurgitation of a food mass bolus. Regurgitation is accomplished by taking a breath (inspiration) with a closed glottis (opening to the trachea). The thoracic cavity enlarges without lung inflation and the intrapleural pressure decreases. The lowered intrapleural pressure is accompanied by a similar lowering of pressure in the mediastinal space and in the organs located within it (e.g., the esophagus, as it relates to regurgitation). The cardia (submerged in mixed rumen content) opens and, because of the lower pressure within the esophagus, the rumen content is aspirated into the esophagus. Reverse peristalsis is initiated in the esophagus, and the food mass bolus is quickly carried to the mouth. The passage of the food bolus can be observed on the left side of the neck. The reticulum contracts just before regurgitation to ensure a rumen mixture in the region of the cardia. It

also aids in clearing the cardia of recently swallowed boluses.

Immediately after the regurgitated bolus arrives in the mouth, the liquid is squeezed from it and swallowed. Remastication and reinsalivation occur simultaneously, and remastication is thorough and deliberate. The number of chews given to each bolus varies depending on diet. For example, an all-roughage diet is remasticated more thoroughly and can be chewed 100 or more times before swallowing. During remastication, saliva might be swallowed 2 or 3 times. Redeglutition (reswallowing) occurs at an appropriate time, and the next cycle of rumination begins in about 5 seconds. Actual tracings showing the sequence of several regurgitation events are shown in Figure 10.40.

The time spent in rumination each day varies with species and diet. Generally, the coarseness of the ration influences the time for rumination—cattle on a hay diet average about 8 h/d. All the rumination is not done at one time, but is spread out into periods (e.g., up to 14 periods/24 h), with the periods being distributed rather evenly. Rumination time in sheep can be reduced from 9 to 5 h/d by changing the ration from long or chopped dried grass to ground dried grass. When only concentrates are fed, rumination time can be reduced to about 2½ h/d.

Gas Production and Eructation

The gases produced in the rumen as a result of fermentation are mainly carbon dioxide and methane. Nitrogen, oxygen, and hydrogen might be present in trace amounts, but only briefly, because they are intermediaries for other reactions. Carbon dioxide is evolved during the fermentation of carbohydrates and the deamination of amino acids. Carbon dioxide can be produced also from salivary bicarbonate when it neutralizes the fatty acids produced from microbial fermentation of lipids. Methane is formed by the reduction of carbon dioxide by methane-producing bacteria. In cattle, carbon dioxide comprises about 60 to 70% of the rumen gas, and methane comprises about 30 to 40%. The volume of gas produced in the ruminoreticulum in a dairy cow is about 0.5 to 1 L/min. It is not known how much gas is absorbed into the blood and lymph across the wall of the rumen and reticulum, but it is thought that most of the carbon dioxide and methane produced in the stomach is eliminated by eructation.

Eructation is the process by which gas from the forestomach is removed by way of the esophagus to the pharynx. Eructation occurs about once each minute. An eructation center exists in the medulla that receives afferent fibers from mechanoreceptors located in the dorsal sac of the rumen and around the cardia. The primary stimulus for eructation is the presence of gas in the dorsal sac. If gas is artificially placed into the dorsal rumen, the frequency and volume of eructation increases. A condition of tympanism or bloating occurs when the eructation mechanism fails. Two general types of bloat are recognized: (1) feedlot or grain bloat, which occurs in cattle as the result of feeding a high-concentrate diet, and (2) legume bloat, which can occur when cattle feed on lush, rapidly growing alfalfa or clover pastures. It is believed that these dietary bloats occur because the gas becomes trapped in tiny bubbles (frothy bloat) and the normal free gas bubble cannot accumulate on top of the ingesta in the dorsal sac of the rumen. The mechanoreceptors are covered effectively and the presence of gas is thus not detectable, which ordinarily would initiate the eructation reflex. Tiny bubbles are formed because the surface tension of the rumen fluid has been lowered. Several agents can be used to increase the surface tension effectively and eliminate bubble formation.

The normal occurrence of eructation requires that the cardia be clear of any ingesta. The cardia is reflexly closed when in contact with liquid rumen contents.

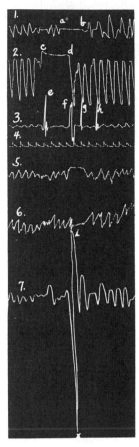

Figure 10.40. Tracings showing the mechanism of regurgitation in rumination. The writing points were vertically placed. The cow regurgitated at X. **1.** Movements of air in the nostrils. Note closure of the glottis from *a* to *b*. **2.** Movements of the jaw in mastication. Note the pause from *c* to *d*. **3.** Movements of boluses in the cervical part of the esophagus: *e*, the masticated bolus; *f*, the regurgitated bolus; *g, h,* the swallowed liquid pressed out of the regurgitated bolus. **4.** Time tracing showing 1-s intervals. **5.** Movements of the thoracic wall. **6.** Rectal pressure. It is not elevated during regurgitation. **7.** Pressure changes in the trachea. A sharp fall coincident with regurgitation is seen. The rise of pressure at *I* is caused by the momentum of the liquid (bromoform) used in the recording manometer. From Bergman HD, Dukes HH. An experimental study of the mechanism of regurgitation in rumination. J Am Vet Med Assoc 1926;69:600–612.

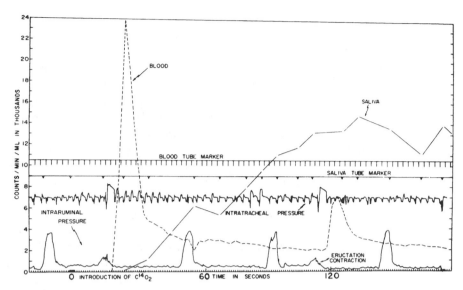

Figure 10.41. Radioactivity in blood and saliva of the goat after intraruminal insufflation with CO_2. From Dougherty RW, Mullenax CH, Allison MJ. Physiological disposition of ^{14}C-labeled rumen gas in sheep and goats. Am J Physiol 1964;207:1185.

Conditions that clear the cardia occur when the dorsally located gas bubble is moved cranially and ventrally toward the cardia by simultaneous contractions in the rumen of the dorsal sac, cranial pillar, and caudal pillar. At the same time, the reticulum relaxes to accommodate the forward-moving rumen content (Fig. 10.36).

A similar expulsion of gas from the stomach in humans produces a sound; the process is characteristically referred to as a belch. Such a sound does not accompany eructation in ruminants. This might have evolved as a protective measure for ruminants in their natural environment, so that their whereabouts would be discovered less readily by predators. The force of evacuation is lessened because a nasopharyngeal sphincter (in the pharynx) contracts which assists in directing part of the eructated gas into the trachea. Subsequent inspiration moves eructated gas into the lungs. It is thought that over half of the eructated gas is directed into the lungs rather than being expelled through the nose to the outside. The inhaled carbon dioxide and methane might provide a source of carbon to be reused in biochemical reactions. Labeled carbon in the form of $^{14}CO_2$ that was inhaled in this manner has appeared in plasma and other body fluids (Fig. 10.41).

Flavors that appear in milk from certain foods (e.g., wild onion, beet tops) are sometimes called off-flavors. They arise as volatile substances from rumen fermentation and become part of the eructated gas. The characteristic flavors get into the milk only if they are inhaled when eructated. When the eructated gas containing the off-flavor is experimentally directed away from the pharynx by a tracheal fistula, its inhalation is prevented and the off-flavor does not occur.

Chemistry and Microbiology of the Rumen

Fermentation that occurs in the rumen and reticulum of ruminants is accomplished by the action of bacterial and protozoan microorganisms. Bacteria account for about

80% of the rumen metabolism (about 10^{11} bacteria/ml of content). Protozoa account for about 20% of the rumen metabolism (about 10^6 protozoa/ml of rumen content). These microorganisms are anaerobic, meaning that they thrive in the absence of oxygen.

Both bacteria and protozoa produce short-chain VFAs, carbon dioxide, and methane from their fermentation of foodstuffs. The principal VFAs are acetic, propionic, and butyric acids (Fig. 10.35). These are mostly absorbed from the rumen before the ingesta reaches the duodenum. The usual proportions of VFAs in the rumen are about 60 to 70% acetic acid, 15 to 20% propionic acid, and 10 to 15% butyric acid. The concentration of propionic acid increases when the diet contains large quantities of soluble sugars or starch and decreases when animals are fed poor-quality hay. The acetic acid concentration varies in an inverse direction. The propionate:acetate ratio is increased by the presence of certain substances. For example, monensin, an antibiotic, inhibits certain organisms (H_2 producers) and favors others (succinate producers), and the propionate to acetate ratio increases.

The products of the fermentation of most carbohydrates are simple mixtures of VFAs with carbon dioxide. The rumen epithelium can absorb glucose as well as VFAs, so that some ingested glucose or intermediary might be absorbed before fermentation. It seems likely, however, that most of the glucose yields VFAs.

The microorganisms of the rumen are also involved in the hydrolysis of protein. Hydrolysis occurs through the breakdown of peptides of decreasing chain length to free amino acids, which are largely destroyed by fermentative deamination with the production of carbon dioxide, ammonia, and VFAs. Some peptides and amino acids pass directly into bacterial cells, but it seems that many of the rumen bacteria can synthesize their nitrogenous cell constituents using ammonia as a principal source of nitrogen. Ammonia is the principal soluble nitrogenous constituent of rumen fluid. The ammonia can be derived from dietary protein, urea from saliva, and urea that diffuses through the rumen wall. Rumen fluid has urease activity, so that urea entering rapidly hydrolyzes to ammonia and carbon dioxide.

Triglycerides undergo hydrolysis in the rumen to glycerol and fatty acids. The hydrolysis is caused by rumen microorganisms and the glycerol is fermented further, mostly to propionic acid. The fatty acids continue into the duodenum for further digestion. Some of the unsaturated fatty acids might be hydrogenated in the rumen to saturated fatty acids.

Rumen bacteria can synthesize the B-complex vitamins. B-vitamin deficiencies are not observed in adult ruminants, except for vitamin B_{12}. Vitamin B_{12} requires cobalt for its synthesis—thus, a cobalt deficiency can result in vitamin B_{12} deficiency.

The types of digestion accomplished by microorganisms for ruminants are also carried out in the large intestine of nonruminant herbivores (see previous section; Microbial Digestion in the Large Intestine). Its occurrence in the forestomach of ruminants instead of the large intestine has certain advantages:

1. Microbial products of value to the host (VFAs and B vitamins) are presented to efficient absorptive sites, both in the rumen and small intestine.
2. Ammonia and substances metabolized to ammonia are used by microbes to synthesize high-quality microbial protein, which is subsequently subjected to abomasal and small intestine digestion and absorption.
3. Selective retention of particles at the reticulo-omasal orifice and the added opportunity for mechanical breakdown of fibers during rumination enhance digestion of coarse foods.
4. The large quantities of gas that are produced can be readily released from the system by eructation.

5. The large input of saliva provides a buffered fluid that permits effective mixing by rumen contractions.

6. Some toxic dietary substances can be rendered nontoxic by fermentation in the rumen, and small intestine absorption of toxin is thereby prevented.

Disorders of Ruminant Digestion and Metabolism

Several indispensable uses for glucose in the body include its function as the principal source of energy for the brain. Glucose also serves as a precursor for glycerol (needed for the synthesis of fats) and as a reducing agent (in the formation of the reduced form of nicotinamide-adenine dinucleotide phosphate, or NADPH) in the degradation of fats. In addition, muscle glycogen is formed from glucose, which serves as an anaerobic energy source during exercise. Liver glycogen present in newborn animals is derived from maternal glucose, and milk sugar (lactose) and milk fat require glucose (glycerol derived from glucose for milk fat) for their synthesis during lactation.

In ruminants, dietary carbohydrates (including cellulose) are fermented in the rumen to VFAs (acetic, propionic, and butyric acids), and only small amounts of glucose are absorbed. To provide glucose for the uses previously mentioned, glucose must be formed (glucogenesis) from nonhexose (nonsugar) sources. In ruminants, about 85% of the glucose is formed in the liver from nonhexose sources. The principal nonhexose sources for glucogenesis in ruminants are propionate (a VFA), glycerol, lactate, and protein (via amino acids). Propionate is the only VFA that can be used for glucogenesis. It is the major source of glucose and glycogen in the ruminant (accounting for about 70%). Protein is the next most important source, accounting for about 20% under normal conditions and up to about 50% during starvation (in which propionate can be absent). A metabolic scheme showing the pathways for glucose and glycogen formation from these four sources is shown in Figure 10.42.

Two major stages are involved in the process by which energy becomes available to an animal: (1) a preliminary conversion of the proteins, carbohydrates, and fats of

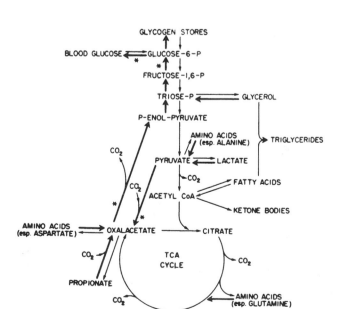

Figure 10.42. Major metabolic pathways in the ruminant liver. Because insufficient glucose is absorbed, one of the main functions of the liver is gluconeogenesis. These reactions are shown by heavy arrows; four major pacemaker reactions are indicated by asterisks (*TCA,* tricarboxylic acid). From Bergman EN. Disorders of carbohydrate and fat metabolism. In: Swenson MJ, Reece WO, eds. Dukes' physiology of domestic animals. 11th ed. Ithaca, NY: Cornell University Press, 1993.

the diet either to acetyl-CoA or to an intermediate of the tricarboxylic acid (TCA) cycle; and (2) the subsequent oxidation of these relatively simple compounds. The second stage is represented by the TCA cycle, also known as the Krebs cycle or citric acid cycle (Fig. 10.43). Propionate can either enter the TCA cycle as an intermediate or it can be glucogenic (Figs. 10.42 and 10.43). The other VFAs (acetate and butyrate) are not glucogenic, but they provide energy by entering the TCA cycle as acetyl-CoA. Acetate and butyrate (and any other substrates that enter the TCA cycle as acetyl-CoA) cannot enter the TCA cycle unless sufficient oxaloacetate is present for condensation with acetyl-CoA to become citrate. Oxaloacetate is derived from three-carbon (3-C) compounds such as propionate and pyruvate or from other intermediates in the cycle. When not enough 3-C compounds are available for the formation of oxaloacetate, or if the production of acetyl-CoA is excessive (e.g., in excess oxidation of fat for glucose or energy), acetyl-CoA accumulates as acetoacetyl-CoA, which is subsequently degraded to aceto-

acetate, β-hydroxybutyrate, and acetone (Fig. 10.43). The latter three compounds are referred to as ketone bodies; accordingly, acetate and butyrate are considered to be potentially ketogenic. The condition in which excess ketone bodies are formed is referred to as ketosis.

In ruminants, ketosis and an associated hypoglycemia (low blood sugar level) occur most frequently in high-producing dairy cows (usually within 6 weeks after calving), in which it is called acetonemia, and in late-gestation pregnant ewes, in which it is called pregnancy toxemia. In cows, there is a sudden or gradual loss of appetite, a rapid decrease in condition, and usually a marked decrease in milk flow. While the onset is usually sudden, there may be a history of unthriftiness or a gradual loss in condition or milk production over a period of 1 to 4 weeks.

The treatment of ketosis in cattle is directed toward increasing the blood concentration of glucose. This can be done by intravenous infusion of glucose. The feeding of sucrose (table sugar) is usually ineffective because it is quickly fermented (first

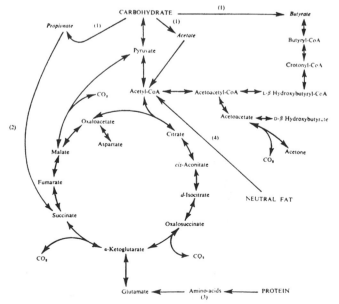

Figure 10.43. Tricarboxylic acid (Krebs) cycle in relation to ruminant metabolism. Only major intermediates are shown. *1*, Produced by ruminal fermentation; *2*, pathway established in rumen epithelium; *3*, arginine, proline, hydroxyproline, and histidine probably enter the TCA cycle after conversion to glutamate; aspartate gives rise to oxaloacetate by transamination; *4*, the glycerol arising from the breakdown of neutral fat is metabolized by the glycolytic pathway. From Annison EF, Lewis D. Metabolism in the rumen. New York: John Wiley & Sons, 1959. Copyright © 1959 John Wiley & Sons, Inc.

to glucose and fructose and then to VFAs). Some benefit might be obtained from absorbed glucose before its further fermentation and from propionate, a VFA obtained from its fermentation. Acetate and butyrate, however, would aggravate ketosis because they are ketogenic. The rationale for administering glucocorticoid (as injections) is that it stimulates gluconeogenesis (production of new glucose) from protein sources. The glucose formed or infused is degraded to pyruvate and then carboxylated to oxaloacetate, so that more acetyl-CoA can enter the TCA cycle and reduce the excess concentrations of ketone bodies (Fig. 10.42). Feeding of sodium propionate might be of some value, but it seems to be unpalatable.

As long as the gas produced in the rumen and reticulum is permitted to collect in the dorsal part of the rumen without frothing, and as long as the eructation mechanism is functioning, no problem arises from gas production, even at high rates. Problems occur when gas cannot be eliminated and a condition known as acute tympany, or bloat, ensues. Bloat does not occur because of any change in the gas composition or because of any increase in the rate of gas production, but because of a failure of the eructation mechanism.

Bloat has been variously described as being caused by the highly soluble protein content of the rumen, mucin in saliva, insufficient amount of saliva, bacterial slime, the high saponin content of ingested plants, and specific eructation inhibitors. It seems that bloat might have several causes. Eating alfalfa or clover pastures (legumes) often causes bloat. Birdsfoot trefoil, however, a leguminous plant, does not cause bloat.

AVIAN DIGESTION

Differences in the anatomy of the digestive tract were noted among the domestic mammalian species, and, although there are general similarities of the domestic avian digestive tracts to those of mammals, there are major differences. The digestive tract of a turkey is shown in Figure 10.44 and it is similar to that of a chicken.

Inasmuch as birds do not have teeth, the mechanical breakdown of their ingested food is accomplished by their beak and by their muscular gizzard. Salivary glands are present in birds and are well-developed in those that eat dry foods. Taste buds are located on the tongue and other parts of the mouth as in mammals.

The esophagus is divided into precrop and postcrop segments. It is comparatively larger in diameter than in mammals to accommodate the swallowing of large food items that would have been divided by teeth. Mucous glands are abundant in the esophagus to provide lubrication for food being swallowed. The crop is a dilatation of the esophagus and has a food storage function.

The proventriculus is located between the postcrop esophagus and the gizzard. The gastric secretions HCl and pepsinogen, and mucus are secreted by the proventriculus. Food does not stay in the preventriculus but rather continues into the gizzard where gastric secretion activity (proteolysis) occurs.

The gizzard is a muscular organ and is adapted for the mechanical reduction of food that has been ingested.

The small intestine has a well-defined duodenum with the pancreas located between its loops (as in mammals), but distinction between jejunum and ileum is not apparent. The yolk sac vestige (Meckel's diverticulum) is noticeable and is located about midway on the small intestine. One of the liver hepatic ducts proceeds directly to the duodenum, another goes directly to the gall bladder. Gall bladders are present in chickens, turkeys, ducks, and geese. The mucosa of the small intestine is similar to that of mammals, except the villi have well-defined blood capillaries but no central lacteal.

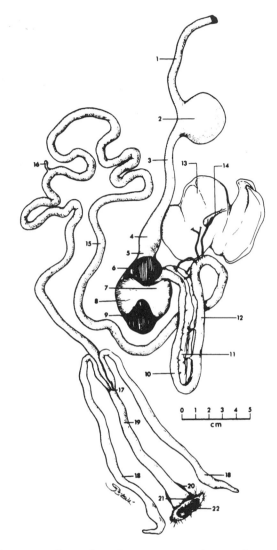

Figure 10.44. Digestive tract of a turkey. *1,* precrop esophagus; *2,* crop; *3,* postcrop esophagus; *4,* glandular stomach (proventriculus); *5,* isthmus; *6–9,* muscular stomach (gizzard); *10,* proximal duodenum; *11,* pancreas; *12,* distal duodenum; *13,* liver; *14,* gallbladder; *15,* ileum; *16,* Meckel's diverticulum (remnant of yolk sac); *17,* ileocecocolic junction; *18,* ceca; *19,* colon; *20,* bursa of Fabricius; *21,* cloaca; *22,* vent. See text for description of the various parts. From Duke G. Avian digestion. In Swenson MJ, Reece WO, eds. Dukes' physiology of domestic animals. 11th ed. Ithaca, NY: Cornell University Press; 1993:428–436.

The ceca, which are paired structures, are located at the junction of the small and large intestine. Not all of the food eaten by chickens and turkeys enters the ceca, and the ceca appear to have lesser importance in domestic fowl as compared to wild fowl. The most noticeable function of the ceca is related to the microbial digestion of cellulose. This is of greater importance for the energy needs of some wild species. Urine that has entered the colon from the cloaca may pass into the ceca via antiperistalsis (oral direction). Antiperistalsis is the most striking feature of colonic motility and is believed to occur almost continuously. Because of antiperistalsis, the ceca are filled. A circular muscular ring of the ileum projects into the colon, and its contraction (sphincter like action) effectively prevents reflux of colonic material into the ileum. In the ceca, the uric acid present in the urine becomes a nitrogen source for the microflora associated with cellulose digestion. Also, water reabsorption from the refluxed urine is another important function of the ceca.

The digestive tract ends with the cloaca, the site that is common to the digestive, reproductive, and urinary systems. The caudal opening to the exterior is known as the vent. The bursa of Fabricius is a dorsal diverticulum of the cloaca and is associated with the development of humoral immunity (see Chapter 6). It is an important site for the preprocessing of B lymphocytes.

The upper ileum is the most important site for absorption of the end-products of digested fats, carbohydrates, and proteins. Heat stress and cold stress can be factors affecting absorption. This may be caused by altered mesenteric blood flow (to the intestines), whereby mesenteric blood flow is decreased about 50% in chickens when the ambient temperature is 37°C (heat stress).

STUDY AIDS—DIGESTION AND ABSORPTION

The Digestive Tract

1. Know the order of the principal parts of the digestive tract. What are the accessory organs of the digestive tract?
2. What are the components of a dental formula? How do you read a dental formula?
3. Define the various exposed surfaces of a tooth.
4. How do points develop on the upper and lower arcades of cheek teeth in the horse (Fig. 10.2)?
5. What is meant by the terms "full mouth," "in wear," and "smooth mouth" when determining the age of a horse by examination of its teeth?
6. What is the unique characteristic of muscle fiber direction in the tongue? What purpose is served?
7. What function is served by the papillae of the tongue? What sensory organs are located in the vicinity of certain papillae?
8. What is the principal tissue of the esophagus? Describe its principal features (consider accommodation of a large bolus or other object)? On what side of the neck could a bolus in the esophagus be observed?
9. What are the glandular regions of the stomach and what are their secretions?
10. Note the extent of the esophageal region (Fig. 10.6). Is it glandular?
11. What are the forestomachs of the ruminant? What is their function?
12. What part of the small intestine receives the pancreatic and bile duct?
13. For those animals not requiring extensive fermentation of their food, where does most of the digestion and absorption take place?
14. Study Figures 10.8, 10.9, 10.10, 10.11, and 10.12. These explain and illustrate the functional aspects of small intestine morphology. Read the text that accompanies the above figures.
15. How is the surface of the small intestine amplified?
16. How are epithelial cells for the villi renewed? What is their replacement time?
17. How does blood and lymph return from the intestines differ?
18. Is fermentation common to the large intestine of all animals? What is the location difference for fermentation between ruminant and non-ruminant herbivores?
19. Are the microbes of fermentation available for their own digestion in both ruminant and non-ruminant herbivores?

20. Note the differences of the digestive tract between the cecum and transverse colon among the domestic animals. Which animals have an ansa spiralis? Which animal has the double horseshoe (ventral and dorsal large colon)?

21. What is the function of the sacculations (haustra) in the cecum and colon of the pig and horse?

22. What is the rectum?

23. What are the names of the three pairs of salivary glands? Where are their openings? How are their secretions described?

24. Describe the location of the pancreas. What are its secretions?

25. Which animal has clearly visible connective tissue septa surrounding each lobule of the liver?

26. Study the triad of vessels and ducts present in a liver lobule (Fig. 10.20). What is the name of the large phagocytic cells that line the sinusoids of the liver lobules?

Composition of Foodstuffs

1. From a diet standpoint, what is the difference between roughages and concentrates?

2. How are carbohydrates classified?

3. What are the principal monosaccharides and disaccharides?

4. What are the polysaccharides that are important to animals? How do they differ?

5. What are the products of complete protein hydrolysis?

6. How are amino acids linked to form a protein? Differentiate between dipeptides, oligopeptides, polypeptides, and proteins.

7. Differentiate between neutral fats, phospholipids and cholesterol. What happens to most of the cholesterol formed in the body?

8. Are water, minerals, and vitamins proper foods or accessory foods? What distinguishes proper food from accessory foods?

Physical and Mechanical Factors

1. What is meant by prehension? What are the principal prehensile structures?

2. Why are cattle prone to tongue injuries? What assists sheep in their ability to graze close to the ground?

3. Observe how different animals drink water. What is an important prehensile organ in the horse?

4. What is accomplished by mastication?

5. Is there a voluntary phase to deglutition? Can an anesthetized or sleeping animal swallow?

6. How can Figure 10.28 be improved (if it is possible) to better visualize the swallowing reflexes? Talk through the events of swallowing.

7. Study Figure 10.29 and review nerve impulse transmission to understand changes in intestinal motility.

8. What is the basic difference between segmentation and peristalsis? How would you define peristalsis?

9. Would peritonitis (i.e., from hardware disease in cattle) inhibit intestinal activity?

10. How do gastrin, cholecystokinin, and secretin affect G-I motility?

11. How do the stomach parts serve their mechanical functions?

12. How do the parasympathetics increase the number of contractions?

13. Does a hyperosmotic solution in the stomach become isotonic by withdrawal of water from the blood?

14. What factors delay gastric emptying?

15. What animals vomit easily? Is there a vomiting center? What interferes with vomition in the horse? Why isn't "upchucking" observed in cattle?

16. Why must the flow of contents in the small intestine be controlled? Where does the greatest delay occur?

17. What are the functions of the large intestine? Is greater time required for these functions?

18. Why is increased colonic activity associated with constipation and decreased activity associated with diarrhea?

19. Why is the reabsorption of water from the intestine an important function? Where are the major sites for this to occur?

20. Note the frequency of defecation in cattle, horses, and carnivores. Note the transit times of food in pigs, horses, and cattle.

Digestive Secretions and Their Functions

1. What is an approximate volume for salivary secretion in a cow?

2. What function of saliva is served in ruminants?

3. Is salivary amylase an important component of domestic animal saliva?

4. In addition to mucus, what are the gastric secretions?

5. What is the function of pepsin?

6. Why would the pH of blood increase (become more alkaline) after ingestion of food? Where is the situation reversed?

7. What factors regulate gastric secretions?

8. Contrast the pancreatic flow rates between the horse and dog. Why is there a difference?

9. How is trypsinogen activated? Where does this occur? What activates the other proenzymes?

10. What stimulates the secretion of secretin and CCK? What is the effect of their secretion?

11. What is bile? Are bile salts a component of bile? What is meant by recirculation of bile salts? What is the relationship of bile salts to cholesterol? What are gallbladder stones (gallstones)?

12. What controls the contraction of the gallbladder and relaxation of the sphincter of Oddi?

13. Is bicarbonate from the liver (biliary bicarbonate) an important source for the intestine of some species?

14. What substances from bile emulsify fats?

15. Study Figure 10.34 for summary of G-I hormones and association with gastric, pancreatic, and biliary secretions.

16. Are disaccharides absorbed from the intestine?

17. How are glucose, galactose, and fructose absorbed?

18. What is the limit to peptide size for their absorption? What electrolyte is involved?

19. What are the products of triglyceride digestion? How are they absorbed?

20. What are chylomicrons? Where are they formed? How do they get to the blood?

21. Is there enzymatic digestion in the large intestine of mammals? What accounts for the digestion that does occur in the large intestine?

22. What are the end products of microbial digestion?

23. What happens to the microorganisms associated with large intestine digestion?

24. What is the importance of large intestine microbial digestion in dogs and cats?

The Ruminant Stomach

1. How does the camel and llama stomach differ from that of sheep and cattle?

2. What kind of epithelium lines the forestomachs of the ruminant?

3. Which side of the cow would be used to detect rumen motility or observe rumen distention from tympanites?

4. Why is bloat a hazard to breathing?

5. Which stomach compartment is largest in newborn calves? In adult ruminants?

6. At what age do calves begin ruminating (assuming they have access to roughage)?

7. Where are boluses first deposited when they enter the rumen? Why are ingested, pointed, hardware items a hazard?
8. What is the function of the reticular groove?
9. How many contractions of the rumen ought to be observed each minute? Where can the contractions be felt?
10. What was the name of the Jersey steer that made the rumen fistula famous?
11. What are functions of the ruminant stomach compartments?
12. What are the four phases of the rumination cycle?
13. How is regurgitation accomplished?
14. How many chews might be associated with remastication of a roughage bolus?
15. How does diet influence rumination time?
16. What are the two principal gases produced during ruminant fermentation? Which one predominates? What is the rate of gas production?
17. What is the stimulus for eructation and where are the receptors located for its detection?
18. How are the eructation receptors related to the condition known as bloat?
19. Is all of the eructated gas expelled into the environment? If not, how is it directed elsewhere?
20. How do off-flavors occur in milk?
21. What comprises the microbial population in the rumen?
22. What are the VFAs produced by microbial fermentation and where are they absorbed?
23. What happens to glucose in the rumen?
24. What happens to protein in the rumen?
25. What happens to lipids in the rumen?
26. What vitamins are synthesized in the rumen? Which vitamin requires cobalt?
27. Note the advantages of "up front" fermentation.
28. What are the principal nonhexose sources of glucose for ruminants? Why do they need nonhexose sources? Why do they need glucose?

29. Study energy production, entry routes of the VFAs into the TCA cycle, ketone production and treatment rationale for ketosis.
30. What is a summary statement for why bloat occurs?

Avian Digestion

1. What structures in birds provide for the mechanical breakdown of their ingested food?
2. Do birds have salivary glands and taste buds?
3. Where is the crop located and what is its function?
4. What are the secretions of the proventriculus?
5. What is the function of the gizzard?
6. Do the common domestic birds have gall bladders?
7. What is the most noticeable function of the ceca?
8. What is the most striking feature of colonic motility?
9. What prevents colonic material from entering the ileum during antiperistalsis?
10. What is the function of the bursa of Fabricius?
11. What part of the digestive tract accounts for most of the end-products of digestion?
12. How does heat stress interfere with absorption?

SELF-EVALUATION—DIGESTION AND ABSORPTION

1. The following dental formula for the sheep, 2(0/4-0/0-3/3-3/3), would indicate that:
   a. the sheep has 8 incisors in the lower jaw of its mouth
   b. the sheep has 16 teeth in its mouth
   c. there are 4 canine teeth on each half of the lower jaw

2. A "smooth mouth" in a horse:
   a. indicates that it is about 5 years old
   b. is represented by 2 complete enamel rings
   c. is seen when the inner enamel ring disappears in all of the lower incisors and is replaced by the dental star (occurs 13 to 15 years of age)
   d. has nothing to do with wear characteristics

3. Mobility of the tongue of domestic animals is facilitated by
   a. 3-directional muscle fibers
   b. greater innervation
   c. the taste buds
   d. greater mental concentration

4. Fermentation in the gastro-intestinal tract of the cat and dog:
   a. never occurs
   b. takes place in the stomach
   c. would occur in the large intestine
   d. causes gas formation only

5. Segmental contractions are noted for their ability to:
   a. mix intestinal contents
   b. propel intestinal contents towards the anus

6. Replacement of intestinal epithelium:
   a. does not occur (they are there for life)
   b. originates from the crypts and migrates to the tip of the villi
   c. originates from the tips of the villi and migrates to the crypts
   d. occurs in cycles

7. The microbes of fermentation are digested in both ruminant and non-ruminant herbivores.
   a. true
   b. false

8. Amino acids can be coupled by peptide linkages to form:
   a. glycogen
   b. triglycerides
   c. cellulose
   d. proteins

9. Seizing and conveying food to the mouth is known as:
   a. apprehension
   b. tension
   c. prehension
   d. pension

10. When a bolus of food is swallowed:
    a. the soft palate is folded over the glottis
    b. the epiglottis is elevated, closing the nasal cavity from the pharynx
    c. respiration is inhibited

11. Parasympathetic stimulation to the intestine:
    a. lowers the resting membrane potential (more negative) thus decreasing motility
    b. raises the resting membrane potential (less negative) thus decreasing motility
    c. lowers the resting membrane potential thus increasing motility
    d. raises the resting membrane potential thus increasing motility

12. Vomition is often observed in horses and cattle.
    a. true
    b. false

13. Where does most of the water and electrolyte reabsorption occur?
    a. stomach
    b. duodenum
    c. ileum
    d. large intestine

14. No further digestion is required for the absorption of: (select the one where all are correct):
    a. glucose, sucrose, galactose
    b. glycerol, fatty acids, monoglycerides
    c. amino acids, polypeptides
    d. glycerol, fatty acids, triglycerides

15. Among the domestic animals, bicarbonate for the gastrointestinal tract is secreted:
    a. only by the salivary glands
    b. only by the bile ducts
    c. only by the exocrine pancreas
    d. by salivary glands, exocrine pancreas, and bile ducts

16. Which one of the following hormones is best known for its association with stimulation of pancreatic enzyme secretions and contraction of the gall bladder?
    a. cholecystokinin
    b. secretin

17. Which one of the following is associated with the sequence of flooding of the cardia, opening of the cardia, inspiration with a closed glottis, entrance of rumen content into the esophagus, and reverse peristalsis of the esophagus?
    a. redeglutition
    b. eructation
    c. regurgitation
    d. rumen contractions

18. A good estimate for the volume of saliva produced by an adult cow in 24 hours is:
    a. 30 gallons
    b. 30 pints
    c. 30 quarts
    d. 30 cups

19. Bloat in cattle is caused by:
    a. an increase in the volume of gas produced
    b. a failure of the eructation mechanism

20. What begins the digestion of protein in the stomach?
    a. rennin
    b. pepsinogen
    c. HCl
    d. pepsin

21. Which one of the following is best associated with the milk coagulating enzyme of calves?
    a. bile, formed in liver
    b. renin, formed in kidney
    c. rennin, formed in abomasum
    d. enterokinase, formed in intestine

22. Which one of the following statements is **NOT** a characteristic of bile?
    a. released from gall bladder under the influence of cholecystokinin
    b. important for digestion because of presence of bile salts

c. contains digestive enzymes
d. emulsifies fat and assists transport of monoglycerides and free fatty acids to epithelial cells for absorption

23. Protein digestion begins in the stomach because of the enzymatic action of:
    a. HCl
    b. pepsinogen
    c. rennin
    d. pepsin

24. Cellulose, starch, and glycogen are classified according to which one of the following?
    a. protein, polypeptide
    b. lipid, triglycerides
    c. carbohydrate, polysaccharides
    d. carbohydrate, disaccharides

25. Which one of the following best describes prehension?
    a. movement of food through the intestines
    b. seizing and conveying food to the mouth
    c. fear
    d. emptying of the stomach

26. Which one of the following best describes the digestion of carbohydrates in the small intestine?
    a. accomplished in the intestinal lumen by carboxypeptidase A and B, trypsin, chymotrypsin and elastase
    b. conversion to glucose, galactose, and fructose occurs in the lumen
    c. pancreatic amylase is produced by the intestinal epithelium
    d. sucrose, maltose, and lactose are degraded to monosaccharides by enzymes in the brush border of the intestinal epithelium

27. Which one of the following salivary functions is either non-existent or insignificant in ruminants?
    a. enzymes for digestion
    b. chemical buffers for rumen
    c. bacterial growth media enhancement
    d. prevention of froth

28. Which one of the following is **NOT** characteristic of large intestine function?
    a. water conservation occurs because incompletely digested foodstuffs are further digested and absorbed
    b. microbial digestion does occur
    c. there is considerable digestion by mammalian enzymes
    d. the large intestine is a major site for water reabsorption

29. Which hormone is responsible for the secretion of the pancreatic digestive enzymes and precursors of enzymes?
    a. secretin
    b. cholecystokinin
    c. oxytocin
    d. antidiuretic hormone

30. Which one of the following best describes trypsinogen and chymotrypsinogen?
    a. precursors of proteolytic enzymes secreted by the intestinal epithelium
    b. precursors of lipolytic enzymes secreted by the intestinal epithelium
    c. proteolytic enzymes secreted by the intestinal epithelium
    d. precursors of proteolytic enzymes secreted by the pancreas

31. Which one of the following does **NOT** characterize the small intestine?
    a. it contains two smooth muscle layers, one arranged circularly and the other longitudinally
    b. the presence of villi, crypts, brush borders on cells, and folds combine to increase surface area
    c. digestion is accomplished by microbial enzymes rather than by mammalian enzymes
    d. it is composed of the duodenum, jejunum, and ileum, in that order from cranial to caudal

32. Which one of the following is most likely to be resynthesized to its beginning form and enter the central lacteals of the intestinal villi for its entry to the circulation?
    a. monoglycerides and fatty acids
    b. amino acids

    c. monosaccharide
    d. fruit cake

33. Which one of the following is a component of rumination?
    a. defecation
    b. vomiting
    c. eructation
    d. regurgitation

34. Bloat in ruminants is caused by a change in the composition of the gas produced.
    a. true
    b. false

35. Ketosis occurs in ruminants because there is not enough acetyl CoA to direct acetic and butyric acid (two of the VFAs) into the Kreb's cycle.
    a. true
    b. false

36. Where would one find chylomicrons?
    a. gall bladder
    b. pancreas
    c. central lacteal
    d. intestinal lumen

37. Which one of the following is not a function of HCl in the stomach?
    a. lowers pH
    b. kills bacteria
    c. converts trypsinogen to trypsin
    d. converts pepsinogen to pepsin

38. The principal end-product(s) of dietary carbohydrates in ruminants is/are:
    a. volatile fatty-acids
    b. triglycerides
    c. glucose
    d. amino acids

39. The hepatic portal circulation:
    a. receives blood from the kidneys
    b. is that which perfuses the hypothalamus
    c. receives blood that arises from the capillaries of the stomach, spleen, small and large intestine, and this blood then perfuses the liver sinusoids before entering the hepatic vein
    d. has to do with concentrating the urine

40. The reactions and conversions necessary to provide energy, build tissues, and synthesize secretions are collectively known as:
    a. digestion
    b. absorption
    c. intermediary metabolism

41. Which one of the following age brackets is characterized by equine incisors being "in wear"?
    a. 3 to 5 years
    b. 7 to 10 years
    c. 13 to 15 years

42. The conical and filiform papillae at the tip of the tongue:
    a. render it more mobile
    b. serve as a plunger for transport of food from the mouth to the esophagus
    c. provide traction for movement of food in the mouth and for grooming hair
    d. discriminate between harmful and proper foods

43. Which one of the following structures is elevated during deglutition to prevent food entrance into the nasal cavity?
    a. soft palate
    b. epiglottis
    c. glottis
    d. larynx

44. For those animals not requiring extensive fermentation of their food, where does most of the digestion and absorption take place?
    a. cecum
    b. small intestine
    c. colon
    d. stomach

45. Which one of the following is the smallest division of intestinal surface amplification?
    a. microvilli (brush border)
    b. intestinal folds (plications)
    c. villus

46. Foods containing a high percentage of cellulose with low digestibility are classified as:
    a. concentrates
    b. roughages
    c. junk foods
    d. fast foods

47. Complete protein hydrolysis yields:
    a. monosaccharides
    b. amino acids
    c. glycerol and fatty acids
    d. peptides

48. The tongue is more important as a prehensile organ in the:
    a. cow
    b. pig
    c. horse
    d. dog

49. Intestinal contractions initiated by distention, which stimulates activity cranial to and inhibits activity caudal to the distention, thus moving contents and propagating the reflex, are called:
    a. twitches
    b. spasms
    c. segmentation
    d. peristalsis

50. Which one of the autonomic divisions depolarizes gastrointestinal smooth muscle, increases spiking, and results in more vigorous gastrointestinal activity?
    a. parasympathetic
    b. sympathetic

51. A hyperosmotic solution in the stomach becomes isotonic before it is evacuated into the duodenum.
    a. true
    b. false

52. Reabsorption of electrolytes and water and microbial digestion are characteristic of:
    a. stomach
    b. small intestine
    c. large intestine

53. A defecation frequency of 10 times per day would be considered diarrhea in:
    a. the horse
    b. the cow
    c. the dog
    d. all of the above

54. Which salivary function is most important for ruminants?
    a. provision of evaporative water for cooling
    b. provision of amylase (conversion of starch to maltose)
    c. provision of bicarbonates and phosphates for buffering

55. Pancreatic fluid flow is continuous in the:
    a. horse
    b. dog
    c. both horse and dog

56. Which one of the following is activated by enterokinase in the intestine so that the active form can then activate the other proteolytic proenzymes?
    a. trypsinogen
    b. chymotrypsinogen
    c. elastase
    d. carboxypeptidase A

57. Contraction of the gall bladder and relaxation of the sphincter of Oddi are initiated by:
    a. CCK
    b. secretin
    c. gastrin

58. Deglutition, regurgitation, and eructation (assuming distention of the esophagus) could all be observed on the left side of the cow.
    a. true
    b. false

59. The presence of gas stimulates receptors in the region of the cardia and initiates:
    a. regurgitation
    b. eructation
    c. defecation
    d. flatulence

60. Rumen contractions can be observed in the left paralumbar fossa and should approximate:
    a. 1 to 2 each minute
    b. 5 to 10 each minute
    c. 5 to 10 each hour
    d. TNTC

61. Regurgitation is facilitated by:
    a. inspiration with a closed glottis (decreases mediastinal pressure)
    b. expiration (mediastinal pressure increased)
    c. salivation
    d. thorough mastication

62. Which vitamin synthesized in the rumen requires cobalt for its structure?
    a. vitamin B_{12}
    b. vitamin K
    c. vitamin A
    d. vitamin C

63. Which one of the following VFAs is the least likely to be productive of ketosis in ruminants?
    a. acetic acid
    b. propionic acid
    c. butyric acid

64. Which one of the avian digestive tract structures secretes HCl and pepsinogen?
    a. crop
    b. proventriculus
    c. gizzard
    d. ceca

65. Which one of the avian digestive tract structures is very muscular and serves to grind or break down food?
    a. crop
    b. proventriculus
    c. gizzard
    d. ceca

66. Which avian digestive tract structure provides for the microbial digestion of cellulose?
    a. gizzard
    b. ileum
    c. ceca
    d. cloaca

67. It is possible for uric acid to go from the cloaca to the ceca.
    a. true
    b. false
68. The avian vent:
    a. ventilates the cloaca
    b. serves as an opening for the passage of feces, feces mixed with urine, and eggs
69. The bursa of Fabricius:
    a. is a part of the small intestine
    b. is associated with humoral immunity
    c. produces erythrocytes
    d. is a site for water reabsorption from the cloaca
70. Heat stress associated with ambient temperatures of 37°C
    a. has no effect upon absorption from the ileum
    b. decreases mesenteric blood flow and thereby reduces absorption
    c. increases turkey intelligence

Suggested Readings

Adams DR. Canine anatomy: a systemic approach. Ames, IA: Iowa State University Press, 1986.

Allison MJ. Microbiology of the rumen and small and large intestines. In: Swenson MJ, Reece WO, eds. Dukes' physiology of domestic animals. 11th ed. Ithaca, NY: Cornell University Press, 1993:417–427.

Annison EF, Lewis D. Metabolism in the rumen. New York: John Wiley & Sons, 1959.

Argenzio RA. Digestion and absorption of carbohydrate, fat and protein. In: Swenson MJ, Reece WO, eds. Dukes' physiology of the domestic animals. 11th ed. Ithaca, NY: Cornell University Press, 1993:362–375.

Argenzio RA. Intestinal transport of electrolytes and water. In: Swenson MJ, Reece WO, eds. Dukes' physiology of domestic animals. 11th ed. Ithaca, NY: Cornell University Press, 1993:376–386.

Argenzio RA. Gastrointestinal motility. In: Swenson MJ, Reece WO, eds. Dukes' physiology of domestic animals. 11th ed. Ithaca, NY: Cornell University Press, 1993:336–348.

Argenzio RA. General functions of the gastrointestinal tract and their control and integration. In: Swenson MJ, Reece WO, eds. Dukes' physiology of domestic animals. 11th ed. Ithaca, NY: Cornell University Press, 1993:325–335.

Argenzio RA. Secretory functions of the gastrointestinal tract. In: Swenson MJ, Reece WO, eds. Dukes' physiology of domestic animals. 11th ed. Ithaca, NY: Cornell University Press, 1993:349–361.

Bergman EN. Disorders of carbohydrate and fat metabolism. In: Swenson MJ, Reece WO, eds. Dukes' physiology of domestic animals. 11th ed. Ithaca, NY: Cornell University Press, 1993:492–502.

Dougherty RW, Allison MJ, Mullenax CH. Physiological disposition of ^{14}C-labeled rumen gases in sheep. Am J Physiol 1964;201:1181.

Dougherty RW, et al. Physiological mechanisms involved in transmitting flavors and odor to milk. I. Contribution of eructated gases to milk flavor. J Dairy Sci 196245:472..

Dougherty RW, Mullenax CH, Allison MJ. Physiological phenomena associated with eructation in ruminants. In: Dougherty RW, et al, eds. Physiology of digestion in the ruminant. Washington, DC: Butterworth, 1965:159–170.

Duke GE. Avian digestion. In: Swenson MJ, Reece WO, eds. Dukes' physiology of domestic animals. 11th ed. Ithaca, NY: Cornell University Press, 1993:428–436.

Duke GE. Alimentary canal: anatomy, regulation of feeding, and motility. In: Sturkie PD, ed. Avian physiology. 4th ed. New York: Springer-Verlag, 1986.

Dukes HH. The physiology of domestic animals. 7th ed. Ithaca, NY: Cornell University Press, 1955.

Dyce KM, Wensing CJG. Essentials of bovine anatomy. Philadelphia: Lea & Febiger, 1971.

Engel HH, St. Clair, LE. Anatomy. In: Leman AD, et al, eds. Diseases of swine. 6th ed. Ames, IA: Iowa State University Press, 1986:3–26.

Fawcett DW. Bloom & Fawcett: A textbook of histology. 11th ed. Philadelphia: WB Saunders, 1986.

Frandson RD, Spurgeon TL. Anatomy and physiology of farm animals. 5th ed. Philadelphia: Lea & Febiger, 1992.

Guyton AC. Textbook of medical physiology. 8th ed. Philadelphia: WB Saunders, 1991.

Ham AW. Histology. 7th ed. Philadelphia: JB Lippincott, 1974.

Jurgens MH. Animal feeding and nutrition. 7th ed. Dubuque, IA: Kendall/Hunt, 1993.

Smith F. Manual of veterinary physiology. 5th ed. Chicago: Alexander Eger, 1921.

Sisson S, St. Clair LE. Equine digestive system. In: Getty R, ed. Sisson & Grossman's anatomy of the domestic animals, Vol. 1. 5th ed. Philadelphia: WB Saunders, 1975:454–497.

Vander AJ, Sherman JH, Luciano DS. Human physiology. The mechanisms of body function. 6th ed. New York: McGraw-Hill, 1993.

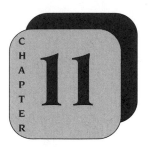

Body Heat and Temperature Regulation

The chemical reactions of the body—and therefore the body functions—depend on body temperature. An elevation of temperature accelerates the reactions, and a lowering of temperature depresses the reactions. To avoid fluctuations of function caused by temperature, mammals and birds have developed a means whereby body temperature is maintained relatively constant regardless of the temperature of the surroundings. Mammals and birds are classified as homeotherm, or warm-blooded, animals. Poikilotherm (cold-blooded) animals have a body temperature that varies with the temperature of the environment.

BODY TEMPERATURE

An average body temperature is associated with each domestic animal species. These temperatures are shown in Table 11.1,

along with their commonly observed ranges. The temperatures were obtained by rectal insertion of a thermometer in resting animals. A number of conditions can influence body temperature, including exercise, time of day, environmental temperature, digestion, and drinking of water.

Gradients of Temperature

Different parts of the body can differ in temperature because of differences in metabolic rate, blood flow, or distance from the surface. For example, the liver and the brain can have a temperature that is higher than that of the blood, and they are therefore cooled by blood circulation. The deep body temperature, or core temperature, is higher than the temperature of the limbs or even higher than the temperature observed rectally. Rectal temperature represents a true steady state of temperature, however, because it reaches equilibrium more slowly.

TABLE 11.1. Average Rectal Temperatures of Various Species

Animal	Average		Range	
	° C	° F	° C	° F
Stallion	37.6	99.7	37.2–38.1	99.0–100.6
Mare	37.8	100	37.3–38.2	99.1–100.8
Donkey	37.4	99.3	36.4–38.4	97.5–101.1
Camel	37.5	99.5	34.2–40.7	93.6–105.3
Beef cow	38.3	101	36.7–39.1	98.0–102.4
Dairy cow	38.6	101.5	38.0–39.3	100.4–102.8
Sheep	39.1	102.3	38.3–39.9	100.9–103.8
Goat	39.1	102.3	38.5–39.7	101.3–103.5
Pig	39.2	102.5	38.7–39.8	101.6–103.6
Dog	38.9	102	37.9–39.9	100.2–103.8
Cat	38.6	101.5	38.1–39.2	100.5–102.5
Rabbit	39.5	103.1	38.6–40.1	101.5–104.2
Chicken daylight	41.7	107.1	40.6–43.0	105.0–109.4

From Andersson BE. Temperature regulation and environmental physiology. In: Swenson MJ, Reece WO. Dukes' physiology of domestic animals. 11th ed. Ithaca, NY: Cornell University Press, 1993.

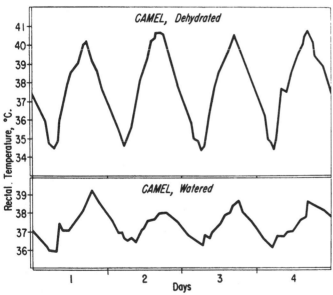

Figure 11.1. Diurnal temperatures in the watered and dehydrated camel. The rectal temperature elevations (heat storage) occur during the day and the reductions occur at night. From Schmidt-Nielsen K. Osmotic regulation in higher vertebrates. In: The harvey lectures, 1962–1963. Series 58. London: Academic Press, Inc., 1963:53–93.

Diurnal Temperature

Variations in temperature related to the time of day are designated as diurnal temperatures. Animals that are active during the day and sleep at night have body temperatures that are lower in the morning than in the afternoon. The opposite is true for nocturnal (night-active) animals. Also, as a water conservation measure, the body temperature of the camel is permitted to increase during the day so that the excess heat can be dissipated at night when the desert air is cool; this is known as heat storage. The temperature of a normal camel, watered every day and fully hydrated, varies by less than 2°C, between about 36 and 38°C (more water available for evaporation and less need for heat storage). When the camel is deprived of drinking water, however, its morning temperature can be as low as 34°C, and its highest temperature, in the late afternoon, can be nearly 41°C (Fig. 11.1).

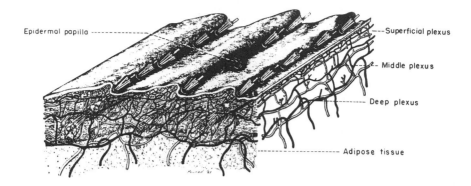

Figure 11.2. Schematic section of dog skin showing the extensive network of blood vessels and the location of insulating adipose tissue. From Lovell JE, Getty R. The sense organs and integument. In: Miller ME, Christensen GC, Evans HE, eds. Anatomy of the dog. Philadelphia: WB Saunders, 1964.

PHYSIOLOGIC RESPONSES TO HEAT AND COLD

Responses to Heat

Circulatory Adjustments

Inasmuch as circulating blood is a distributor of body heat, heat can be lost from the blood if blood is brought to the skin surface and exposed to a gradient for loss to the environment. A schematic section of the skin of the dog (Fig. 11.2) illustrates the extensive network of blood vessels to the skin. The amount of blood circulating to the skin is controlled by sympathetic vasoconstrictor fibers to the blood vessels. An increase in tone results in constriction of blood vessels and diversion of blood from the surface, thereby conserving heat. A decrease in tone lets more blood go to the surface. A stimulus for a decrease in tone, so that more heat can be lost from the body, is the temperature of the blood circulated to the brain. Thermosensitive cells in the anterior hypothalamus respond to warming by activating physiologic and behavioral heat loss mechanisms (Fig. 11.3). Similarly, cooling of the same region stimulates other thermosensitive cells to evoke thermoregulatory responses for heat gain. Reflexes to inhibit vasoconstric-

tor tone also arise from thermoreceptors in the skin and other parts of the body. Special receptors for heat (corpuscles of Ruffini) and receptors for cold (Krause end-bulbs) are illustrated in Figure 2.1.

Evaporative Heat Loss

Evaporation of water results in cooling. Loss of water by evaporation is referred to as insensible water loss; this includes water lost from the skin surfaces and water lost in the heated exhaled air. Normally, about 25% of the heat produced in an animal at rest is lost when water is lost by insensible means.

Evaporative heat losses are increased by sweating and panting. The relative importance of sweating as a heat loss mechanism varies among species. Generally, the function of sweat glands as dissipaters of body heat is less effective in domestic animals than in humans.

There are two types of sweat glands: apocrine and eccrine. Eccrine sweat glands are those typically found in humans but are sparse among domestic animals. In the dog and cat, they occupy only the foot pad location. This area does not subserve thermoregulation; it provides for a moist surface and subsequent improved traction.

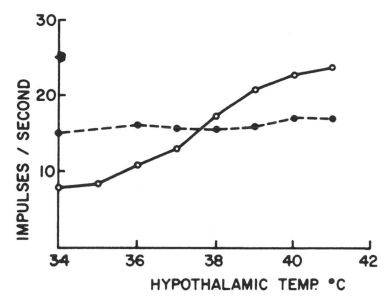

Figure 11.3. Response of warmth-sensitive neurons (*solid line*) in the anterior hypothalamus of the cat to increasing hypothalamic temperature. Neurons insensitive to warmth (*dashed line*) do not increase their activity. From Nakayama T, Hammel HT, Hardy JD, Eisenman JS. Thermal stimulation of electrical activity of single units of the preoptic region. Am J Physiol 1963;204:1122.

Horses, cattle, sheep, dogs, and cats have apocrine sweat glands disseminated over the body surface (Fig. 11.4). The composition, volume, stimulus for secretion, and function of apocrine sweat varies among species. In the dog, and perhaps in other species, apocrine sweat is a proteinaceous, white, odorless, milky fluid that is formed slowly and continuously. On the skin surface, it mixes with sebum from the sebaceous glands to form a protective emulsion that acts as a physical and chemical barrier. Characteristic animal odors arise from bacterial flora action on apocrine secretions. Heat loss from sweating (thermoregulatory function) is probably greatest in the horse, followed (in order) by cattle, sheep, dogs, cats, and swine.

The panting mechanism is effective in dissipating the heat load because greater amounts of air are made to go over moist surfaces. Panting is most effective in the dog, but it is also observed in other domestic animals. Essentially, panting is an increase in dead space ventilation without change in respiratory alveolar ventilation. A decreased tidal volume is associated with the increased respiratory frequency of panting; in this way, hyperventilation of the alveoli is prevented.

In cattle, panting is accompanied by increased salivation, and the salivary secretion promotes cooling by evaporation. Salivary secretion loss by evaporation and drooling (physical loss to the exterior of the body) can result in metabolic acidosis because of loss of bicarbonate and phosphate buffers contained in ruminant saliva.

Increases in sweating and panting are brought about by increased blood temperature, subsequent adjustments by the hypothalamus, and reflexes produced by local heating of the skin.

Responses to Cold

Cold activates body heating mechanisms, just as excess heat activates body cooling mechanisms. With excess cooling, heat is either conserved by reducing heat loss or is generated to compensate for that which is lost. The physiologic responses to cold are activated by blood temperature and local reflexes, as are the responses to heat.

Reduction of Heat Loss

In an attempt to reduce heat loss, animals instinctively curl up when they lie down. This behavioral response reduces the surface area exposed to the cold. To increase the insulation value of their hair or fur, piloerection occurs. In this process, the hair becomes more erect by the arrector pili muscle of the hair follicle (Fig. 11.4).

With sustained exposure to cold, the hair coat thickens and the amount of subcutaneous fat increases.

In contrast to vasodilation, which occurs to accommodate heat loss, the peripheral vessels are constricted by an increase in vasoconstrictor tone.

Heat is also conserved by the arrangement of the deep blood vessels that supply the legs of animals. Blood returning in the veins from the colder legs is close to the warmer blood in the arteries going to the legs. Because of the temperature differences, heat is transferred from the arteries to the veins; this decreases the gradient for heat loss from the arterial

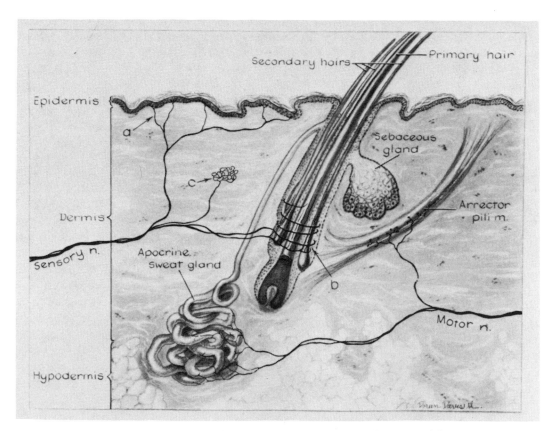

Figure 11.4. Schematic representation of nerve supply and glands of section of dog skin. The blood supply is not shown. *a, b,* Elements of the dermal and hair follicle nerve network; *c,* specialized sensory organ (typical for cold or heat). Contraction of the arrector pili muscle erects the hair follicle. From Muller GH, Kirk RW, Scott DW. Small animal dermatology. 4th ed. Philadelphia: WB Saunders, 1989.

blood to the environment. This arrangement of blood vessels is known as a countercurrent system.

Increase of Heat Production

When the ability to reduce heat loss is not adequate to maintain a normal body temperature, heat must be produced. The temperature to which body temperature falls before heat generation begins is known as the critical temperature. Among farm animals, cattle and sheep have the lowest critical temperature, which means that they are better suited to withstand cold.

Shivering is one means by which heat is generated for withstanding cold. Shivering is a generalized rhythmic contraction of muscles. Because about 75% of the energy of muscle contraction is converted to heat, the seemingly spasmodic contraction of muscle serves a useful purpose.

Other means are recruited to generate heat in addition to shivering. Epinephrine and norepinephrine are both released in increased amounts in the cold. Brown fat is an important source of thermogenesis (see Brown Fat versus White Fat later in this chapter). Epinephrine and norepinephrine are the stimuli for increased metabolism of brown fat. In addition to hibernating animals, brown fat is also found in newborn mammals. Epinephrine and norepinephrine have calorigenic effects with other cells as well, and the calorigenic effects are potentiated by the thyroid hormone. Thyroid hormone is secreted in increased amounts during periods of cold.

Responses to Extreme Environmental Temperatures

Different animal species differ in their ability to withstand heat. The humidity of the air becomes a factor—as humidity increases, evaporation from insensible losses is reduced and less cooling occurs.

Out of all domestic animals, cattle and sheep appear to be the most able to withstand extremes of heat. Open mouth panting and sweating occur as the temperature rises, and these animals can withstand temperatures as high as 43°C (109°F) with the humidity above 65%.

The pig cannot tolerate a temperature above 35°C (95°F) with a humidity above 65%. The intolerance of pigs to heat is recognized by transporters of livestock. During periods of heat, the transport of pigs is usually delayed until night, and they often are hosed with water. Pigs do not sweat copiously, and their small mouth makes them ineffective panters. In addition, they often have substantial subcutaneous fat.

When the relative humidity is above 65%, the cat cannot withstand prolonged exposure to an environmental temperature of 40°C (104°F) or higher. In addition to panting, the cat can increase evaporative losses by spreading saliva over its hair coat.

Because the dog is an effective panter, it can withstand extreme environmental temperatures better than the cat, but it is in danger of collapse when its rectal temperature reaches 41°C (106°F).

In birds, the air sacs are extensions of their lungs, which extend into the body cavities. The body temperature of birds is about 41°C (106°F). Ventilating air is more likely to cool the body of birds than that of mammals because of the larger gradient and because of the closeness of the air to the body organs. It appears that prolonged exposure of a hen to an air temperature of 38°C (100°F) is unsafe if the relative humidity is above 75%. A rectal temperature of 45°C (113°F) is the upper limit of safety in the chicken.

HIBERNATION

Hibernation is the act of resting in a dormant state in a protected burrow. This definition has recently returned to favor. Formerly, it was proposed that "Hibernation is the assumption of a state of greatly reduced core temperature by a mammal or a bird which has its active body temperature near 37°C, meanwhile retaining the capability of spontaneously rewarming back to the normal homeothermic level without absorbing heat from its environment" (Menaker M. Hibernation—hypothermia: an annual cycle of response to low temperature in the bat *Myotis lucifugus*. J Cell Comp Physiol 1962;59:16–174). According to the second definition, bears were not considered to be true hibernators because their core body temperature was not greatly reduced. The core body temperature of bears is reduced by only 6.8°C during their dormancy, as opposed to a reduction of 20 to 30°C by animals that are considered to be true hibernators. The lesser reduction in body temperature of the bear is now believed to be a biologic protection for hibernating bears; accordingly, they are considered true hibernants. Because of their large body mass, it is thought that too much time would be involved in their revival to activity if their body temperature was lowered by 20 to 30°C. The longer revival time would make them an easy victim to another cannibalistic bear that had revived.

Characteristics of Hibernation

The characteristics of hibernation are as follows:

1. Hibernation is a process of warm-blooded animals.
2. The process is autonomous—the animal induces and reverses hibernation by some self-contained mechanism.
3. The process is radical—changes involve not only overt physiologic functioning, but also cellular and subcellular changes.
4. All physiologic functions continue, but at a reduced rate.

5. During the process, body temperature is lowered significantly to a level compatible with survival for the species.

Awakening from Hibernation

Hibernating animals awake from their dormant state periodically. For example, the kidneys continue to form urine and the animal has a need to urinate. A protective mechanism against profound cooling also exists in winter hibernants. If the body temperature declines to levels near freezing, the animal awakes and rapidly rewarms.

Brown Fat Versus White Fat

The ability of hibernators to elevate their body temperature from reduced levels to the temperature necessary for arousal is facilitated by their depots of brown fat. Brown fat differs from white fat, not only in color, but also in metabolic characteristics. When brown fat cells are stimulated, they consume oxygen and produce heat at a high rate. Brown fat tissue is located mainly between the shoulder blades, and its temperature during arousal is among the highest of any part of the body.

HYPOTHERMIA AND HYPERTHERMIA

Reduction of the deep body temperature below normal in nonhibernating homeotherms is known as hypothermia; hyperthermia is the reverse.

Hypothermia can readily occur during central nervous system anesthesia because the hypothalamic response to cold blood is depressed. It normally occurs as a result of prolonged exposure to cold, coupled with an inability of the heat-conserving and heat-generating mechanisms to keep pace. Tolerance to lowered body temperatures varies among species. In dogs, death can occur when the rectal temperature approximates 25°C (77°F). Hypothermia in any animal can become life-threatening unless environmental conditions improve or external heat is provided.

Hyperthermia

Fever

Fever is an elevation of deep body temperature that is brought on by microorganism-caused disease. Fever is usually beneficial because immunologic mechanisms are accelerated and the high temperature induced is detrimental to the microorganisms; but fever can be damaging if it is allowed to go too high. In fever, the set point of the hypothalamus is elevated and the body senses that the blood is too cold, so heat-conserving and heat-generating mechanisms are recruited. Shivering and a feeling of coolness are characteristics of beginning fever. Fever is generally self-limiting; maximum temperatures of 41°C (106°F) can be approached.

Heat Stroke and Impaired Evaporation

Hyperthermia exclusive of fever can be associated with heat stroke. In this condition, heat production exceeds the evaporative capacity of the environment. Hyperthermia can also develop when the evaporative mechanisms become impaired as a result of loss of body fluid or reduced blood volume. Antipyretic drugs are ineffective in reducing the body temperature in these conditions, and relief is obtained only by whole-body cooling.

STUDY AIDS—BODY HEAT AND TEMPERATURE REGULATION

Body Temperature

1. Does a rectal temperature reading represent the temperature throughout the body?

2. What is meant by diurnal temperature?
3. Give an example of heat storage in an animal. What advantage is served by heat storage?
4. What is an approximate value for rectal temperature in the common domestic animals?

Physiologic Responses to Heat and Cold

1. How can the diversion of blood to the skin result in loss of body heat? How can heat loss by this means be regulated?
2. What is the stimulus for allowing heat to be lost via the skin?
3. Where are thermosensitive cells located in the brain?
4. Are there any reflexes associated with heat gain or heat loss?
5. What percent of the heat produced in the body is normally lost by insensible means?
6. What type of sweat glands predominate in animals?
7. What is the principal function of the apocrine sweat glands?
8. Is sweating an important mechanism for heat loss among domestic animals? Which one of the domestic animals represents the greatest use of this means? The least?
9. What function is accomplished by panting? What is panting? How is hyperventilation prevented while panting? Is panting only observed in the dog?
10. How are responses to cold activated?
11. What is accomplished by the countercurrent flow of blood in the limbs of animals?
12. What are some behavioral responses to reduce heat loss?
13. What is piloerection?
14. Which farm animals have the lowest critical temperature?

15. What is accomplished by shivering?
16. What is the role of thyroid hormone in adaptation to cold?
17. Which domestic animals are most able to withstand extremes of heat?
18. What factors are associated with the pig's intolerance to heat?
19. How does the cat increase evaporative heat loss?
20. What is an approximate body temperature of birds? Why is ventilation more likely to cool the body of birds than that of mammals?

Hibernation

1. What is the definition of hibernation? Is a greatly reduced core temperature a necessary component of hibernation?
2. Is the bear considered to be a true hibernant?
3. Is hibernation characteristic of homeotherms or poikilotherms?
4. What prevents hibernants from freezing? Is there periodic awakening from hibernation?
5. What is brown fat?

Hypothermia and Hyperthermia

1. What is hypothermia?
2. How can hypothermia occur in anesthetized animals?
3. What is fever? What are its beneficial effects?
4. Where is the need for fever sensed?
5. What are characteristics of heat stroke? How can its associated hyperthermia be relieved?

SELF-EVALUATION—BODY HEAT AND TEMPERATURE REGULATION

1. A true hibernant:
   a. is not represented by the bear
   b. abandons homeothermy in cold weather but will awaken if body temperature approaches freezing or some other higher set point
   c. abandons homeothermy in the cold and may freeze if body temperature becomes lower than freezing
   d. maintains a constant body temperature even while it sleeps through cold weather
2. The average rectal temperature in a healthy cow should be about:
   a. 98.6 °F
   b. 101.5 °F
   c. 104.0 °F
   d. 106.5 °F
3. What part of the brain has a temperature regulating center?
   a. medulla
   b. thalamus
   c. hypothalamus
   d. cerebral cortex
4. Which sweat gland type predominates among the domestic animals?
   a. eccrine
   b. apocrine
5. The countercurrent flow of blood to the limbs of animals assists in warming the limbs.
   a. true
   b. false
6. Which domestic animal(s) is/are best able to withstand cold?
   a. horse
   b. dog
   c. pig
   d. cattle and sheep
7. Which one of the following animals has the greatest heat loss from sweating?
   a. sheep
   b. cats
   c. dogs
   d. horses
   e. pigs
8. Increased blood flow to the skin would increase heat loss.
   a. true
   b. false
9. White fat is more productive of heat production than brown fat.
   a. true
   b. false

10. Which one of the following is characterized by greater heat production than
the capacity for heat dissipation?
a. fever
b. heat stroke

Suggested Readings

Al-Bagdadi F. The integument. In: Evans HE. Miller's anatomy of the dog. 3rd ed. Philadelphia: WB Saunders, 1993.

Andersson BE. Temperature regulation and environmental physiology. In: Swenson MJ, Reece WO, eds. Dukes' physiology of domestic animals. 11th ed. Ithaca, NY: Cornell University Press, 1993:886–895.

Folk GE, Jr. Textbook of environmental physiology. 2nd ed. Philadelphia: Lea & Febiger, 1974.

Folk GE, Jr, Larson A, Folk MA. Physiology of hibernating bears. Proceedings of the third international conference on bear research and management, June 1974. In: Pelton MR, Lentfer JW, Folk GE, eds. Bears—their biology and management. Morges, Switzerland: International Union for Conservation of Nature and Natural Resources, 1976:373–380.

Muller GH, Kirk RW, Scott DW. Small animal dermatology. 4th ed. Philadelphia: WB Saunders, 1989.

Schmidt-Nielsen K. Osmotic regulation in higher vertebrates. In: The harvey lectures, 1962–1963. Series 58. London: Academic Press, Inc., 1963:53–93.

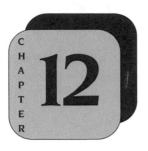

Male
Reproduction

The reproductive functions of the male involve the formation of sperm and the deposition of the sperm into the female. Sperm are produced in the seminiferous tubules of the testes and are then transported through the rete testes to the epididymides, where they are stored and matured. The production of sperm is a continuous process once it has been initiated. However, it can change in rate at times in some species, depending on the amount of daylight (photoperiod). The introduction of semen into the female is preceded by erection of the penis so it can enter the tubular genitalia of the female. Entrance is followed by emission of sperm into the penile urethra, along with stored secretions of the accessory glands. Actual transport of semen through the penile urethra to the region of the cervix or into the uterus of the female is accomplished by ejaculation. The process of male reproduction is assisted by hormones and by the autonomic nervous system.

PARTS OF THE MALE REPRODUCTIVE SYSTEM

Testis

The two testes produce spermatozoa. Although they vary somewhat in size, shape, and location among species, they share a similar structure. The bull testicle and its associated genitalia are shown in Figures 12.1 and 12.2. The seminiferous tubules are convoluted and occupy the greatest portion of each testicle. The spermatozoa are produced within them. The testicle is surrounded by a connective tissue capsule called the tunica albuginea. Support of the seminiferous tubules is provided by connective tissue extensions (septa or trabeculae) into the testis from the tunica albuginea. A cross section of the testicle (Fig. 12.3) shows the relationship of the seminiferous tubules to each other and to their connective tissue support (interstitial tissue).

In addition to spermatozoa in various stages of development, two other impor-

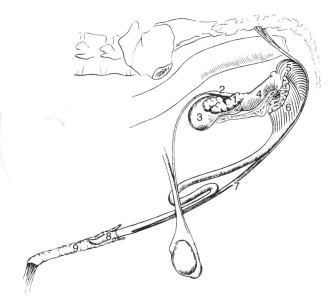

Figure 12.1. Genital organs of the bull. *1,* Seminal vesicle; *2,* ampulla of vas deferens; *3,* bladder; *4,* urethral muscle surrounding pelvic urethra; *5,* bulbospongiosus muscle; *6,* ischiocavernosus muscle; *7,* retractor penis muscle; *8,* glans penis; *9,* preputial membrane and cavity. From Roberts SJ. Veterinary obstetrics and genital diseases (theriogenology). 3rd ed. Woodstock, VT: Stephen J. Roberts, 1986.

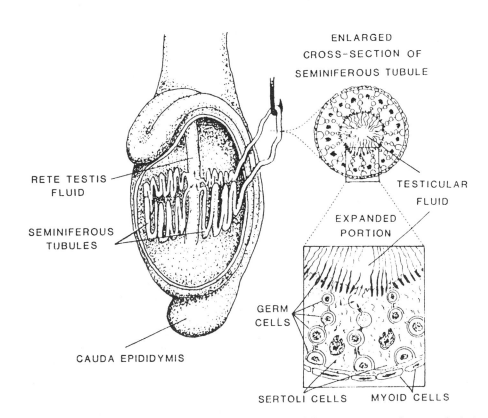

Figure 12.2. Detailed structure of the testicle. Only two of the many seminiferous tubule loops are shown. Testicular fluid is secreted by Sertoli cells into the lumen of the seminiferous tubules. Myoid cells are contractile cells contained within the basement membrane. From Hafez ESE. Reproduction in farm animals. 6th ed. Philadelphia: Lea & Febiger, 1993.

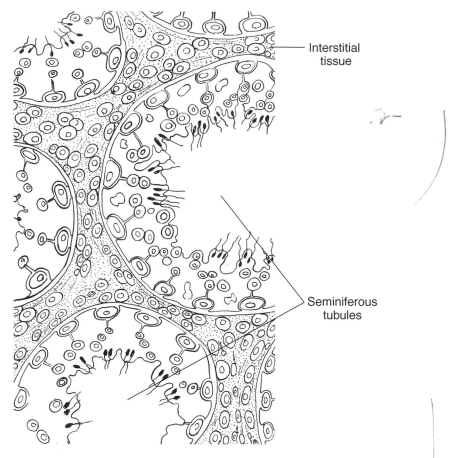

Interstitial
tissue

Seminiferous
tubules

Figure 12.3. Relationship of the seminiferous tubules to each other and to the interstitial tissue. The interstitial tissue is occupied not only by the usual blood vascular network but also by Leydig cells (interstitial cells) and by connective tissue septa (provides support for seminiferous tubules) from the connective tissue capsule (tunica albuginea) of the testis.

tant cell types are the Sertoli cell (sustentacular cell) and the Leydig cell (interstitial cell). The Sertoli cell provides a "nurse" function for developing spermatozoa. Processes from Sertoli cells surround spermatids and spermatocytes and provide intimate contact with all stages of spermatozoa production; in this respect, they are known as sustentacular (supporting) cells. The arrangement of Sertoli cells and the details of seminiferous tubule compartments are shown in Figure 12.4. The Sertoli cells have their base at the periphery of the seminiferous tubules and extend toward the center. The basal junction (tight junction) with adjacent Sertoli cells forms a blood-testis barrier that permits control of the environment within the tubule and also prevents spermatozoa from entering the interstitium. The Sertoli cells divide the seminiferous tubules into two compartments: (1) the basal compartment, which communicates with interstitial fluid and provides space for germinal epithelial cells; and (2) the adluminal compartment, which is the space between Sertoli cells that communicates centrally with the lumen of the tubule. Division of a germi-

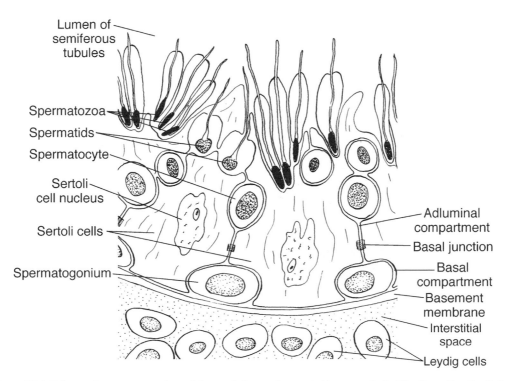

Lumen of semiferous tubules

Spermatozoa
Spermatids
Spermatocyte
Sertoli cell nucleus
Sertoli cells
Spermatogonium

Adluminal compartment
Basal junction
Basal compartment
Basement membrane
Interstitial space
Leydig cells

Figure 12.4. Schematic representation of the periphery of a seminiferous tubule. The Sertoli cells divide the seminiferous tubule into adluminal and basal compartments at their basal junction (tight junction). Leydig cells are in the interstitial space. The basal junction forms a blood-testis barrier whereby the tubule environment is controlled and spermatozoa are prevented from entering the interstitium.

nal epithelial cell (spermatogonium) in the basal compartment provides a replacement cell and another cell, which must move through the Sertoli cell junction to enter the adluminal compartment. Here, further divisions occur and spermatozoa are finally formed. The Sertoli cells secrete a fluid into the adluminal compartment; its composition favors the developing spermatozoa.

Epididymis

The epididymis is a collection and storage tubule for the testis (Fig. 12.5). It begins at the pole of the testis in which blood vessels and nerves enter; this is known as the head of the epididymis. The head continues along one side of the testis as the body of the epididymis, which terminates before making a turn upward as the tail of the

epididymis. The head of the epididymis receives sperm and adluminal fluid through efferent ducts from the rete testis (the intratesticular network of straight tubules that receives content from the convoluted seminiferous tubules). Spermatozoa move to the epididymis by the flow of fluid into the lumen of the seminiferous tubules from the adluminal spaces. Storage in the epididymis allows the spermatozoa to reach maturity and become motile. Reabsorption of much of the seminiferous tubular fluid occurs in the head of the epididymis.

Ductus Deferens

The ductus deferens (Fig. 12.1), sometimes called the vas deferens, is the continuation of the duct system from the tail of the epididymis to the pelvic urethra. As the ductus deferens leaves the testis, toward the abdomen, it is enclosed along with the testicular artery, vein, and nerve, lymphatic vessels, and internal cremaster muscle within the visceral layer of the tunica vaginalis (tunica vaginalis propria). This combination of structures is known as the spermatic cord (Fig. 12.6). The visceral layer of the tunica vaginalis also envelops the testis and epididymis. It is derived from abdominal peritoneum of embryonic origin, when the testes descended to the scrotum. After the spermatic cord passes through the internal and external inguinal rings (slits in the tendinous attachments of the two flat abdominal muscles to the pelvis), the ductus deferens separates from the spermatic cord to proceed to the pelvic urethra (Fig. 12.1). The ductus deferens terminates with an enlarged, glandular area (variable size among species), known as the ampulla of the ductus deferens (absent in the boar). The relationship of the terminal ductus deferens to the urinary bladder, accessory glands, and pelvic urethra is also shown in Figure 12.1.

Scrotum

The scrotum is a cutaneous sac containing the testes. The scrotum contains a subcutaneous layer of smooth muscle fibers, the tunica dartos, which contracts in cold weather and holds the testes closer to the abdominal wall. The scrotum is lined with the parietal layer of the tunica vaginalis, which is a continuation of parietal peritoneum into the scrotum.

Tunica Vaginalis

Describing the lining of the scrotum and covering of the testis in more detail is helpful because it explains the origin of

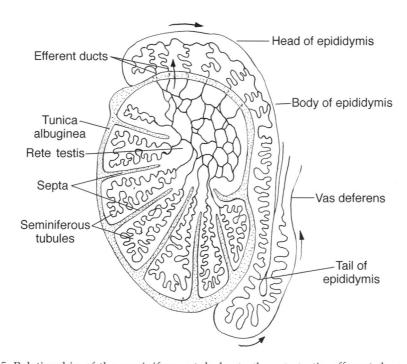

Figure 12.5. Relationship of the seminiferous tubules to the rete testis, efferent ducts, epididymis, and vas deferens. The rete testis is a network of straight tubules connecting convoluted seminiferous tubules with the highly convoluted epididymal tubule via efferent ducts (extratesticular). The flow of spermatozoa with their fluids is shown by the arrows.

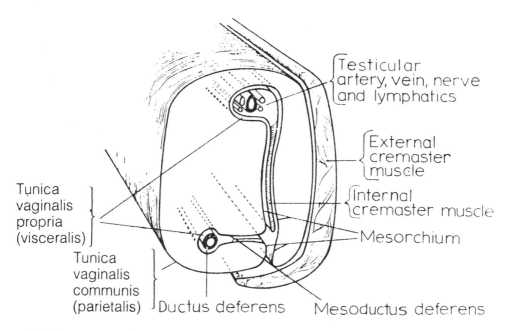

Figure 12.6. Spermatic cord of mammals. From Frandson RD, Spurgeon TL. Anatomy and physiology of farm animals. 5th ed. Philadelphia: Lea & Febiger, 1992.

scrotal or inguinal hernias frequently encountered in pigs. During embryonic development, the testis is intra-abdominal but is outside the peritoneum. It has not yet entered the scrotum, but it has a fibrous connection to the scrotum known as the gubernaculum testis. As development and growth progress, the gubernaculum testis pulls the testis through the inguinal canal (a slit-like passage between the two flat abdominal muscles associated with the inguinal rings) into the scrotum through a double-walled tube of peritoneum, the vaginal process, which preceded the descent of the testis (Fig. 12.7). The vaginal process grew downward through the inguinal canal to the bottom of the scrotum and was accompanied by an inguinal extension of the gubernaculum testis that provided the testicular pull. The testis, epididymis, ductus deferens, internal cremaster muscle, and testicular vessels are enveloped by the inner tube of peritoneum known as the tunica vaginalis propria (visceral tunic). The vessels, nerves, internal cremaster muscle and ductus deferens are the components of the spermatic cord (Fig. 12.6). The outer tube of peritoneum is known as the tunica vaginalis communis (parietal tunic) and it lines the scrotum. The testis and epididymis that are enveloped within the visceral tunic completely fill the scrotal cavity lined by the parietal tunic so that only a narrow space remains between the two tunics (the vaginal cavity). The vaginal cavity is continuous with the abdominal cavity at the vaginal ring (the location where the parietal tunic of the scrotum is continuous with the parietal peritoneum of the abdominal cavity). The spermatic cord passes through the vaginal ring into the abdominal cavity (Fig. 12.7). If the vaginal ring is too large, loops of small intestine may enter the vaginal cavity to constitute what is known as a hernia. The intestinal loops have the potential for strangulation (cutting off of blood-supply)

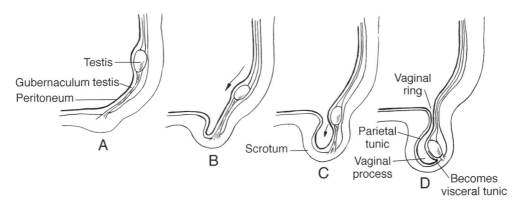

Figure 12.7. The descent of one testis is shown as it is pulled from its retroperitoneal location into the scrotum. The testis shown in D will become enveloped by viscreal tunic that will extend into the abdominal cavity, whereupon an inner tube of peritoneum (the spermatic cord) will be separated from the outer tube that lines the scrotum and peritoneal cavity. The space bewteen the two tubes is the vaginal cavity. A defective vaginal ring predisposes to hernias. See text for details.

or for evisceration (removal from the abdominal cavity) at the time of castration.

Cryptorchid testes are those that fail to descend. This condition appears to be most prevalent in pigs and horses. When the testis is in the inguinal canal, but not in the scrotum, the horse is referred to as a "high flanker." The testis or testes often are retained entirely within the abdominal cavity.

Accessory Sex Glands and Semen

The accessory sex glands provide secretions that empty into the pelvic urethra near their origin (Fig. 12.8). They vary in size and shape among species and can be absent in some. The accessory glands are comprised of the ampullae of the ducti deferentes, the vesicular glands (sometimes called seminal vesicles), the prostate gland, and the bulbourethral glands (sometimes called Cowper's glands). The ampullae (absent in the boar and dog) are enlargements of the terminal part of the ducti deferentes, and their secretion empties into the lumens of the ducti deferentes. The vesicular glands (absent in the dog) are paired glands that empty into the pelvic urethra along with the ducti deferentes. The prostate gland is present in all domestic animals. It is prominent in the dog; it

encircles the urethra. Enlargement can be a cause for obstruction of urine flow through the urethra; this condition is more common in older dogs. Multiple ducts from this gland empty directly into the urethra. The paired bulbourethral glands (absent in the dog) are the most caudal of the accessory glands. At the time of ejaculation, the accessory gland secretions (collectively known as seminal plasma) are mixed with sperm and fluid from the epididymides to form semen.

The seminal plasma provides an environment conducive to the survival of sperm within the female reproductive tract. It is rich in electrolytes, fructose, ascorbic acid, and other vitamins. Whereas fertilization can occur with sperm unaided by seminal plasma, the greatest fertilization potential is achieved with it. Species differ in the composition of seminal plasma, but it seems that each species has solved the same fundamental problems in a different way. One unvarying component among all species, however, is fructose. The advantage of fructose as an energy source might be that it does not require metabolic energy for entrance into the spermatozoa.

Several prostaglandins are present in seminal plasma. It is thought that they aid in fertilization in two ways: (1) prosta-

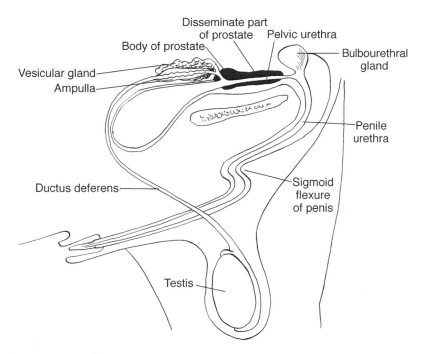

Vesicular gland

Ampulla

Body of prostate

Disseminate part
of prostate

Pelvic urethra

Bulbourethral
gland

Penile
urethra

Ductus deferens

Sigmoid
flexure
of penis

Testis

Figure 12.8. Disposition of the accessory glands that discharge into the pelvic urethra of the bull.

glandins react with cervical mucus and make it more receptive to sperm; and (2) some of the prostaglandins present cause smooth muscle contraction, so it is believed that reverse peristalsis is initiated in the uterus and oviducts to facilitate transport of sperm toward the ovaries.

Most of the sperm in an ejaculate never reach the oviduct. In fact, only a few dozen might reach the vicinity of the ovum, where only one is required for fertilization. Semen collected for artificial insemination is often diluted and is mixed with extenders to obtain the greatest number of insemination units. The number of sperm intended for each artificial insemination varies among species, but it approximates 10 and 125 million, respectively, for cattle and sheep, and 2 billion each for pigs and horses.

Penis

The penis is the male organ of copulation through which urine and semen pass by way of the penile urethra. The appearance

of the penis of several farm animals and its association with other structures is shown in Figure 12.9. The roots (crura) of the penis begin at the caudal border of the pelvic ischial arch. The forward extension from the roots is known as the body and the free extremity is known as the glans. The internal structure (Fig. 12.10) is occupied mostly by cavernous tissue (known more commonly as erectile tissue). Cavernous tissue is a collection of blood sinusoids separated by sheets of connective tissue. The stallion has a large amount of erectile tissue relative to connective tissue (Fig. 12.10B), and greater enlargement is possible during erection than in the bull (Fig. 12.10A), where the ratio of erectile tissue to connective tissue is less. The urethra is on the ventral aspect of the body of the penis (Fig. 12.10).

The ram has a highly visible urethral process (Fig. 12.9B), and sometimes, urethral calculi become lodged in its narrowed extremity. This can be corrected by

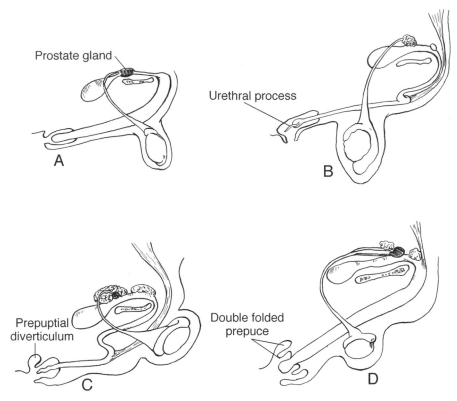

Figure 12.9. Comparative anatomy of the male reproductive organs of various domestic animals. **A**. Dog. **B**. Ram. **C**. Boar. **D**. Stallion. Note the encirclement of the pelvic urethra by the prostate in the dog, urethral process in the ram, preputial diverticulum in the boar, and double folded prepuce in the stallion.

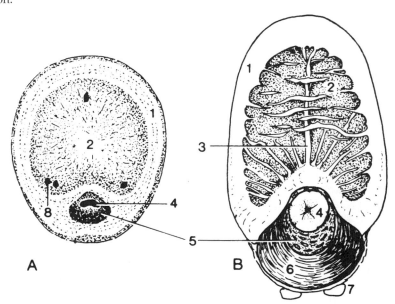

Figure 12.10. Transverse sections of the fibroelastic penis of a bull (**A**) and the musculocavernous penis of a stallion (**B**). *1*, Tunica albuginea; *2*, corpus cavernosum; *3*, septum; *4*, urethra; *5*, corpus spongiosium; *6*, bulbospongiosus; *7*, retractor penis; *8*, large, thick-walled veins. From Dyce KM, Sack WO, Wensing CJG. Textbook of veterinary anatomy. 2nd ed. Philadelphia: WB Saunders, 1996.

amputation of the process. It is speculated that the function of the urethral process in the ram is to spray the cervical area with semen during ejaculation. The free end of such an extension would move in a circular pattern with the emission of fluid under pressure.

The dog has a bulbus glandis at the caudal part of the glans. The enlargement of the bulbus glandis is responsible for prolonged retention of the penis during coitus. Contraction of muscles in the vestibule of the female vagina caudal to the bulbus glandis assists this retention, commonly known as the tie (Fig. 12.11).

The bull, ram, and boar have a sigmoid flexure of their penis, resulting in an S shape when not erect (Figs. 12.8 and 12.9).

Erection causes extension of the flexure as shown for the bull in Figure 12.12.

Prepuce

The prepuce is an invaginated fold of skin that surrounds the free extremity of the penis (Fig. 12.9). The stallion has a double-folded prepuce. Waxy accumulations known as "beans" sometimes form in the outer fold and must be removed manually. The boar has a preputial diverticulum (pouch) on the dorsal wall, which often contains decomposing urine and macerated epithelium. The fluid in the diverticulum also contains a pheromone that causes sows to assume the immobile mating stance.

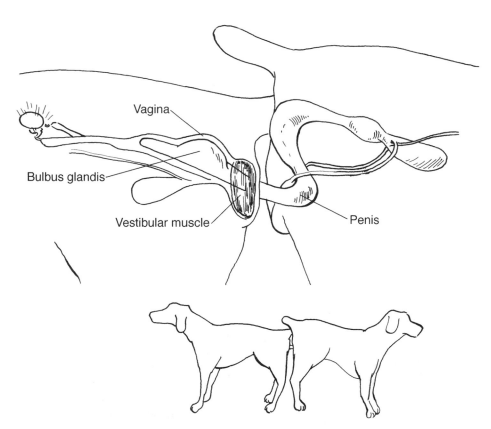

Figure 12.11. "Locking" phase, or "tie" of canine coitus (lateral view). In the dog, erection primarily involves the glans penis. Enlargement of the bulbus glandis and contraction of vestibular muscles during intromission "lock" the dog's penis in the bitch's vagina.

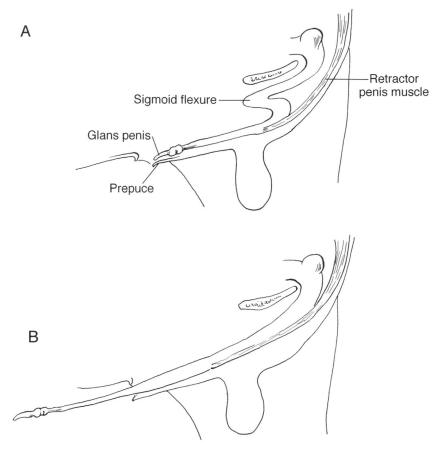

Figure 12.12. Penis of the bull. **A**. Nonerect position with its characteristic sigmoid flexure. **B**. Erect position with elimination of the sigmoid flexure and extension beyond the prepuce. The retractor penis muscle assists return of the penis to its nonerect position.

Muscles of Male Genitalia

The external cremaster muscle is formed from the caudal fibers of the internal abdominal oblique muscle. It passes through the inguinal canal and attaches to the outside of the parietal layer of tunica vaginalis (Fig. 12.6). This muscle pulls the testis up against the external inguinal ring, particularly in cold weather. The cremaster muscles are responsible for the testes being drawn into the abdominal cavity of the elephant, deer, and rabbit during times other than the breeding season. The internal cremaster muscle (Fig. 12.6) is composed of smooth muscle fibers that help to hold spermatic cord structures together.

A skeletal muscle, the urethralis, is the pelvic continuation from the smooth muscle wall of the urinary bladder. Peristaltic action of this muscle assists in the transport of urine or semen through the pelvic urethra.

The bulbospongiosus muscle (Fig. 12.13) is a striated muscle continuation of the urethralis. It continues throughout the length of the penis in the horse but only proceeds for a short distance along the penile urethra in other animals. The bulbospongiosus muscle continues the action of the urethralis in emptying the urethra.

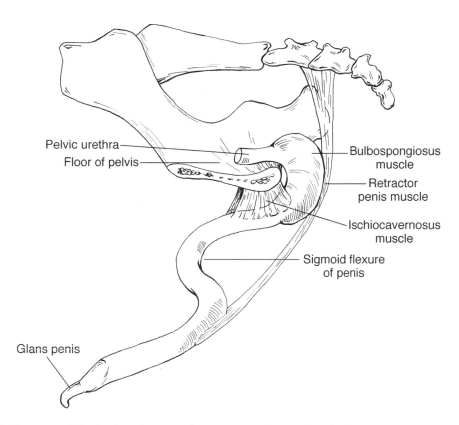

Pelvic urethra
Floor of pelvis
Bulbospongiosus muscle
Retractor penis muscle
Ischiocavernosus muscle
Sigmoid flexure of penis
Glans penis

Figure 12.13. Penis of the bull and some of its associated muscles. The bulbospongiosus muscle assists in emptying the urethra. The ischiocavernosus muscle assists in the erection process and the retractor penis muscle assists in the return of the penis to the prepuce after intromission.

The ischiocavernosus muscles are paired, striated muscles that converge on the body of the penis from their origins on the lateral sides of the ischial arch (Figs. 12.1 and 12.13). When these muscles contract, they pull the penis upward against the floor of the pelvis. Much of the venous drainage from the penis is obstructed because of the location of the veins on the dorsal surface of the penis, and erection is thereby assisted.

The retractor penis muscles are paired striated muscles that originate from the suspensory ligaments of the anus. They continue forward and converge caudal to the body of the penis (Figs. 12.12 and 12.13). After they join on the underside of the penis, they continue forward to the

glans penis. The retractor penis muscles pull the flaccid penis back into the prepuce.

Blood and Nerve Supply

Blood to the testicles is supplied by the testicular arteries. The testicular veins parallel the testicular arteries. Both artery and vein are enclosed within the spermatic cord (Fig. 12.6). A short distance above the testicle, the testicular vein is convoluted (the pampiniform plexus) and is in close association with the convoluted part of the testicular artery (Fig. 12.14). Their closeness, and because they are convoluted and are therefore longer, provides a means whereby blood entering the testis is cooled by the venous blood leaving the testis. The arteries and veins are also close to the surface of

Figure 12.14. Lateral view of the stallion testis with emphasis on the pampiniform plexus. The pampiniform plexus is illustrated by the intertwining of the testicular artery and vein. This intertwining allows the cooler venous blood to cool the warmer arterial blood going to the testis.

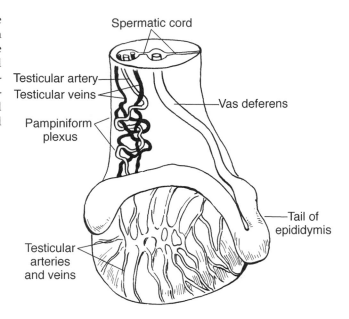

the testes, and so direct loss of heat from the testes is favored. Spermatogenesis requires a cooler temperature than normal body temperature. Arterial blood to the penis provides for filling of the cavernous tissue and provides nutrition to the tissues. The exclusive supply is the artery of the penis, a terminal branch of the internal pudendal arteries. The blood supply to the penis of the horse is slightly different than that of other species and is more extensive.

In addition to autonomic nerve fibers to the testes, penis, and accessory glands, the penis is supplied by a spinal nerve, the pudendal nerve. Terminations of the pudendal nerve are located in the glans penis. Sensory stimulation of the glans provides the afferent side for reflexes associated with erection and ejaculation. Reflex centers for erection and ejaculation are located in the lumbar region of the spinal cord.

SPERMATOGENESIS

Mitosis and Meiosis

The term "spermatogenesis" refers to the entire process involved in the transforma-

tion of germinal epithelial cells (stem cells) to spermatozoa. Mitosis (cell division in which each new cell retains a diploid, or 2n, number of chromosomes) and meiosis (cell division in which each new cell has a haploid, or n, number of chromosomes) occur progressively during spermatogenesis, so that spermatozoa have a haploid number of chromosomes (Fig. 12.15). In the initial stage of the first meiotic division, each chromosome of a chromosome pair forms two chromatids that remain bound together and that have duplicate genes of that chromosome. When a primary spermatocyte divides into two secondary spermatocytes (the first meiotic division), each contains one chromosome (with its two coupled chromatids) of a chromosome pair. In the second meiotic division, two spermatids are formed from each secondary spermatocyte. In this division, the two chromatids of each chromosome separate, forming two sets of duplicate genes with one of the two sets passing into each of the two spermatids. Each spermatid that is finally formed has only half the genes of the original spermatogonium. Similarly, the developing ovum has a haploid number of

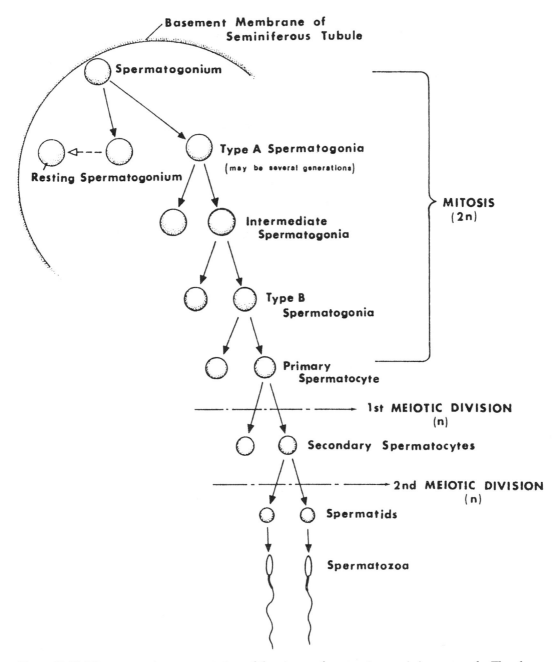

Figure 12.15. Diagrammatic representation of the stages of spermatogenesis in mammals. The chromosome number (*2n,* diploid; *n,* haploid) is also shown for each stage. From Pineda MH. The biology of sex. In: McDonald LE, Pineda MH, eds. Veterinary endocrinology and reproduction. 4th ed. Philadelphia: Lea & Febiger, 1989.

chromosomes, so that the union of spermatozoan and oocyte produces a cell with a diploid number of chromosomes.

Production of Spermatozoa

The stem cells (spermatogonia) are located in the basal compartment of the seminiferous tubules (Fig. 12.4). The mitotic division of a spermatogonium results in one cell being a replacement for the cell that has just divided (it stays in the basal compartment). The other cell becomes a type A spermatogonium, which migrates through the Sertoli cell barrier to the adluminal compartment. Type A spermatogonia undergo mitotic division (sometimes involving several generations) until large numbers (variable among species) of type B spermatogonia have been produced. Type B spermatogonia undergo the last of the mitotic divisions, which results in the formation of primary spermatocytes with 2n chromosome numbers. Primary spermatocytes undergo meiotic division (described previously) to form secondary spermatocytes, which in turn undergo meiotic division to form spermatids (n chromosome numbers). In the bull, 64 spermatids are formed from one type A spermatogonium. Maturation of the spermatids occurs while they are still in the adluminal compartment; it involves a series of nuclear and cytoplasmic changes called spermiogenesis. Spermiogenesis is comprised of a series of nuclear and cytoplasmic changes and a transformation from a nonmotile cell (not able to move) to a potentially motile cell in which a flagellum (tail) has formed. The mature spermatids produced during the final phase of spermiogenesis are released into the lumen of the seminiferous tubules as spermatozoa.

Spermatozoa from several animal species are compared in Figure 12.16. The release of matured spermatids into the lumen of the seminiferous tubules is known as spermiation. The newly formed spermatozoa are essentially immotile. They are transported to the epididymis by fluid secretions into the seminiferous tubules and rete testis and by activity of contractile elements in the testis that direct fluid flow to the head of the epididymis.

Epididymal Transport

The fertilizing ability of an animal is attained progressively during the transit of spermatozoa through the epididymis. Changes include development of unidirectional (as opposed to circular) motility, changes in nuclear chromatin (DNA-protein complex), and changes in the nature of the surface of the plasma membrane.

The major site of sperm storage within the male reproductive tract is the tail (last portion) of the epididymis. About 70% of the total number of spermatozoa in the ducts outside the rete testis (excurrent duct system) are found in the tail of the epididymis.

Many of the spermatozoa formed in the testes are either phagocytized in the excurrent duct system or lost into the urine. About 85% of the daily sperm production in sexually inactive rams are voided in the urine.

Spermatogenic Wave

If all segments of the seminiferous tubules were involved in the same activity at the same time, a continuous supply of spermatozoa would not be produced because about 64 days (in the bull) are required for spermatogenesis (development from spermatogonia to spermatozoa). Mitotic division of stem cells occurs in the bull every 14 days (a cycle); therefore, within an adluminal compartment, spermatogenesis requires 4.6 cycles (64/14). A cycle may be initiated in one segment of the seminiferous tubule on one day and in adjacent segments the next day and continuing, in the case of the bull, through successive segments for 14 days. The adluminal compartments within each segment will undergo 4 to 6 cycles until spermatozoa are released into the

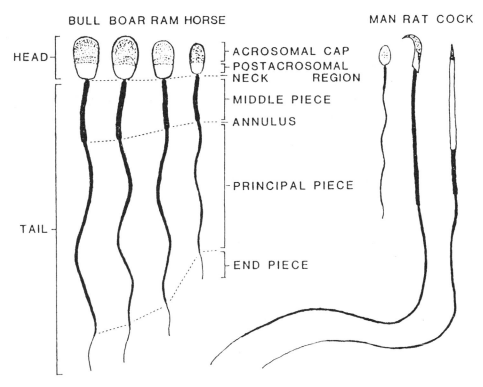

Figure 12.16. Comparison of the spermatozoa of farm animals and other vertebrates. The major structural features are given. Note the differences in the relative size and shape. From Hafez ESE. Reproduction in farm animals. 6th ed. Philadelphia: Lea & Febiger, 1993.

lumen of the seminiferous tubule. A new release will occur daily for each of the successive 14 segments. This continuous presentation of spermatozoa for these 14 segments constitutes a spermatogenic wave, and any one tubule may have as many as 15 waves. The segments progress both ways from the center of each tubule toward the rete testis with the more advanced segments closest to the rete testis. Thus, programming of adjacent segments to cycle at different times provides for a continuous production of spermatozoa. The spermatogenic wave of the rat involves a 12 day cycle and is illustrated in Figure 12.17.

A large number of spermatozoa are produced daily in the normal male animal, about 6.0×10^9 spermatozoa in the bull and about 16.5×10^9 in the boar. In the bull, daily sperm production increases with age, reaching a maximum at about 7 years.

Hormonal Control of Spermatogenesis

Leydig and Sertoli cells are responsible for hormone production within the testes. The production of testosterone by Leydig cells is controlled by the gonadotropin known as luteinizing hormone, LH (sometimes called interstitial cell-stimulating hormone, or ICSH). Low levels of testosterone cause an increase in LH secretion by the anterior pituitary. The increase in LH secretion causes the Leydig cells in the testes to secrete testosterone; when increased, testosterone inhibits the further secretion of LH and testosterone levels are thus stabilized. A subsequent decline in testosterone again stimulates LH secretion, and the cycle is repeated; this is known as a negative feedback system.

The influence of testosterone on spermatogenesis requires that it diffuse from the interstitial tissues into the seminiferous tubules. Within the seminiferous tubules it appears that testosterone maintains spermatogenesis by supporting the meiotic process.

Another gonadotropic hormone, follicle-stimulating hormone (FSH) from the anterior pituitary, stimulates production of an androgen-binding protein (ABP) by the Sertoli cells. ABP is secreted into the lumen of the seminiferous tubules and binds with testosterone and other androgens to stabilize their concentrations and ensure appropriate amounts for spermatogenesis. It is also believed that FSH stimulates the secretion of estrogens by the Sertoli cells. The actual secretion of estrogen might arise from the intracellular conversion of testosterone (originating from Leydig cells) by the Sertoli cells. The Sertoli cells are also the source of a hormone known as inhibin, which inhibits secretion of FSH by the anterior pituitary.

Whereas LH is required continuously for spermatogenesis (testosterone-supported meiosis), FSH is not essential for the maintenance of spermatogenesis once it has been initiated. Initiation of spermatogenesis at puberty and after physiologic or pathologic interruptions requires FSH.

Other Functions of Hormones

Testosterone

In addition to its spermatogenic activity, testosterone fulfills other functions in the peripheral circulation. After secretion of testosterone by Leydig cells into the interstitial space of the testes, a greater amount diffuses into the blood and lymphatic capillaries than that which diffuses into the seminiferous tubules. After entrance into the blood, testosterone is bound loosely with a plasma protein for its transport.

Within 15 to 30 minutes, the testosterone is released from the protein to be fixed to target tissues or to be degraded, mainly by the liver, into inactive products that are subsequently excreted.

Other functions of testosterone include the development and maintenance of libido, secretory activity of the accessory organs, and general body features associated with the male.

Libido refers to sexual drive. It can be eliminated effectively by castration (removal of the testes). Castrated animals usually, but not invariably, lack libido. Small amounts of testosterone from other sources such as the adrenal gland (interconversion

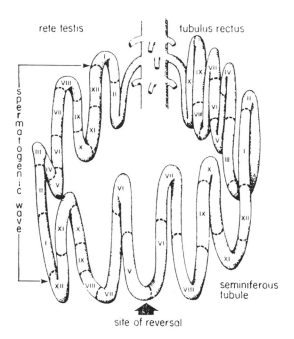

Figure 12.17. Spermatogenic wave for the rat, with a 12-day spermatogenic cycle. The spermatogenic cycle is just beginning in segment I, whereas it is in day 12 of development in segment XII and in day 2 in segment II. Within each segment are four or five developmental forms, with each separated by about 12 days. An actual seminiferous tubule can contain 15 or more spermatogenic waves. From Hafez ESE. Reproduction in farm animals. 6th ed. Philadelphia: Lea & Febiger, 1993.

potential) might be sufficient to provide libido in some animals.

The structural development and physiologic functioning (production of secretions) of the accessory sex glands are influenced by testosterone. In this regard, hyperactive prostate glands (enlargement) can be treated effectively by estrogen administration. The estrogen inhibits the secretion of LH, and testosterone production by the Leydig cells is suppressed. A reduced concentration of testosterone causes the hyperactive prostate gland to reduce its activity, and its size decreases.

General body features associated with the male (secondary sexual characteristics) are influenced by testosterone. These features include increased bone growth (heavier bones), greater muscling, thicker skin, and deeper voice (in the bull). During fetal growth, testosterone directs the descent of the testes. The presence or absence of testosterone determines the respective development of a penis and scrotum or a clitoris and vagina. Before sexual differentiation in the embryo, the structures needed for the development of either sex are present. With normal male hormonal stimulation, the wolffian ducts become tubular portions of the male reproductive system, and the müllerian ducts regress. In the female, the müllerian ducts become tubular portions of the reproductive system, and the wolffian ducts regress.

Metabolically, testosterone has protein anabolic functions that affect the greater muscling potential of males. Probably the thicker skin and laryngeal changes of the male are also related to this function of testosterone. Because of the desirability for more muscle and less fat in meat-producing animals, the current trend is to use noncastrated males for meat production. The protein anabolic effect obtained from testicular testosterone is thereby retained.

Other Androgens

The boar testes secrete large amounts of compounds known as C-16 unsaturated androgens. These androgens act as pheromones when they are excreted in boar saliva, and they cause the sow in heat to adopt the mating posture. When the C-16 unsaturated androgens are excreted in urine, they contribute to the characteristic odor of boar urine. These compounds are also responsible for the undesirable flavor of boar meat, which is known as boar taint.

PHYSICAL CONSIDERATIONS

Erection

An increase in the turgidity of the penis is known as erection. It is caused by an increase of blood pressure within the cavernous sinuses of the penis as a result of greater blood inflow than outflow. The inflow of blood increases through vasodilation of the arteries caused by parasympathetic stimulation. The outflow of blood decreases through compression of the dorsal veins of the penis against the pelvis when the ischiocavernosus muscles contract. Contraction of the ischiocavernosus muscles also compresses the blood in the cavernous sinuses (now a closed system), which also assists erection by increasing blood pressure in the cavernous sinuses (Fig. 12.13).

Complete erection of the glans penis of the horse is delayed until after introduction of the penis into the vagina of the mare. Mounting of the mare compresses the prepuce against the vulva, and venous drainage from the prepuce is impaired. Complete erection of the glans is then possible because venous drainage from the glans is directed to the prepuce.

In animals with a sigmoid flexure, the filling of the cavernous sinuses, coupled with relaxation of the retractor penis muscles, causes the flexure to be eliminated and the penis to be straightened. Even though animals with a sigmoid flexure have a higher ratio of connective tissue to cavernous tissue, the length and diameter of the penis increase somewhat as a result of erection, in addition to penis straightening. As compared to the bull, ram, and boar, the penis of the horse has a lower ratio of connective tissue to cavernous tissue, and a relatively greater increase in the length and diameter of its penis occurs during erection.

Blood pressure within the corpus cavernosum penis of the bull has been measured during coitus. A pressure of approximately 14,000 mm Hg was associated with peak activity, and peak activity was correlated with an increased intensity of ischiocavernosus muscle contraction that furthered compression of blood in the cavernous tissue. Higher pressures have been recorded. It is believed that these high pressures, coupled with cavernous tissue capsule weakness, might be the cause of rupture of the corpus cavernosum penis (hematoma of the penis) in some bulls. The usual rupture site is on the dorsal surface of the distal curve of the sigmoid flexure (Fig. 12.12).

Mounting and Intromission

Mounting is the stance assumed by the male by which the penis is brought into apposition with the vulva of the female. Successful mounting must be preceded by a receptive stance on the part of the female. Failures in mounting are encountered when there are injuries, weakness, or soreness in the hind limbs of the male.

Introduction of the penis into the vagina and its maintenance within the vagina during coitus is known as intromission. Pelvic thrusts assisted by the abdominal muscles assist penetration of the penis into the vagina. The duration of intromission varies among species—it is shortest for the bull and ram and longest for the boar. Failures of intromission occur in some animals; causes include phimosis (constriction of the preputial orifice), hematoma of the penis (as in the bull), and congenital deformities. Final distention of the penis does not occur in the dog until after intromission. It is presumed that intromission is facilitated in the dog by the presence of the os penis (penis bone in the dog).

Emission and Ejaculation

As sexual stimulation increases, a point is reached at which reflex centers in the spinal cord bring about emission and ejaculation. Emission precedes ejaculation. It results from sympathetic innervation whereby sperm and fluids in the vasa deferentia and ampullae are emptied into the urethra along with fluids from the other accessory glands (seminal plasma). The sympathetic innervation provides peristaltic movement for transport to the urethra and constricts the neck of the bladder to minimize reflux (backward flow) of sperm and fluids into the urinary bladder. Once emission has been accomplished, reflex peristalsis of the urethral muscles propels the urethral content toward the external urethral orifice. The latter phase, peristalsis of the urethra, is assisted by contraction of the bulbospongiosus muscle, which in turn compresses the urethra. The combination of pressure and peristalsis forces the semen and fluid from the urethra to the exterior, the process of ejaculation. Stimulation for emission and ejaculation is derived from sensory nerves located in the glans penis.

Sperm and fluids are ejaculated near the opening of the cervix in cattle and sheep, directly into the uterus in swine, and partially into the uterus in the horse.

FACTORS AFFECTING TESTICULAR FUNCTION

Puberty

Testicular function becomes manifest at the onset of puberty. It is believed that puberty is correlated with a decreased sensitivity of the hypothalamus to testosterone, so that LH is secreted in greater amounts. An increased LH concentration stimulates the Leydig cells to secrete testosterone in greater quantities, and all aspects of testosterone function begin to appear. FSH is essential for the initiation of spermatogenesis at puberty.

Photoperiod

In some species, photoperiod (length of daylight) changes have a marked influence on testicular function. Photoperiod is also related to ovarian activity in the female of these same species. The purpose of photoperiod influence is the coordination of birth with favorable weather conditions. Sheep and goats have major periods of testicular regression during increasing photoperiods, which is restored by decreasing photoperiods. In the stallion, a decreasing photoperiod reduces testicular function. Testicular function and photoperiod in cattle and swine are related only to a minor degree. The pineal gland mediates the photoperiod response in the ram and is probably involved in the response of the other species. When spermatogenesis is stopped during photoperiod inhibition, FSH is again required for its initiation.

REPRODUCTION IN THE AVIAN MALE

The paired testes of the male bird are located within the body cavity in contrast to those of most mammals (Fig. 12.18). In this location they are able to function at body temperature (about 41 to 42°C for domestic species). The internal structure is composed of seminiferous tubules, Sertoli cells, stem cells, and Leydig cells similar to that of mammals. The blood supply to the testes does not provide for a pampiniform plexus, which in mammals is present to assist in

cooling the testes. Instead of an epididymis as arranged in mammals, there are tubules (vasa efferentia) conducting sperm from the testis to a short epididymal duct that is continued as the vas deferens. The vas deferens terminates as an enlargement before its opening into the cloaca at a papilla. The vas deferens and the enlargement serve as storage sites for spermatozoa. The accessory organs of the male include the vasa efferentia, epididymides, vasa deferentia, ejaculatory groove, and phallus (penis). Seminal

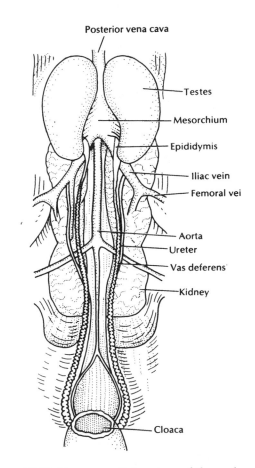

Figure 12.18. The urogenital system of the male chicken (ventral view). The testes are located within the body cavity, and the vasa deferentia conduct spermatozoa to the cloaca. From Sturkie PD, Opel H. Reproduction in the male, fertilization, and early embryonic development. In: Sturkie PD, ed. Avian physiology. 3rd ed. New York: Springer-Verlag, 1976.

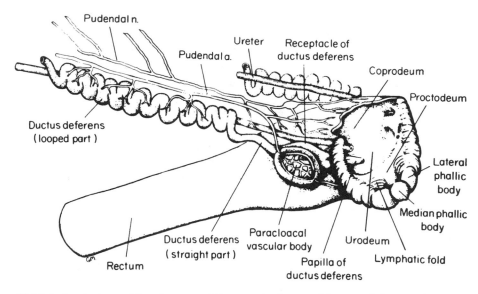

Figure 12.19. Lateral view of the cloaca and the terminal part of the vas deferens (ductus deferens) of the domestic fowl. The ejaculatory groove (not shown) is formed at the time of sexual excitation when the lymphatic folds become engorged with lymph, forming a troughlike structure to direct the flow of semen. The receptacle of the ductus deferens serves as a storage site for spermatozoa. From Lake PE. Male genital organs. In: King AS, McClelland J, eds. Form and function in birds. Vol. 2. San Diego: Academic Press, 1981.

plasma is derived from the seminiferous tubules and vasa efferentia inasmuch as birds do not have a prostate gland, bulbourethral gland, and seminal vesicle. The ejaculatory groove of the erected phallus (Fig. 12.19) is formed at the time of sexual excitation when several folds in the ventral cloaca become engorged with lymph. The engorged folds direct semen through the groove of the erect phallus. The phallus of the male chicken (cock or rooster) and turkey (tom) do not perform intromission but rather transfer semen to the female by touching their phallus to the female vagina, that part of the female reproductive tract terminating at the cloaca. Ducks and geese have sizable penises, and intromission is accomplished at mating.

In the cock, protrusion of the genitalia and forceful expulsion of semen follows external stroking of the base of the tail. Phallic eversion follows similar stimulation in the tom, but semen generally is released only after pressure is applied to the termi-

nal storage depots (terminal enlargements of the vasa deferentia).

The gonadotropic influence of LH and FSH on testicular function is similar to that of mammals, wherein LH acts on Leydig cells to promote their development and testosterone production, and FSH acts on Sertoli cells. Full testicular function results from the combined action of FSH and testosterone.

The collection of semen from cocks and toms is practiced widely. The average volume of cock ejaculate is about 0.5 ml and that of the tom is about 0.3 ml. Sperm concentration of the cock is about four billion/ml and it is about 10 billion/ml for the tom. The chemical composition of seminal plasma varies among birds as well as in mammals. See Figure 12.16 for the comparison of a spermatozoan of the cock with several mammalian species. Spermatozoa of toms are similar to those of cocks. It appears that cock sperm are functionally mature before they leave the testes. Much of the maturation of mammalian spermatozoa occurs in the epididymides.

After mating or artificial insemination, sperm are found in sperm-storage glands of the female that are located in the vagina, near its junction with the uterus. They persist at this location for the fertile period of the female. It is likely that sperm are nourished by the uterovaginal sperm-storage glands and/or are placed into reversible quiescence (quiet period).

STUDY AIDS—MALE REPRODUCTION

Parts of the Male Reproduction System

1. What are the seminiferous tubules?
2. Know the relative location of the Sertoli cells. Are they within the seminiferous tubules?
3. Know the relative location of the Leydig cells. Are they within the seminiferous tubules?
4. Which compartment of the seminiferous tubule provides a home for the spermatogonium. What must it move through to get into the other compartment? What is the name of the compartment where spermatozoa are finally formed?
5. What are the parts of the epididymis?
6. What is accomplished by storage of spermatozoa in the epididymis?
7. What structures comprise the spermatic cord?
8. Read and understand the relationship of scrotal hernias to the visceral and parietal tunica vaginalis.
9. What are cryptorchid testes?
10. What comprises the accessory sex glands? Which one is present in all of the domestic animals? What is its relationship to the pelvic urethra?
11. What is the collective name of the accessory gland secretions? What is the difference between seminal plasma and semen?
12. What function is served by seminal plasma?
13. What function may be served by the prostaglandins present in seminal plasma?
14. Are we talking about big numbers when describing the number of sperm present for each artificial insemination? Give an example.
15. Why is greater enlargement of the penis possible in the stallion than it is in the bull?
16. What is the urethral process of the ram penis?
17. How does the bulbus glandis of the dog penis participate in the "tie" associated with canine coitus?
18. Which domestic species have a sigmoid flexure of their penis?
19. Note the preputial diverticulum (pouch) in the boar and the double folded prepuce in the stallion (Fig. 12.9).
20. Note the functions for the external cremaster muscle, the internal cremaster muscle, the urethralis and bulbospongiosus muscle, the ischiocavernosus muscles, and the retractor penis muscles.
21. What is the function of the pampiniform plexus?

Spermatogenesis

1. Define spermatogenesis.
2. Spermatids undergo nuclear and cytoplasmic changes and develop a tail. What is this maturation phase called?
3. What is spermiation?
4. Where is the fertilizing ability of spermatozoa attained? Where are they stored? What happens to spermatozoa that are not ejaculated?
5. What function is served by the spermatogenic wave?
6. Describe the negative feedback system that relates to the production of testosterone by Leydig cells. Why is luteiniz-

ing hormone called interstitial cell stimulating hormone (ICSH)?
7. What is the role of testosterone in spermatogenesis?
8. What are the assumed roles of FSH in
the male?
9. Aside from spermatogenesis, what are
other functions of testosterone in the
male?
10. What embryonic structures stimulated
by testosterone become tubular portions of the male reproductive system?
11. What metabolic function is served by
testosterone?
12. What are C-16 unsaturated androgens
that are secreted by boar testes?

Physical Considerations

1. How is erection of the penis accomplished?
2. Does erection accomplish straightening
of the sigmoid flexure?
3. What is an approximate blood pressure
within the corpus cavernosum penis of
the bull during coitus? What is
hematoma of the penis?
4. Define intromission. Which domestic
species has the longest duration of
intromission and which one has the
shortest? Can there be intromission
failures?
5. Differentiate between emission and
ejaculation.

Factors Affecting Testicular Function

1. When does testicular function become
manifest?
2. How does puberty begin in the male?
3. What is the purpose of photoperiod
influence upon testicular function?
4. How does increasing photoperiod affect
sheep and goats? Is this different in the
stallion? Are cattle and swine influenced by photoperiod?
5. What gland mediates the photoperiod
response?

Reproduction in the Avian Male

1. Contrast the location of avian testes
with those of mammals.
2. Is there a pampiniform plexus for cooling of the testes in birds as there is for
most mammalian species?
3. How does the avian epididymis differ
from mammals?
4. What are the storage sites for avian
spermatozoa?
5. What structures provide for seminal
plasma?
6. What name is given to the penis of
birds?
7. Describe the route of ejaculated sperm
from the vasa deferentia to the exterior
in the cock and tom.
8. Which domestic birds accomplish intromission at the time of mating?
9. Where is maturation of spermatozoa
accomplished in birds?
10. Is there a long life for spermatozoa once
they are deposited into the female
vagina?

SELF-EVALUATION—MALE REPRODUCTION

1. A scrotal hernia exists when a loop of
intestine:
   a. descends to the scrotum within the
   spermatic cord
   b. descends to the scrotum in the space
   between the visceral tunic and the
   parietal tunic
   c. is in the peritoneal cavity
   d. occupies the pleural cavity
2. Which one of the following cells lines
the periphery of the seminiferous
tubules and provides a "nurse" function for developing spermatozoa?
   a. Leydig cells
   b. spermatid
   c. Sertoli cells
   d. MPS cells

3. Which one of the following hormones is/are found in seminal plasma and is/are thought to assist fertilization by making cervical mucus more receptive to sperm and to facilitate sperm transport by contracting uterine smooth muscle?
   a. prostaglandins
   b. testosterone
   c. estrogen
   d. FSH

4. The pampiniform plexus:
   a. pampers the testicles
   b. assists warming of the testicles
   c. assists cooling of the testicles
   d. is a nerve network to the testicles

5. The maturation phase whereby spermatids undergo nuclear and cytoplasmic changes and develop a tail is known as:
   a. spermatidosis
   b. spermiation
   c. spermatogenesis
   d. spermiogenesis

6. Testosterone is produced:
   a. by Leydig cells in response to stimulation by LH
   b. by Sertoli cells in response to stimulation by FSH
   c. by Leydig cells in response to stimulation by FSH
   d. by Sertoli cells in response to stimulation by LH

7. An approximate blood pressure within the corpus cavernosum penis of the bull during coitus is:
   a. 140 mm Hg
   b. THTM (too high to measure)
   c. 1400 mm Hg
   d. about the same in mm Hg as Pike's Peak is high in feet above sea level

8. Intromission is defined as:
   a. emptying of sperm and fluids from the vas deferens and ampullae into the urethra along with seminal plasma
   b. a time-out between mounting and ejaculation

   c. introduction of the penis into the vagina and its maintenance therein during coitus
   d. the movement of urethral content toward the external urethral orifice

9. Which one of the following choices is an androgen?
   a. testosterone
   b. estrogen
   c. LH
   d. FSH

10. The spermatogenic wave:
   a. is a spectator performance at athletic events
   b. ensures a continuous supply of spermatozoa
   c. is an activity of the epididymis
   d. is a friendly acknowledgement

11. Maturation and storage of spermatozoa occurs in the:
   a. epididymis
   b. seminiferous tubules
   c. prostate gland
   d. urethra

12. The gubernaculum testis plays a role in:
   a. spermatogenesis
   b. erection
   c. descent of the testicles during fetal development
   d. elevation of testicles to inguinal ring

13. Contraction of the ischiocavernosus muscle in the bull:
   a. pulls the testis up against the external inguinal ring
   b. assists in emptying the urethra
   c. pulls the penis upward against the floor of the pelvis, which obstructs venous outflow, thereby assisting erection
   d. pulls the flaccid penis back into the prepuce

14. Which one of the following choices is the principal androgen in the male?
   a. interstitial cell stimulating hormone
   b. testosterone
   c. follicle stimulating hormone
   d. cholesterol

15. The function of luteinizing hormone in the male animal is to:
    a. stimulate the production of estrogen by Sertoli cells
    b. stimulate spermatogenesis
    c. stimulate the production of testosterone by the interstitial cells (Leydig cells)
    d. cool the testicle
16. An intra-abdominal location for avian testes is abnormal.
    a. true
    b. false
17. Cooling of avian testes below body temperature is:
    a. accomplished by their close proximity to the air sacs
    b. accomplished by a vascular arrangement similar to the pampiniform plexus
    c. not necessary for their functional integrity
18. The avian penis is also known as the:
    a. malleus
    b. phallus
    c. incus
    d. organ
19. Intromission is a reproductive component for:
    a. all avian species
    b. cocks (male chickens) and toms (male turkeys)
    c. drakes (male ducks) and ganders (male geese)
    d. cocks, toms, drakes, and ganders
20. When avian semen is inseminated, the spermatozoa:
    a. are short lived (minutes)
    b. perish after a one-time fertilization
    c. have a prolonged life in sperm-storage glands of the female and persist at this location for the fertile period of the female

Suggested Readings

Beckett SD, Waler DF, Hudson RS, et al. Corpus cavernosum penis pressure and penile muscle activity in the bull during coitus. Am J Vet Res 1974;35:761.

Beckett SD, Reynolds TM, Walker DF, et al. Experimentally induced rupture of corpus cavernosum penis of the bull. Am J Vet Res 1974;35:765.

Dyce KM, Sack WO, Wensing CJG. Textbook of veterinary anatomy. 2nd ed. Philadelphia: WB Saunders, 1996.

Fawcett DW. Bloom & Fawcett: A textbook of histology. 11th ed. Philadelphia: WB Saunders, 1986.

Frandson RD. Anatomy and physiology of farm animals. 5th ed. Philadelphia: Lea & Febiger, 1992.

Genuth SM. The reproductive glands. In: Berne RM, Levy MN, eds. Physiology. 2nd ed. St. Louis: CV Mosby, 1988:983–1024.

Hafez ESE. Reproduction in farm animals. 6th ed. Philadelphia; Lea & Febiger, 1993.

Johnson AL. Reproduction in the male. In: Sturkie PD, ed. Avian physiology. 4th ed. New York: Springer-Verlag, 1986.

Pineda MH. The biology of sex. In: McDonald LE, Pineda MH, eds. Veterinary endocrinology and reproduction. 4th ed. Philadelphia: Lea & Febiger, 1989:231–260.

Roberts SJ. Veterinary obstetrics and genital diseases (theriogenology). 3rd ed. Woodstock, VT: Stephen J. Roberts, 1986.

Stabenfeldt GH, Edqvist LE. Male reproductive processes. In: Swenson MJ, Reece WO, eds. Dukes' physiology of domestic animals. 11th ed. Ithaca, NY: Cornell University Press, 1993:665–677.

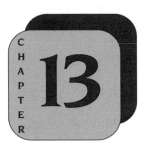

13

Female Reproduction

The reproductive functions of the female are production of oocytes and provision of an environment for growth and nutrition of the fetus that develops after fertilization of a mature oocyte by a spermatozoan. Terminal conditions of the latter function are to give birth at an appropriate time and to continue the nutritional function through lactation.

The complex relationships of hormones and tissue changes are coordinated for the female's role of perpetuating the species.

PARTS OF THE FEMALE REPRODUCTIVE SYSTEM

The female reproductive system consists of the two ovaries, two ovarian tubes, uterus, vagina, and vulva (Fig. 13.1). The mammary glands are an important part of the reproductive system as well, but they are described separately. The location of the reproductive system relative to the rectum and bladder is shown in Figure 13.2 .

Ovaries

The ovaries are paired glands that provide for the development of oocytes and for the production of hormones. Each ovary is located caudal to its respective right or left kidney and is suspended from the dorsal wall of the abdomen by a reflection of the peritoneum, the mesovarium. The mesovarium is part of the broad ligament (Fig. 13.3), an inclusive term that also refers to the suspensions of the uterine tubes (mesosalpinx) and uterus (mesometrium). The rather pendulous suspension of the ovaries provides for easy manipulation by rectal palpation in the cow and horse. The ovaries are described as almond-shaped in most species and as bean-shaped (kidney-shaped) in the mare (Fig. 13.4). In the sow, the ovary resembles a cluster of grapes (berry-shaped) because of the larger number of protruding follicles. Ovulation (release of mature oocytes) occurs throughout the entire surface of the ovary in most species but is confined to an ovulation

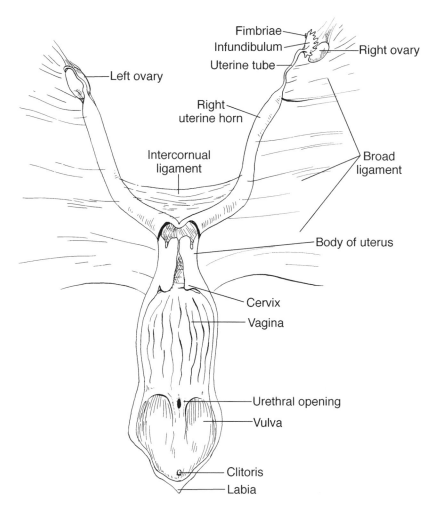

Figure 13.1. Reproductive tract of the cow (dorsal aspect). The body of the uterus, vagina, and vulva (vestibule of the vagina) have been laid open and the right ovary withdrawn from the infundibulum. The broad ligament (a downward reflection of the peritoneum) suspends the reproductive tract from the dorsolateral abdominal wall.

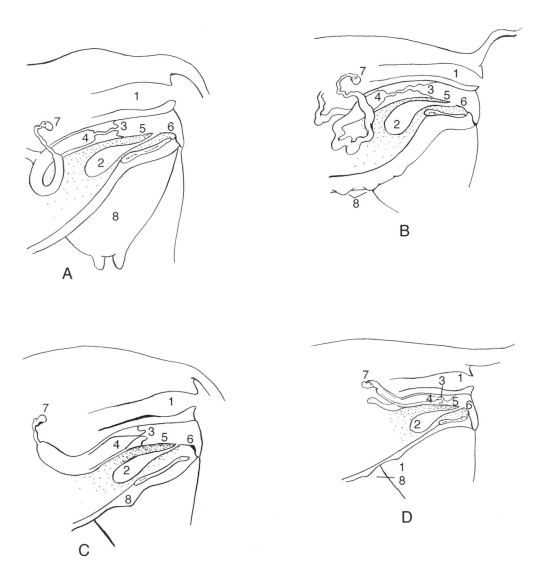

Figure 13.2. Location of reproductive organs relative to the rectum and urinary bladder. **A**. Cow. **B**. Sow. **C**. Mare. **D**. Bitch. Note species differences in anatomy of the cervix and mammary gland(s). *1*, rectum; *2*, urinary bladder; *3*, cervix; *4*, uterus; *5*, vagina; *6*, vulva; *7*, ovary; *8*, mammary gland(s).

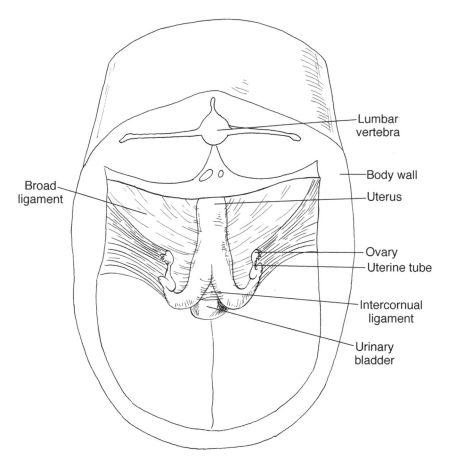

Figure 13.3. Cranial view of bovine female reproductive organs. The broad ligament is the inclusive term for the mesovarium, mesosalpinx, and mesometrium that suspend the ovary, uterine tubes, and uterus, respectively, from the dorsolateral wall of the sublumbar region. The broad ligament is a reflection from the peritoneum.

Figure 13.4. Ovarian differences resulting from species morphology and functional changes. **A.** Sow ovary (berry-shaped). **B.** Cow ovary (almond-shaped) with ripening follicle. **C.** Cow ovary with fully developed corpus luteum. **D.** Mare ovary (kidney-shaped) with ovulation fossa (indentation). From Dyce KM, Sack WO, Wensing CJG. Textbook of veterinary anatomy. 2nd ed. Philadelphia: WB Saunders, 1996.

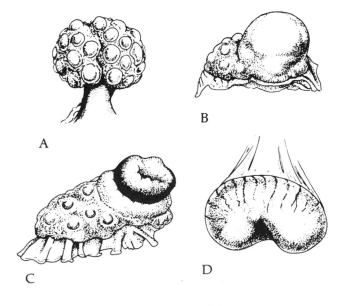

fossa (an indentation) in the mare; this gives the latter its bean shape.

The ovary has a surface or superficial layer of epithelium that is underlaid by the tunica albuginea, a connective tissue covering of the entire ovary. Beneath the tunica albuginea is the cortex, which contains a large mass of follicles in various stages of development. The medulla is centrally located and contains loose connective tissue, blood vessels, lymphatics, and nerves.

The follicles within the cortex are classified as 1) primordial (sometimes called primary) follicles, 2) growing follicles, and 3) graafian follicles (Fig. 13.5). The primordial follicles contain a single oocyte that is surrounded by a single layer of granulosa cells. The granulosa cells are derived from the superficial epithelium, and the oocytes are derived from mitosis of oogonia in the embryonic

genital ridge that then migrate to the ovary. Growing follicles are follicles that have begun growth from the resting stage as primordial follicles but have not developed a thecal layer or antrum (fluid filled cavity; Fig. 13.5). It has two or more layers of granulosa cells surrounding the oocyte. Additional layers are added with continued growth. A zona pellucida that surrounds the oocyte may also be present. The zona pellucida provides pores through which processes of granulosa cells can interact with the oocyte surface. Also, sperm must first recognize and then contact and traverse the zona pellucida to reach the oocyte plasma membrane. Graafian follicles are those in which an antrum is clearly visible. Two layers of thecal cells, theca interna and theca externa, are also present (Fig. 13.5).

Considerable atresia (regression) of the many primordial follicles occurs by birth

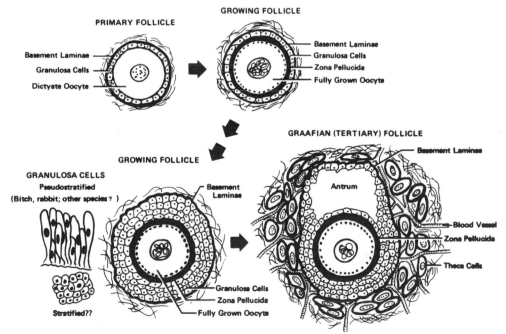

Figure 13.5. Development of an ovarian follicle from its primordial (primary) form to a graafian follicle. Growing follicles are those that have begun growth from the resting stage as primordial follicles but have not developed thecal layers or an antrum. From Pineda MH. Female reproductive system. In: McDonald LE, Pineda MH, eds. Veterinary endocrinology and reproduction. 4th ed. Philadelphia: Lea & Febiger, 1989.

and throughout the reproductive life of the female. At the end of the female's reproductive life, only a few primordial follicles remain, and even these undergo atresia soon thereafter. Growth of some number of primordial follicles does occur after birth and before puberty, but these never reach the graafian follicle stage and regress. The growth that occurs before puberty is not hormone related and is probably controlled by an unknown intraovarian factor. The formation of graafian follicles is hormone dependent and begins at puberty when tonic levels of LH and FSH begin to rise and fall with each estrous cycle. Many of the follicles that undergo growth and maturation with each cycle never ovulate. Therefore, the number of primordial follicles that reach the graafian follicle stage and proceed to ovulation is a very small fraction of the birth number.

The process by which oocytes are formed is known as oogenesis. The oocyte of the primordial follicle is a primary oocyte that is in a quiescent (arrested) stage of meiosis. Meiosis resumes at the time of ovulation. Whereas four spermatozoa arise from one primary spermatocyte, only one oocyte develops from the reduction division of a primary oocyte. A polar body that lacks sufficient cytoplasmic material for viability develops when a primary oocyte divides to form a secondary oocyte. Another polar body is formed by the division of the secondary oocyte at the time of ovulation. The surviving oocyte has a haploid (n) number of chromosomes (similar to a spermatozoan) so that the union of a spermatozoan with an oocyte produces a cell with a diploid (2n) number of chromosomes.

Uterine Tubes

The uterine tubes are also called the oviducts or fallopian tubes. They are paired, convoluted tubes that conduct oocytes from the ovaries to the respective horn of the uterus. The uterine tubes serve as the site for fertilization of released oocytes by spermatozoa in domestic species. The portion of each tube adjacent to its respective ovary expands to form the infundibulum (Fig. 13.1), and fimbriae project from its free edge. The fimbriae assist in directing the oocyte into the infundibulum at the time of ovulation.

The lumen of the oviduct is lined with secretory cells and ciliated cells. These cells provide an environment for the oocytes and they transport the spermatozoa. Both longitudinal and circular smooth muscles are located within the walls of the uterine tubes, which assist in the transport of oocytes and sperm by their contractions. The serous covering of the uterine tubes (Fig. 13.3) is known as the mesosalpinx, which is a continuation of the mesovarium and it is a part of the broad ligament (providing the serous support system for the internal genitalia).

Uterus

The uterus provides a place for development of the fetus, if fertilization has occurred. The uterus consists of a corpus (body), a cervix (neck), and two cornua (horns). The relative proportions of corpus, cornua, and cervix varies among species. The corpus is largest in the mare, less extensive in the cow and sheep, and small in the sow and bitch (Figs. 13.1, 13.2, and 13.6).

The mucous membrane lining the interior of the uterus (endometrium) is highly glandular. The glands are scattered throughout the entire endometrium of the uterus except in ruminants, in which the caruncles (mushroomlike projections from the inner surface that provide attachment for the fetal membranes) are nonglandular (Fig. 13.7). The endometrium varies in thickness and vascularity with hormonal changes in the ovary and with pregnancy.

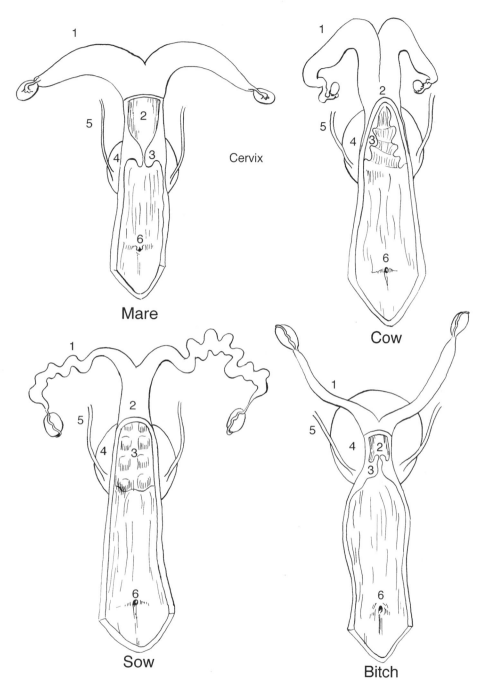

Figure 13.6. Genital tract comparisons among some domestic animals. *1,* uterine horn; *2,* uterine body; *3,* cervix; *4,* urinary bladder; *5,* ureter; *6,* urethral opening. The genital tracts are opened dorsally near the body of the uterus, and the opening is extended caudally to the labia to show the cervix and urethral opening. Note that the relative proportions of uterine horns, uterine body, and cervix varies among species. The illustrations are not drawn to scale and do not compare size.

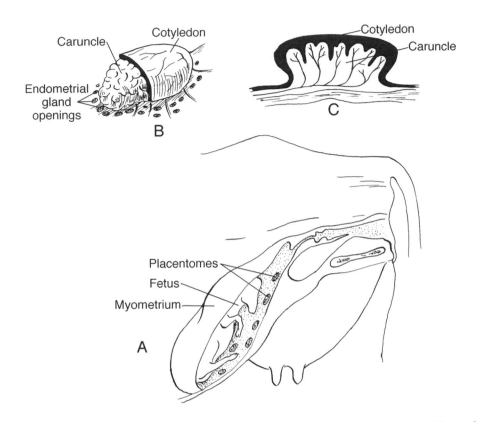

Figure 13.7. Relationship of the bovine fetal placenta to the maternal endometrium. **A**. View of fetus within the uterus showing multiple placentomes. **B**. Magnification of a placentome that is surrounded by a number of endometrial gland openings. Only a part of the fetal cotyledon is shown so that the underlying maternal caruncle and endometrial gland openings can be visualized. **C**. Cross-section of a placentome. The contribution by the fetal placenta is known as the cotyledon and the maternal contribution is known as the caruncle.

The glandular secretion of the endometrium provides nutrients for the embryo before placentation (development of placental membranes), after which nutrition is provided by the mother's blood.

The cervix projects caudally into the vagina (Fig. 13.2). This heavy, smooth muscle sphincter is tightly closed, except during estrus and at parturition (birth of young). The mucus seen at estrus is the secretion of cervical goblet cells. Goblet cell secretion of mucus during pregnancy and its outward flow prevents infective material from entering through the vagina.

The myometrium is the muscular portion of the uterus, comprised of smooth muscle cells. The myometrium hypertrophies during pregnancy, increasing both in cell number and cell size. The principal function of the myometrium is aiding in the expulsion of the fetus at parturition.

The serous covering of the uterus is continuous with the mesosalpinx; in the uterus it is known as the mesometrium. The mesometrium provides a suspensory support, particularly for the nongravid uterus. The gravid (pregnant) uterus enlarges and major support is provided by

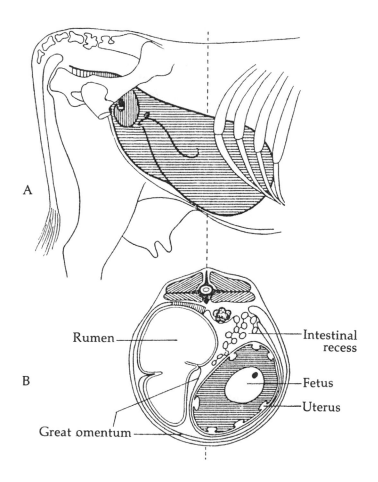

A

B

Rumen

Intestinal
recess

Fetus

Uterus

Great omentum

Figure 13.8. Position of the cow's uterus at the third and sixth month of pregnancy. **A.** Superimposed uterus and ovary (left) (*vertical striping,* uterus; *blackened circle,* ovary) represents the uterus at the third month of pregnancy. **B.** Cross-section of uterus at the sixth month of pregnancy with its contained fetus relative to the adjoining abdominal viscera (rumen on left and uterus on right side of abdomen). From Dyce KM, Wensing CJG. Essentials of bovine anatomy. Philadelphia: Lea & Febiger, 1971.

the abdominal wall (Fig. 13.8). It should be noted that there are two broad ligaments, each extending from the right or left sublumbar region and lateral pelvic wall to their respective ovary, uterine tube, uterine horn, and extending caudally onto the body of the uterus.

Vagina

The vagina is the portion of the birth canal located within the pelvis, between the uterus cranially and the vulva caudally (Figs. 13.1 and 13.2). The vagina serves as a sheath for the male penis during copulation. It is lined with stratified squamous epithelium, which is glandless. The fornix is the space formed cranial to the projection of the cervix into the vagina. In some animals, the fornix is only visible dorsally, whereas in others it can encircle the cervix completely or be entirely absent (as in the pig).

Vulva

The vulva is the caudal portion of the female genitalia that extends from the vagina to the exterior. The external urethral orifice (opening) is the landmark junction of vagina and vulva. The vestibule of the vagina (Fig. 13.9) is another name for the vulva. It is that part of the tubular genitalia between the vagina and the labia (lips of the vulva). The clitoris (female vestigial counterpart of the penis) is concealed by the lowest part of the vulva. The clitoris is supplied with erectile tissue and sensory nerve endings.

The external part of the vulva is its vertical opening, the labia (Fig. 13.1).

Blood Supply of Female Genitalia

The ovary and oviduct receive their blood supply from the ovarian artery and the vagina receives its blood supply from the vaginal artery (Fig. 13.10). The major blood supply to the uterus comes from the uterine artery (formerly called the middle uterine artery). The cranial part of the uterus is also supplied with blood from the ovarian artery, and the caudal part of the uterus receives blood from the vaginal artery. During pregnancy, the blood supply to the uterus increases dramatically. When the uterine artery is palpated, a vibration of the blood within it can be felt. This is called fremitus and is considered to be a good indicator of pregnancy. The ovarian artery is coiled and adheres closely to the uterine vein (Fig. 13.11). Such an arrangement is important for the diffusion of the hormone prostaglandin $F_{2\alpha}$ ($PGF_{2\alpha}$) from the uterine vein to the ovarian artery in some species (e.g., cow and ewe—perhaps others). Early transport by this arrangement avoids the general circulation, where much of it would be inactivated by vascular endothelial cells in the lungs. Production requirements are lower because most of the $PGF_{2\alpha}$ produced goes only to the target organ (ovary) and avoids general circulation (and subsequent inactivation) to all body parts. $PGF_{2\alpha}$ at the ovarian site initiates luteolysis (termination of the corpus luteum).

HORMONES OF FEMALE REPRODUCTION

Estrogens

Estrogens occur naturally and synthetically. The important estrogens in mammals are steroids, produced by the ovary (granulosa cells of follicles), placenta, and the adrenal cortex. A common synthetic estrogen is diethylstilbestrol, which is not

Figure 13.9. Species variations in position of the vestibule of the vagina. **A.** Cow. **B.** Mare. **C.** Bitch. The vulva, and hence the vestibule of the vagina, extends caudally from the external urethral orifice. *1,* vagina; *2,* bladder; *3,* urethra; *4,* suburethral diverticulum; *5,* vulva. From Dyce KM, Sack WO, Wensing CJG. Textbook of veterinary anatomy. 2nd ed. Philadelphia: WB Saunders, 1996.

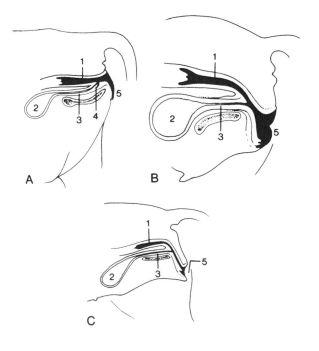

a steroid, but a complex alcohol with estrogenic properties. The chemical structures of diethylstilbestrol and estradiol-17β (a steroid) are compared in Figure 13.12 . Regardless of production site, steroids share a common biosynthetic pathway (Fig. 13.13).

Estradiol-17β and estrone are estrogens that predominate in domestic nonpregnant and pregnant animals, respectively. Generally, the principal function of the estrogens is to cause cellular proliferation and growth of the tissues related to reproduction. Tissue responses caused by estrogens include 1) stimulation of endometrial gland growth, 2) stimulation of duct growth in the mammary gland, 3) increase in secretory activity of uterine ducts, 4) initiation of sexual receptivity, 5) regulation of secretion of luteinizing hormone (LH) by the anterior pituitary gland, 6) possible regulation of $PGF_{2\alpha}$ release from the nongravid and gravid uterus, 7) early union of the epiphysis with the shafts of long bones, whereby growth of long bones cease, 8) protein anabolism, and 9) epitheliotropic activity. The protein anabolic effect of estrogens is less pronounced than that associated with testosterone. Their effect is probably associated more specifically with the sex organs rather

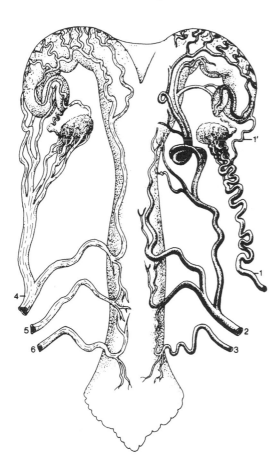

Figure 13.10. Blood supply to the reproductive tract of the cow. The arteries are shown on the right side and the veins on the left. *1,* ovarian artery; *1'* uterine branch; *2,* uterine artery; *3,* vaginal artery; *4,* ovarian vein; *5,* uterine vein; *6,* vaginal vein. From Dyce KM, Sack WO, Wensing CJG. Textbook of veterinary anatomy. 2nd ed. Philadelphia: WB Saunders, 1996.

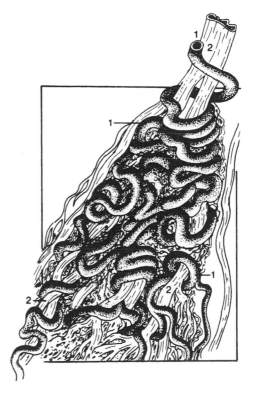

Figure 13.11. Relationship of the ovarian artery of a ruminant and its branches (1) to those of the uterine vein (2). The intertwining ensures a large area of contact. From Dyce KM, Sack WO, Wensing CJG. Textbook of veterinary anatomy. 2nd ed. Philadelphia: WB Saunders, 1996.

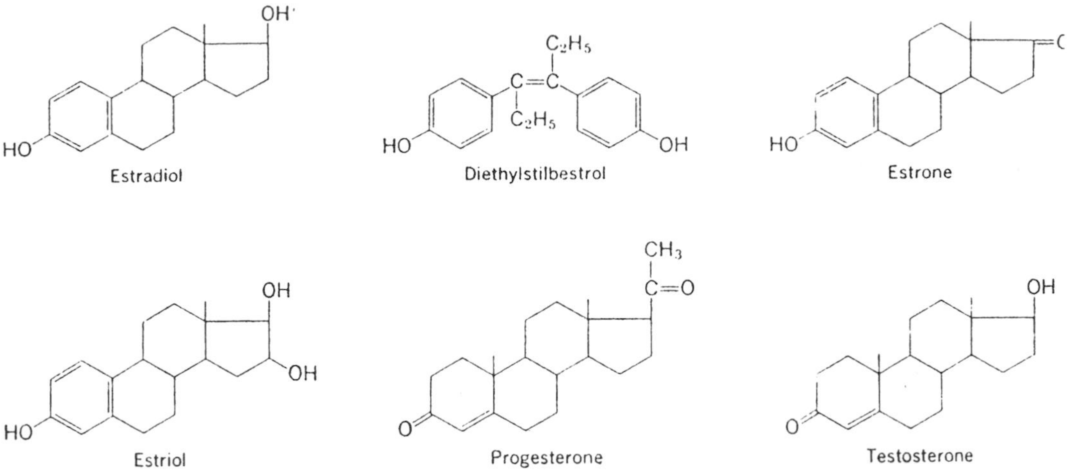

Figure 13.12. Chemical structure of some steroid hormones and diethylstilbestrol. From McDonald LE. Veterinary endocrinology and reproduction. 4th ed. Philadelphia: Lea & Febiger, 1989.

than with a generalized effect. The epitheliotropic function manifests at estrus when the epithelium in the vagina proliferates and cornification is more prevalent.

Progesterone

Progesterone, like the estrogens, is a steroid hormone produced by the corpus luteum (CL) of the ovary, placenta, and adrenal cortex. Its place in the common biosynthetic pathway scheme is shown in Figure 13.13.

The activities associated with progesterone are often performed in concert with estrogens and usually require previous estrogen priming. The functions of progesterone include: 1) promotion of endometrial gland growth, 2) stimulation of secretory activity of the oviduct and endometrial glands to provide nutrients for the developing embryo prior to implantation, 3) promotion of lobuloalveolar growth in the mammary gland, 4) prevention of contractility of the uterus during pregnancy, and 5) regulation of secretion of gonadotropins.

The interrelationships of the estrogens, progesterone, and gonadotropins are described later in the discussions of the estrous cycle and pregnancy.

Gonadotropins

Follicle-stimulating hormone (FSH) and luteinizing hormone (LH) are collectively referred to as the gonadotropins because of their role in stimulating cells within the ovary and testis (the gonads). FSH and LH are hormones secreted by cells within the anterior pituitary. Both are classified chemically as glycoproteins. A glycoprotein consists of chains of amino acids linked together by peptide bonds and chains of carbohydrates linked to the polypeptides (Fig. 13.14).

The main function of FSH in the female is promotion of the growth of follicles. LH is important for the ovulatory process and the luteinization of the granulosa, an essential aspect of CL formation.

Apparently, FSH and LH concentrations exist in the plasma at a tonic or basal level. These levels are controlled by negative feedback from the gonads. Tonic levels are increased by estrogen and decreased by progesterone.

The release of FSH and LH from the anterior pituitary is controlled by a releas-

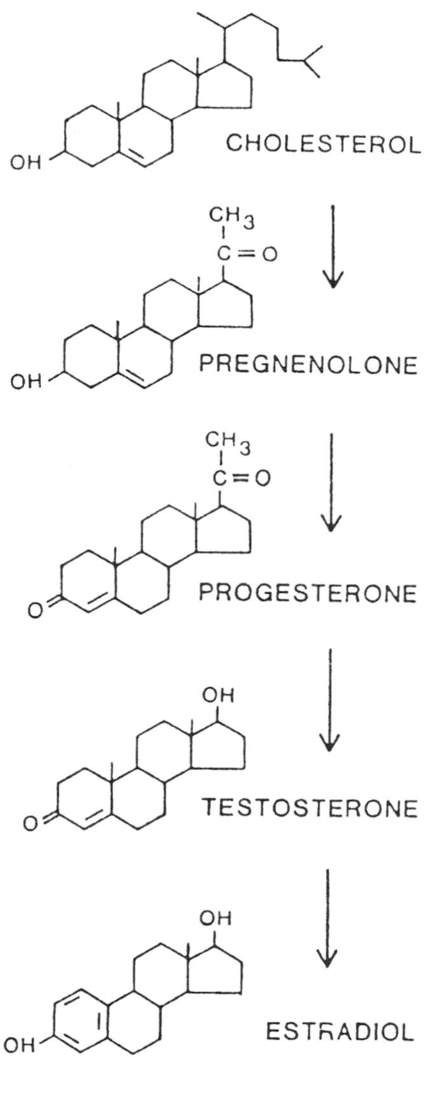

CHOLESTEROL

PREGNENOLONE

PROGESTERONE

TESTOSTERONE

ESTRADIOL

Figure 13.13. Biosynthesis of steroid hormones from cholesterol. From Hafez ESE. Reproduction in farm animals. 6th ed. Philadelphia: Lea & Febiger, 1993.

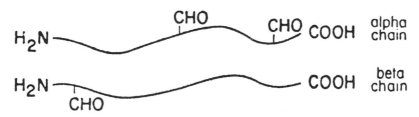

Figure 13.14. Diagrammatic representation of the α and β subunits of luteinizing hormone (a glyco-protein). Shown is the approximate position of the polysaccharide units. (CHO) The peptide bonds linking the amino acid chains are not shown. From Hafez ESE. Reproduction in farm animals. 6th ed. Philadelphia: Lea & Febiger, 1993.

382 Female Reproduction

ing hormone from the hypothalamus. The circulatory system involved is known as the hypothalamic-hypophyseal portal system (Fig. 13.15). A portal system begins with capillaries and terminates with capillaries. The hypothalamic capillaries receive a secretion from sensing cells in the hypothalamus known as luteinizing hormone-releasing hormone (LHRH) (sometimes called gonadotropin-releasing hormone, GnRH). LHRH is secreted in response to low levels of LH or FSH and is then followed by secretion of LH or FSH. It appears that LH release is more responsive to LHRH than FSH release; some doubt exists as to whether LHRH controls FSH.

The concentrations of estrogens and progesterone also influence the amount of LH or FSH secretion. Generally, an increasing concentration of estrogen causes an increase in sensitivity of the anterior pituitary to LHRH and results in an increased release of gonadotropins. Progesterone decreases sensitivity of the anterior pituitary to LHRH, and LH and FSH concentrations decrease. These influences, particularly that of estrogen, depend on gradually increasing concentrations of estrogen over a period of time, which results in the preovulatory surge of LH release. Conversely, when estrogen concentration is basal and of short duration, LH and FSH secretions are suppressed.

OVARIAN ACTIVITY AND FOLLICULAR GROWTH

Follicular Growth

Puberty is defined as the beginning of reproductive life, which in the female is usually marked by the beginning of ovarian activity. The formation of graafian follicles from growing follicles is hormone dependent and begins at puberty when tonic levels of LH and FSH begin to rise and fall with each estrous cycle. Interstitial

cells begin to surround the basement membrane of the granulosa cells to form the theca, which differentiates into a theca interna and externa. As the thecal cells are formed around the follicle, a capillary bed develops among them. These thecal capillaries increase in size and are concentrated in the theca interna close to the basement membrane that separates the theca interna cells from the granulosa cells (Fig. 13.16). LH receptors form on the cells of the theca interna, and receptors for FSH and estrogen form on the granulosa cells.

During the hormone dependent stage, under the influence of LH, androgens are produced by cells of the theca interna. The androgens diffuse from the theca interna to the granulosa cells. Under the influence of FSH, the granulosa cells convert the androgens to estrogens. The estrogens produced

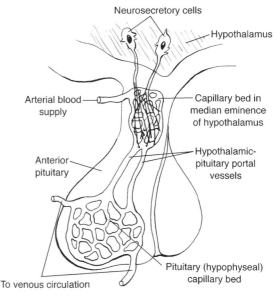

Figure 13.15. The hypothalamic/hypophyseal portal circulation involved with the secretion of anterior pituitary hormones. Cell bodies in the hypothalamus sense the need for a hormone and secrete a releasing hormone into the hypothalamic capillary bed. The releasing hormone enters the hypophyseal capillary bed and diffuses to specific cells, causing them to secrete their specific hormone.

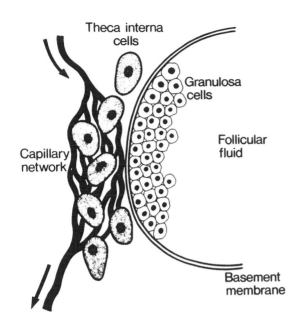

Figure 13.16. Formation of a graafian follicle from a growing follicle. Wall structure. The theca interna cells are well supplied with blood. The basement membrane deprives granulosa cells of blood supply. From Baird DT. Reproductive hormones. In: Austin CR, Short RV. Reproduction in mammals, Book 3. Cambridge, England: Cambridge University Press, 1972.

cause growth and division of the granulosa cells and, together with FSH, cause the granulosa cells to produce secretions that effect separation of the granulosa cells and formation of a space filled with fluid (liquor folliculi), called an antrum (Fig. 13.16). Also, FSH stimulates the formation of LH receptors on the granulosa cells. A surge of LH output (preovulatory surge) occurs about 24 hours before ovulation. In addition to its role in ovulation and formation of a corpus luteum, the LH surge causes a reduction in the number of FSH receptors on granulosa cells, so that the output of estrogen by the granulosa cells decreases.

Ovarian Hormone Cycle

Events in the ovary associated with a cycle of hormone changes can be summarized as follows:

1. After regression of the CL (luteolysis caused by $PGF_{2\alpha}$), FSH and LH secretion increases (because of a decrease in the concentration of progesterone).
2. LH stimulates secretion of androgens by the theca interna cells, which diffuse into the granulosa cells.
3. FSH stimulates conversion of androgen to estrogen by the granulosa cells, and the estrogen concentration gradually increases.
4. FSH stimulates the formation of LH receptors on the granulosa cells.
5. Estrogen-rich fluid formed by the granulosa cells separates the granulosa cells and forms a pocket known as an antrum.
6. The gradually increasing estrogen concentration causes a preovulatory surge of LH release.
7. The LH surge promotes the maturation of oocytes by resuming meiosis through the first polar body stage.
8. The LH surge promotes the intrafollicular production of prostaglandins A and E (PGA and PGE), which are associated with rupture of the follicle.
9. Concomitant with PGA and PGE production is the formation of multivesicular bodies (MVB), which form as outpockets of the exposed theca externa.
10. MVBs appear to secrete proteolytic enzymes that digest ground substance cementing the theca externa

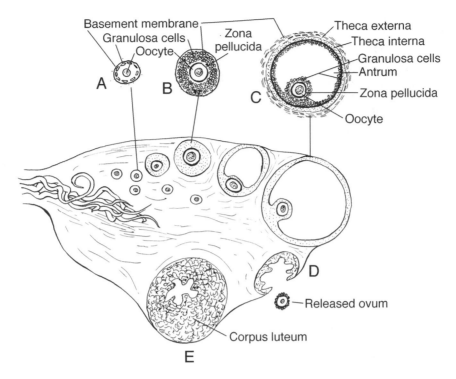

Figure 13.17. Sagittal section of an ovary. **A**. Primary follicle. **B**. Growing follicle. **C**. Graafian follicle. **D**. Ruptured follicle. **E**. Corpus luteum. This schematic representation shows in sequence the origin, growth, and rupture of a graafian follicle and a corpus luteum that develops from the remains of the ruptured follicle.

fibroblasts, allowing for the escape of the oocyte (ovulation).

11. The LH surge causes reduction in number of FSH receptors on the granulosa cells, so the rate of conversion of androgen to estrogen diminishes.

12. LH attaches to granulosa cell LH receptors and begins the conversion of the granulosa from estrogen secretion in the follicular phase to progesterone secretion in the luteal phase.

13. At some point in the latter stages of these events, ovulation occurs, and the cavity previously occupied by the mature follicle becomes a corpus luteum.

14. The corpus luteum secretes progesterone, which causes a decrease in the output of FSH and LH by the anterior pituitary.

15. The corpus luteum regresses and the output of progesterone begins to decrease.

16. A decrease in the level of progesterone causes FSH and LH secretion to increase, and the cycle is repeated.

The ovarian events are illustrated in Figure 13.17 .

Ovulation

When the oocyte is released into the abdomen from its protruding follicle, it is covered by those granulosa cells that immediately surrounded it just before ovulation; these are known as the corona radiata. The oocyte and granulosa cells are evacuated with an enveloping viscous (gelatinous) follicular fluid. At ovulation, the oocyte, together with its surrounding cells and gelatinous mass, is swept into the uterine tubes by motility of the fimbriae. The relationship of ovulation to estrus for domestic animals, and other factors involved in female reproduction, is given in Table 13.1.

Ovulation is spontaneous (no stimulation needed) in all the domestic species except the cat. The cat and other nonspontaneous ovulators (e.g., mink, rabbit, ferret) are reflex ovulators, in that coitus is required for ovulation to occur. Coital contact apparently brings forth an LH surge.

The selection of follicles for ovulation appears to occur primarily by chance. It is usually associated with the largest actively growing follicles present when the previous CL regressed (i.e., when progesterone decreased and FSH and LH output began to increase). Follicles continue to grow and develop during all phases of the ovarian cycle, with some impairment during the luteal phase, and the LH surge is necessary for ovulation to occur. Follicles close to full development, but without adequate LH receptors, do not ovulate in response to the LH surge and become atretic.

Corpus Luteum

Formation

Formation of the CL involves luteinization of the granulosa, by which the granulosa is converted from estrogen secretion to progesterone secretion (LH receptors on the granulosa cells were previously induced by

TABLE 13.1. Factors Related to Female Reproduction

Animal	Onset of Puberty (mo)	Age First Service (average)	Length of Estrous Cycle (d)	Length of Estrus	Gestation Period (d)
Mare	18 (10 to 24)	2 to 3 yr.	21 (19 to 21)	5 d (4.5 to 7.5 d)	336 (323 to 341)
Cow	4 to 24	14 to 22 mo	21 (18 to 24)	18 h (12 to 28 h)	282 (274 to 291)
Ewe	4 to 12 (first fall)	12 to 18 mo	16½ (14 to 20)	24 to 48 h	150 (140 to 160)
Sow	3 to 7	8 to 10 mo	21 (18 to 24)	2 d (1 to 5 d)	114 (110 to 116)
Bitch	6 to 24	12 to 18 mo	6 to 12 mo	9 d (5 to 19 d)	63 (60 to 65)

	Time of Ovulation	Optimum Time for Service	Advisable Time to Breed After Parturition
Mare	1 to 2 d before end of estrus	3 to 4 d before end of estrus or 2nd or 3rd d of estrus	About 25 to 35 d or second estrus; about 9 d or first estrus only if normal in every way
Cow	10 to 15 h after end of estrus	Just before middle of estrus to end of estrus	60 to 90d
Ewe	12 to 24 h before end of estrus	18 to 24 h after onset of estrus	Usually, following fall
Sow	30 to 36 h after onset of estrus	12 to 30 after onset of estrus	First estrus 3 to 9 d after weaning pigs
Bitch	1 to 2 d after onset of true estrus	2 to 3 d after onset of estrus; or 10 to 14 d after onset of proestrus bleeding	Usually first estrus or 2 to 3 mo after weaning pups

From Frandson RD, Spurgeon TL. Anatomy and physiology of farm animals. 5th Ed. Philadelphia: Lea & Febiger, 1992.

FSH). The process is initiated by the preovulatory LH surge. The cavity of the ruptured follicle and the fibrin clot within serve as the framework on which the granulosa cells develop. Blood vessels from the theca externa invade the developing CL, so that it becomes vascularized. Maintenance of the CL is provided for by LH derived from the LH surge and by the basal circulating levels of LH. In the sheep, prolactin, a gonadotropin hormone for some species, is required to maintain the CL, in addition to LH.

Regression

The uterus (endometrium) plays a major role in controlling the life span of the CL in nonpregnant mares, cows, sows, ewes, and does (goats), but it is not active in CL regression in the bitch (dog) and queen (cat). $PGF_{2\alpha}$ is released by the nonpregnant uterus about 14 days after ovulation and is considered to be the natural luteolytic substance (causes regression of the CL). The venous return of uterine blood to the right heart and from there to the lung before transport of arterial blood to the ovary results in inactivation by the vascular endothelium of about 90% of $PGF_{2\alpha}$. To ensure that enough $PGF_{2\alpha}$ is delivered directly to the ovary for luteolysis, the anatomic arrangement of the uterine vein and ovarian artery is such that $PGF_{2\alpha}$ can diffuse from the vein to the artery and ovarian perfusion of $PGF_{2\alpha}$ can occur before circulation through the lungs (Fig. 13.18). For $PGF_{2\alpha}$ to be effective when it enters the general circulation, it must either be secreted by the uterus in larger amounts, be more resistant to degradation in the lungs, or both. Survival of $PGF_{2\alpha}$ for the general circulation is more important in the sow and mare.

The reason for final regression of the CL in the bitch and queen (bitch, 75 d; queen, 35 d) is not known. An acute lytic process does not occur.

Persistent Corpus Luteum

Prolongation of the luteal phase beyond 14 d to perhaps 1 to 5 mo is known as persistent corpus luteum. The presence of a persistent CL prevents a return to the follicular phase and its next ovulation. The immediate reason for persistent CL is the failure of the endometrium to synthesize $PGF_{2\alpha}$. The failure often is caused by an acute or chronic endometrial inflammation.

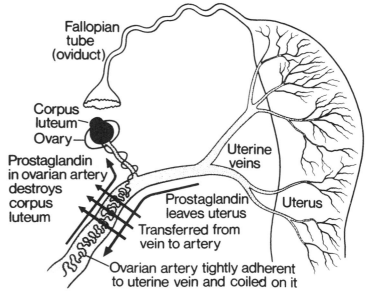

Figure 13.18. Postulated route by which prostaglandin secreted by the progesterone-primed uterus can enter the ovarian artery and destroy the corpus luteum in the ewe, and possibly other species. From Short RV. Role of hormones in sex cycles. In: Austin CR, Short RV. Reproduction in mammals, Book 3. Cambridge, England: Cambridge University Press, 1972.

SEXUAL RECEPTIVITY

If copulation is to occur near ovulation, the female must be receptive to the male. Initiation of sexual receptivity in all animals requires estrogen derived from the antral follicles. Also, in some species (e.g., bitch, ewe, sow, cow), progesterone acts synergistically with estrogen for manifestation of receptivity. Neurons associated with a "sex center" are located diffusely in the hypothalamus and are critical in initiating the mechanisms of sexual behavior as a response to hormones. It appears that progesterone (tonic levels) acts as a primer for the hypothalamic sexual centers, so that estrogen becomes effective. During the postpartum (after parturition) period in some cows and sows, the low progesterone concentration fails to prime the sexual centers of the hypothalamus, and they are not sexually receptive at the time of the first postpartum ovulation. In sheep, the priming of the hypothalamus with progesterone is essential, after their seasonal anestrus, before sexual receptivity is manifested. Accordingly, ewes do not show sexual receptivity in conjunction with the first ovulation of the breeding season.

During proestrus in the bitch, when estrogen levels increase, sexual receptivity is absent even though they might be sexually attractive. It is only when the LH surge occurs near ovulation that sexual receptivity occurs. Preovulatory progesterone from the LH surge (luteinized granulosa cells) can be sufficient to prime the hypothalamus. Before proestrus, a long period of sexual inactivity (anestrus) occurs, during which progesterone levels are either low or nonexistent.

Some evidence has shown that LHRH has a role in the manifestation of sexual receptivity. Injection of LHRH without estrogen causes sexual posturing in some animals. Also, the onset of sexual receptivity is correlated closely with the preovulatory LH surge as caused by LHRH release.

Progesterone is not synergistic with estrogen in manifesting sexual receptivity in the doe, queen, and mare.

Estrous Cycle and Related Factors

The term "estrous cycle" refers to the rhythmic phenomenon observed in all mammals involving regular but limited periods of sexual receptivity (estrus) that occur at intervals characteristic of a species. One cycle interval is defined as the time from the onset of one period of sexual receptivity to the next (the ovulatory interval).

Animals are usually classified as monestrous or polyestrous. Monestrous animals are characterized by experiencing estrus once each year. Most wild carnivorous mammals are monestrous and, with some variation, the bitch is usually considered to be monestrous. Polyestrous animals, including most domestic species, have more than one period of estrus in a year. A seasonally polyestrous animal is one that has repeated estrous cycles within a physiologic breeding season (some part of a year), followed by a period of anestrus until the next breeding season.

The estrous cycle can be divided into several stages, according to behavioral or ovarian changes:

1. Estrus—the time of sexual receptivity, sometimes referred to as "heat." Ovulation usually, but not always, occurs at the end of estrus.
2. Metestrus—the early postovulatory period, during which the CL begins development.
3. Diestrus—the period of mature luteal activity, which begins about 4 days after ovulation and ends with regression of the CL.
4. Proestrus—the period beginning after CL regression and ending at the onset of estrus. During proestrus, rapid follicle development leads to ovulation and to the onset of sexual receptivity.

The follicular periods (proestrus and estrus) are characterized by estrogen dominance. From the behavioral standpoint, the estrus-sexually receptive period encompasses estrus, and the diestrus-sexually non-receptive period includes metestrus, diestrus, and proestrus.

Photoperiod

Among the domestic animals, the seasonal breeders are considered to be the queen, doe, ewe, and mare. These animals are sexually inactive during certain times of the year. The resumption of sexual activity is correlated with conception, so that birth occurs when environmental conditions are more conducive to survival of the young.

The most important factor associated with seasonal breeding is photoperiod (relative lengths of alternating periods of lightness and darkness). Both the queen and mare become anestrous (without estrous cycles) late in the fall (turn-off time) because of decreasing light, and ovarian cycles are resumed in late winter or early spring (turn-on time) by increasing light.

The phenomenon in the ewe and doe is opposite to that of the queen and mare, in that the ovarian cycle has a turn-on time associated with a decrease in daylight and a turn-off time associated with an increase in daylight. Not only do differences in photoperiod response among species exist but so do those within species as a result of genetic (breed) differences. Intraspecies difference is most apparent among sheep breeds and probably relates to their origin and related environmental differences. A representation of photoperiod influence on ovarian activity is shown for the queen, mare, ewe, and doe in Figure 13.19. Approximate dates of turn-on and turn-off vary according to distance from the equator and associated differences in photoperiods.

Nutrition

The influence of nutrition on the estrous cycle is most apparent at puberty and on reestablishment of the estrous cycle after parturition. Animals ingesting sound nutritional regimens reach puberty at an earlier age than nutritionally deprived animals.

Figure 13.19. Effects of photoperiod on ovarian activity in the cat, horse, sheep, and goat at a latitude of 38.5° north (California). The open bars represent periods of ovarian inactivity (anestrum). The transition from anestrous to estrous (often erratic) is shown by the cross-hatched portion of the bars for the horse, sheep, and goat. From Stabenfeldt GH, Edqvist L. Female reproductive processes. In: Swenson MJ, Reece WO, eds. Dukes' physiology of domestic animals. 11th ed. Ithaca, NY: Cornell University Press, 1993.

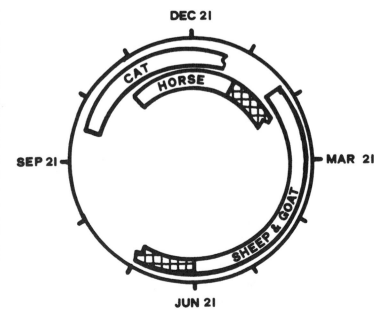

Consequently, breeding seasons can be delayed if calves are deprived of adequate nutrition. After parturition and during early lactation, cows can have a negative metabolic balance, which can result in an increased interval between parturition and resumption of ovarian activity.

Species Characteristics

Whereas the general pattern of the estrous cycle is similar among the domestic species, differences are noted in duration, not only in the cycle, but also for stages within the cycle. Duration of the cycle and for estrus is shown in Table 13.1 for domestic animals. The age of puberty onset also varies, and for some species it is affected by the breeding season for that species.

Cow

Smaller breeds of cows usually reach puberty at an earlier age than larger breeds (Jersey, 8 mo; Holstein, 11 mo). Behavioral changes associated with estrus include restlessness, mounting activity, standing to be mounted, being more alert to other animals, and decreased appetite. At the same time, decreased milk production, mucus discharge from the vulva, and redness and relaxation of the vulva are noted. It is important to detect estrus so that the correct time for artificial insemination can be determined.

Most domestic animals ovulate toward the end of estrus, but the cow ovulates 12 to 14 hours after estrus. The most successful artificial insemination occurs when it is performed about 12 hours after the beginning of estrus. In the cow, therefore, insemination precedes ovulation, and optimum fertilization is coupled with expected sperm and oocyte life and with capacitation. Capacitation refers to a modification of ejaculated or inseminated sperm within the female reproductive tract, enabling the sperm to fertilize oocytes. The fertile life for bovine sperm (time in female genitalia) is 30 to 48 hours, and for bovine oocytes (after ovulation) is 20 to 24 hours. The effect of time of insemination on conception rate in cattle is shown in Figure 13.20.

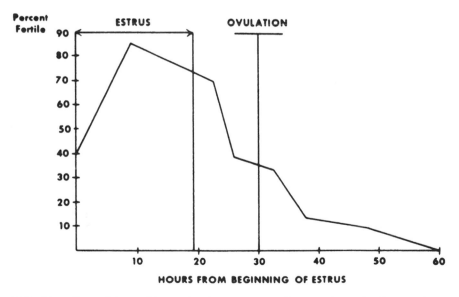

Figure 13.20. The effect of time of insemination on conception rate in cattle. Conception rate is best when insemination occurs about 10 hours from the beginning of estrus. From Stabenfeldt GH, Edqvist L. Female reproductive processes. In: Swenson MJ, Reece WO, eds. Dukes' physiology of domestic animals. 11th ed. Ithaca, NY: Cornell University Press, 1993.

Mare

The onset of puberty in the mare occurs during the breeding season after birth. If the interval between birth and the next breeding season is short (e.g., summer birth), puberty can be delayed for 12 months. A wide range of age for puberty is seen in the mare, from 12 to 18 months.

The transition from winter anestrus to estrus in late winter or early spring is often erratic, in that follicles might be grown but not ovulated. This results in prolonged estrous periods. After the first ovulation, the length of the estrous cycle stabilizes, and the duration of estrus is 5 to 6 days.

Ovulation occurs about 24 hours before the end of estrus and causes the end of estrus, which is a good indication that ovulation has occurred. Signs of estrus in the mare are elevation of the tail, standing with the hind legs apart, squatting and urinating, and rhythmically erecting the clitoris.

Ewe

Where lambs are normally born between December and March (in the northern hemisphere), puberty onset occurs the following fall, at about 8 to 9 months of age.

The estrous cycle in sheep is shorter than in the other domestic species because the antral phase of follicle growth is 3 to 4 days shorter. The physiologic breeding season lasts 6 to 7 months, during which repeated estrous cycles are observed in the absence of pregnancy.

A prominent sign of estrus is fluttering of the tail. Also, females separated from males by a barrier often assume a close proximity to the barrier.

Sow

Pigs born at any time of the year reach puberty at 6 to 7 months of age. Ovulation rates are more pronounced at the third estrus after puberty.

Signs of estrus include swelling of the vulva, restlessness, and decreased appetite. Application of pressure on the sow's back during estrus brings forth the rigidity reflex that occurs during natural mating with a boar.

Ovulation occurs from both ovaries, and 14 to 16 oocytes can be released. Because of the large number of follicles or corpora lutea at any one time, the sow ovaries often appear to be lobulated (Fig. 13.4).

Doe

The breeding season and gestation periods are similar for goats and sheep, and puberty is reached at about the same age (8 to 9 months). Breeding is often delayed, however, until the next breeding season.

Signs of estrus in the doe are similar to those in the ewe. When mating occurs, intromission and ejaculation are accomplished rapidly, usually within several seconds.

Pseudopregnancy is a condition in which a female has most signs of pregnancy but is not pregnant. Enlargement of the uterus occurs as a result of fluid accumulation. This phenomenon occurs in the goat and is believed to be caused by prolongation of the CL (see previous section, Persistent Corpus Luteum). The injection of $PGF_{2\alpha}$ results in CL regression and discharge of the accumulated uterine fluid.

Bitch

The onset of puberty in the bitch occurs 2 to 3 months after she reaches adult size. Among breeds it ranges from 6 to 12 months of age.

The bitch has an unusually long period of ovarian inactivity (anestrus) that is unrelated to photoperiod or nutrition. Because of this she is sometimes considered to be monestrous. Estrous cycles are common at all times of the year. The stages of the estrous cycle are different from those of the other species in that each is longer. Proestrus and estrus are each of 7 to 10 days duration, and diestrus is prolonged, lasting 70 to 80 days.

The LH surge occurs at the end of proestrus, followed by ovulation within 24 to 48 hours. The bitch might be sexually attractive during proestrus but is not sexually receptive until after the LH surge. Progesterone secretion thereafter is essential for receptivity and, even though the estrogen level declines, sexual receptivity is maintained for 7 to 10 days.

Vaginal cytologic changes seem to be more pronounced in bitches than in other domestic species and have been correlated with each estrous cycle stage. Vaginal smears are useful for assessing the stage of estrus and for predicting the most suitable time for breeding. The principal cytologic changes are 1) thickening and cornification of the vaginal epithelium, 2) loss of leukocytes because of the thickened epithelium, and 3) appearance of erythrocytes from the developing vascular system of the endometrium.

Among those animals that exhibit pseudopregnancy, it is most often seen in the bitch. In the absence of pregnancy, the corpus luteum persists, and during the exaggerated diestrus, progesterone continues to be produced for 50 to 80 days. This is a normal phenomenon in bitches because the uterus is not active in CL regression (production of $PGF_{2\alpha}$). The endometrium hypertrophies and endometrial glands develop, even though no fetus is present. Some bitches have no other signs of the prolonged elevation of progesterone concentration, but others have mammary gland enlargement and relaxation of the pelvis. Occasionally, a maternal attitude develops that leads to nest building. Rarely, lactation begins and the bitch shows signs of labor.

The long period of progesterone dominance (long diestrus), coupled with the relatively long period of regression of the endometrium after luteolysis of the CL, predisposes the endometrium to pyometra

(pus in the uterus). Pyometra is common in older bitches.

Queen

Cats born in the spring and summer months reach puberty in the following breeding season, at about 6 to 8 months of age. Cats born in the fall and early winter have their puberty delayed for 1 year until the next breeding season. The breeding season is considered to be January to October in the northern hemisphere.

If the queen does not have coitus, ovulation does not occur, and no luteal phase intervenes until the next cycle. The 8-day follicular phase is followed, however, by an 8-day period of ovarian inactivity. If queens have coital contact but fail to conceive, a luteal phase prolongs the onset of the next proestrus, with a minimum time of 42 days between estrus. Pseudopregnancy occurs in queens if a luteal phase occurs without pregnancy. Development of the uterus, mammary glands, and abdomen is not as marked as in the bitch, and nest building and lactation seldom occur.

Signs of estrus in queens include an increase in affection, which can be shown to almost any object—humans, table legs, or other pieces of furniture. They also crawl with their thorax against the floor, roll about, and vocalize for prolonged periods.

Several coital contacts might be made, with intromission and ejaculation occupying only 10 to 15 seconds each time. A refractory period or lack of sexual receptivity occurs for 10 to 15 minutes after each intromission. During the first hour of contact, four or five intromissions and ejaculations might occur.

PREGNANCY

Pregnancy is the condition of the female in which unborn young are contained within the body. Pregnancy is also called gestation

and its length is frequently known as the gestation period, extending from fertilization
through birth. Its length for various domestic
animals is shown in Table 13.1. Pregnancy
begins with fertilization, ends with parturition, and includes the essential aspects of
implantation and placentation. Before fertilization, the oocyte and sperm are transported to appropriate sites in the oviducts.

Transport of Oocyte and Spermatozoa

At ovulation, the fimbriae of the oviducts
(Fig. 13.3) are in close contact with the
ovaries. The contractile activity of the fimbriae directs the shed oocyte into the funnel-shaped opening of the oviduct. Within
the oviduct the oocyte is directed toward
the uterus by cilia and by oviduct motility.

The ejaculated spermatozoa are transported to the oviducts by increased motility

within the uterus caused by the release of
oxytocin at the time of coitus and by the
presence of prostaglandins in semen. The
oxytocin is effective because of the uterus
being primed by estrogen. Another factor
that assists in transport is thought to be the
presence of a negative pressure (vacuum) in
the uterus. Many spermatozoa are transported rapidly to the oviducts after ejaculation, but it is believed that these are not the
ones destined for fertilization. Their presence
might be coincidental with the spread of
accessory fluids throughout the tubular genitalia. The spermatozoa destined for fertilization are transported more slowly from their
sites of deposition (cervical canal, uterus,
vagina) to sperm reservoirs. The cervix of
ruminants has prominent ridges and
mucosal crypts that provide an extensive
secretory surface (Fig. 13.21). The cervical

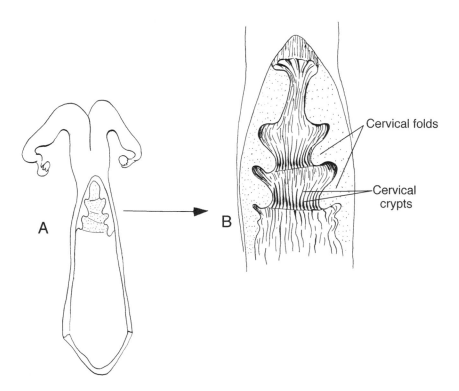

Figure 13.21. Dorsal view of the ruminant cervix. **A**. The cervix has been cut open and its lateral walls
reflected to show the folds and crypts. **B**. Magnified view of the cervix. A mucous covering assists
physical entrapment of spermatozoa destined for fertilization. The folds and crypts serve as sperm
reservoirs and allow for capacitation of spermatozoa.

crypts and their mucous covering aid in the physical entrapment of spermatozoa and serve as sperm reservoirs. Another important sperm reservoir is located at the junction of the uterine body with the uterine tubes.

Within the sperm reservoirs, the spermatozoa undergo changes necessary for later penetration of the zona pellucida and fertilization of the oocyte. These changes, known as capacitation, require several hours. One important change involves the acrosome, in which channels are established for the escape of hyaluronidase and a proteolytic enzyme; these substances are essential for penetration of the ovum. Capacitated spermatozoa are released slowly from the sperm reservoirs and proceed to the ampulla of the oviduct (dilated portion near infundibulum) for fertilization. Ovulation occurs after the onset of estrus, so that insemination is accomplished before ovulation. This allows enough capacitation time and, because the fertilizing life span is twice as long in spermatozoa as in oocytes, large numbers of spermatozoa are usually ready for fertilization at the time of ovulation. Oocytes retain viability for about 12 to 18 hours after ovulation in most domestic animals and spermatozoa retain their fertilizing ability for 24 to 48 hours in the cow, ewe, and sow, for up to 90 hours in the bitch, and for 120 hours (5 days) in the mare.

Fertilization

Fertilization is the fusion of male and female gametes to form one single cell, the zygote. The first step in fertilization is penetration of the zona pellucida by the spermatozoon. This involves not only the enzymes hyaluronidase and acrosin (proteolytic enzyme from acrosome), but also sperm motility. Motility ceases once contact with the oocyte has been made. In most domestic species, the second maturation division (meiosis) occurs when a spermatozoan penetrates the zona pellucida,

whereas the first meiosis occurred a few hours before ovulation. The zona reaction occurs after penetration of the zona pellucida and protects the oocyte from further penetration by other spermatozoa. Penetration by more than one spermatozoa (polyspermy) is deleterious to normal development of the zygote.

Pronuclei develop from the nuclei of the sperm and ovum. For each pronucleus, this involves the appearance of a number of nucleoli, which coalesce, and the development of a nuclear membrane around their respective periphery. Fertilization is complete after the pronuclei have disappeared and are replaced by chromosome groups united in prophase of the first cleavage division. The processes of fertilization are presented in Figure 13.22.

Zygotes usually remain in the uterine tube for 3 to 4 days before being transferred to the uterus. Uterine motility is unfavorable for zygote survival, and estrogen dominance at estrus must be changed to progesterone dominance, which occurs with the formation of the corpus luteum. Progesterone has a quieting influence on the uterus and promotes development of a glandular endometrium that can secrete "uterine milk," a nutrient medium for the embryo preceding its implantation. Cell division produces a 16- to 32-cell structure known as the morula. A cavity forms within the morula by 6 to 8 days of age, and the cell mass is called a blastocyst.

The period of the oocyte ends when the blastocyst attaches to the endometrium. This is the beginning of the embryonic period. The embryonic period is characterized by rapid growth—major tissues, organs, and systems develop and the major features of external body form become recognizable. The fetal period extends from this time until birth, and begins at about day 45 of gestation in the cow.

The nutritive requirements of the developing blastocyst are satisfied by diffusion from yolk in the ovum and by secretions of

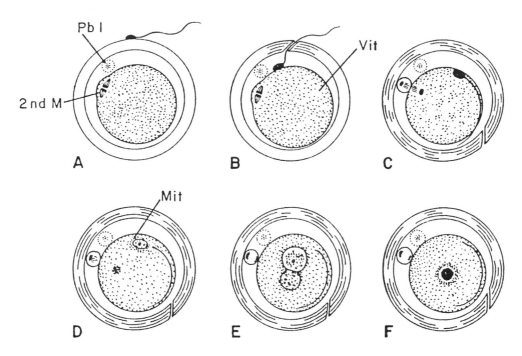

Figure 13.22. Processes occurring during fertilization in swine. **A.** The sperm is in contact with the zona pellucida. The first polar body (*Pb1*) has been extruded; the nucleus of the ovum is undergoing its second meiotic division (*2nd M*). **B.** The sperm has penetrated the zona pellucida and is now attached to the vitellus (*Vit*). This evokes the zona reaction, which is indicated by shading as it passes around the zona pellucida. **C.** The sperm has now been taken almost entirely within the vitellus. The head is swollen. The vitellus has decreased in volume and the second polar body has been extruded. The zona has rotated relative to the vitellus. **D.** Male and female pronuclei develop. Mitochondria (*Mit*) gather around the pronuclei. **E.** The pronuclei are fully developed and contain many nucleoli. The male pronucleus is larger than that of the female. **F.** Fertilization is complete. The pronuclei have disappeared and been replaced by chromosome groups, which have united in the prophase of the first cleavage division. From Hafez ESE. Reproduction in farm animals. 6th ed. Philadelphia: Lea & Febiger, 1993.

the oviduct and uterus ("uterine milk"), until it becomes fixed in position in the uterus. Implantation of the embryo occurs when it becomes fixed in position and forms a physical and functional contact with the uterus. It occurs 2 to 5 weeks after fertilization. The interval is shortest for the cat (2 weeks) and longest for cattle and horses (5 weeks).

Placentation

Because the embryo continues to grow, the central mass of cells becomes further removed from the surface. Diffusion of nutrients is no longer adequate and membranes develop, concurrent with a circulatory system, that provide for receiving nutrients from the dam. The development of extraembryonic membranes is known as placentation, and the collective name for the membranes is the fetal placenta, which consists of the chorion, allantois, and amnion. The relationship of the fetal membranes to the fetus is shown in Figure 13.23. The chorion is the outermost membrane and is the one most intimately associated with the endometrium. The amnion envelops the fetus and contains amniotic

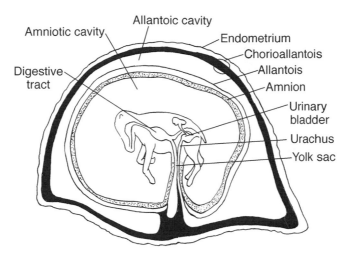

Figure 13.23. Fetus of horse within the placenta. The chorioallantois is the combination of the outer allantois with the chorion. Umbilical arteries and veins (not shown) occupy the space between the outer allantois and chorion. The chorion is associated intimately with the endometrium. The inner allantois is fused with the amnion.

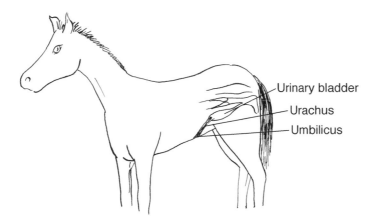

Figure 13.24. Diagrammatic view of persistent urachus in a foal. Failure of urachus closure at birth results in a continuous drip of urine at its umbilical exit.

fluid in the amniotic sac. The amniotic fluid is derived from fetal urine from the urethra, from secretions from the respiratory tract and oral cavity, and from the maternal circulation. The amniotic fluid protects the fetus from external shock, prevents adhesion of fetal skin with amniotic membrane, and assists in dilating the cervix and lubricating the birth passage at parturition. The allantois outer layer is fused to the chorion and the inner layer of allantois is fused to the amnion. The space between the two layers of allantois is called the allantoic sac. It is continuous with the cranial extremity of the urinary bladder by way of the urachus, which passes through the umbilical cord. When the urachus fails to close at birth, a continuous drip of urine is observed from the navel, a condition known as persistent urachus (Fig. 13.24).

Allantoic fluid originates from fetal urine and from secretory activity of the allantoic membrane. The fluid brings the chorioallantoic membrane into close apposition with the endometrium during early attachment and stores fetal excretory products. Branches of umbilical arteries and veins are distributed between the outer layer of allantois and the chorion.

The yolk sac is connected to the fetal intestine (the remnant after birth is known as Meckel's diverticulum). It serves as a nutrition source early in development.

When the attachment (extension of chorionic villi) of fetal membranes to the endometrium is continuous throughout the entire surface of the fetal membranes, it is known as a diffuse placenta. A diffuse type of placenta is found in the horse and pig (Fig. 13.25A). Ruminants have a cotyledonary placenta, in which attachment occurs only at the many mushroom-like projections from the endometrium (Fig. 13.25B). The fetal cotyledons are attached to the maternal caruncles, a combination known as a placentome. The fetal placentas of the dog and cat are attached by a girdle-like band that encircles the placenta, called a zonary placenta (Fig. 13.25C). The human placenta attachment is confined to a disk-shaped area and is called a discoidal placenta (Fig. 13.25D).

Hormones

Pregnancy is maintained as a result of the predominance of progesterone. During gestation, progesterone is produced by the placenta and CL. The contribution from placental and luteal sources and the duration of their contribution varies among species. The CL source is needed by all species during early pregnancy, but it is not needed by the mare and ewe after about days 100 and 60, respectively. A CL is needed for most of pregnancy in the cow, bitch, and queen and for the entire pregnancy in the sow and doe. Even though

progesterone from the CL is not needed by the ewe, regression of the CL does not occur and luteal production continues, but placental production is dominant. Regression of the CL occurs in the mare about midway,

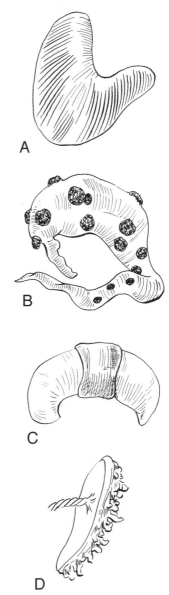

Figure 13.25. Placental types according to the distribution of chorionic projections (villi) on the endometrium. **A.** Diffuse placenta of the horse and pig. **B.** Cotyledonary placenta of ruminants. **C.** Zonary placenta of the dog and cat. **D.** Discoid placenta of the human and monkey.

and the placenta is the sole source of progesterone for the maintenance of pregnancy.

In the mare, endometrial cups begin to be formed at about day 35 of gestation within the endometrium from cells migrating from the placenta. The cups begin to secrete a hormone known as pregnant mare serum gonadotropin (PMSG) at about 35 days, which continues until about 130 days of gestation. PMSG helps to form new follicles, which ovulate and provide for additional corpora lutea. A greater supply of luteal progesterone is thereby ensured until the endometrial supply of progesterone is adequate for maintenance. All corpora lutea regress by about 150 days. Early pregnancy in the mare can be diagnosed by analyzing for the presence of PMSG.

Diagnosis

It often is of economic importance to determine whether an animal is actually pregnant. Pregnancy is obvious during the late stages when the size of the fetus, uterus, and fetal fluids have increased to the point where the abdomen has enlarged and definite dropping of the abdominal wall has occurred (known as "bellying down"). Rectal palpation is a useful procedure for detecting earlier signs of pregnancy, particularly in the cow. The hand is inserted into the rectum and structures located outside the rectal wall can be felt.

Early pregnancy by rectal palpation in the cow is suggested if a corpus luteum is present and if one horn of the uterus is larger than the other. This condition can be apparent at 30 to 45 days. At about 3 months, the fetal membranes can be felt to slip away from the grasp when the uterus is lifted, and small caruncles in the uterine wall are palpable. Also at 3 months, a vibration or "buzzing" of blood in the uterine artery is palpable, known as fremitus. At 5 to 7 months, the weight of the fetus causes the uterus to slip over the brim of the pelvis, and the cervix becomes taut. The

ovaries and fetus are difficult to palpate when this occurs because of their distance from the palpator, but definite caruncles are palpable.

After the fetus has descended over the brim of the pelvis in the cow, it can be possible to detect pregnancy by an external technique known as ballottement. Pressure is exerted on the lower right abdominal wall (Fig. 13.9) with the fist or knee in an inward and upward direction and then released, causing the fetus to rise and fall in its suspending fluids. The fall should be felt by the manipulator.

The use of radiography for the diagnosis of pregnancy has had limited application in veterinary medicine. Penetration of the rays is restricted in large animals and exposure of the film is difficult. In small animals, such as the dog, exposure is adequate, but differentiation of a fetus is not possible until calcification of bones is adequate for contrast. This does not occur until about 45 days in the dog, and other means, such as palpation and observation, are often more useful for earlier diagnosis of pregnancy.

A biologic test for the detection of pregnancy can be performed in the mare, based on the production of PMSG by the endometrial cups (see previous text). Injection of serum taken from a mare at 40 to 130 days of pregnancy into a female rabbit that has been isolated from male rabbits for at least 30 days brings forth ovarian follicles that rupture and form reddened corpora hemorrhagica about 48 hours after injection. The corpora hemorrhagica can be seen when the rabbit is butchered or observed by other procedures when placed under anesthesia. Because the rabbit does not ovulate and form corpora hemorrhagica unless coitus occurs, only the injected PMSG could have caused the ovulation.

Human chorionic gonadotropin (HCG) is excreted in the urine of pregnant women. It is detectable about 8 days after ovulation, which is 1 day after implantation. Early detection of pregnancy in women is possible by diagnostic tests that use the presence of HCG in urine. Functionally, HCG is the signal from the placenta for the corpus luteum to be maintained and thus sustain pregnancy.

PARTURITION

Parturition, sometimes called labor, is the physiologic process by which the pregnant uterus delivers the fetus and placenta from the mother.

Signs of Approaching Parturition

Throughout pregnancy, the abdomen continues to enlarge and its maximum size is reached just before parturition. The mammary glands also continue to enlarge and, within a few days of parturition, begin to secrete a milky material. Other signs include swelling of the vulva and a discharge of mucus from the vulva. The abdominal muscles relax, which causes the belly to drop and the rump to sink on both sides of the tail head. It is believed that the hormone relaxin, in association with the rising level of estrogen of late pregnancy, causes the relaxation of ligaments to enable the birth canal to enlarge. Also, it is thought that $PGF_{2\alpha}$ helps to relax the cervix. In addition to these physical signs, certain behavioral signs are characteristic, such as restlessness, frequent lying down and getting up, and frequent urination. The bitch and sow often attempt to build elaborate nests.

Respiratory rates are better indicators than milk let-down that sows are close to farrowing. Respiratory rates increase steadily and peak 6 hours before farrowing in almost all sows. In contrast, some sows produce colostrum as long as 3 to 4 days before farrowing. An example of the respiratory rate index can be obtained from the following data:

1. Respiratory rates average 54 breaths/minute during the 12 to 24 hour period before farrowing.
2. From 12 to 4 hours before farrowing respiratory rates are the highest, averaging 91 breaths/minute.
3. The lowest respiratory rates are recorded between 6 and 18 hours after birth of the last piglet, averaging 25 breaths/minute.

Rectal temperature changes have also been studied as indicators of impending parturition under the assumption that certain hormones influence body temperature. For example, progesterone raises the basal body temperature because it causes an increase in the basal metabolic rate. The temperature index is most dramatic and reliable in the bitch, in which a drop (loss of progesterone) of 2 to 3°C (4 or 5°F) might be observed 6 or 8 hours before parturition. Temperature index has not been found to be a reliable indicator in other species.

Hormone Changes

An important hormone change that occurs just before parturition is an increase in the production of estrogen. Estrone is produced by the fetoplacental unit as maturity of the fetus increases (approximately 3 to 4 weeks prepartum in the cow). The increase in production of cortisol by fetal adrenal cortices, concurrent with maturity of the fetus, initiates the prepartum increase in estrogen production. The secretion of estrogen assists in the production of uterine muscle contractile proteins before parturition. Estrogen might also be the signal for the secretion of $PGF_{2\alpha}$ that occurs in the immediate prepartum period (24 to 36 hours prepartum in the cow). $PGF_{2\alpha}$ initiates regression of the corpus luteum (if present) and subsequent lowering of progesterone levels. The increase in estrogen and decrease in progesterone levels convert the uterus from a state of quiescence to a state of potential contractility. The increase in estrogen level varies among domestic animals as to time of occurrence before parturition (Fig. 13.26). The length of increase is longest for the cow and shortest for the ewe.

Changes in maternal hormonal levels do not seem to play a major role in parturition in the mare. At parturition the mare has relatively high levels of progestogens and low levels of estrogens. $PGF_{2\alpha}$ level increases, however, during foaling. The progesterone concentration does not decrease in the mare after $PGF_{2\alpha}$ secretion because no corpus luteum is present after about 150 days of pregnancy.

$PGF_{2\alpha}$ is also believed to increase the contractility of the uterus by permitting greater mobility of sarcoplasmic calcium. These early contraction increases might be important in positioning the fetus for delivery (presentation) through the pelvic canal. The presence of the fetus in the pelvic canal causes oxytocin to be released from the posterior pituitary. In the presence of an estrogen-primed uterus, the muscle contractions increase in intensity to assist in expelling the fetus. $PGF_{2\alpha}$ also increases the sensitivity of the uterus to oxytocin, which enhances the rhythmic contractions of the uterine musculature during delivery.

The uterus can only assist in the expulsion of the fetus and must have the coordinated contraction of the abdominal muscles. The presence of the feet in the pelvic canal and the consequent stimulation of the vagina provides for reflex contraction of the abdominal muscles, similar to the straining that occurs when one attempts to replace a prolapsed uterus. The abdominal and uterine muscle contraction, coupled with relaxed pelvic ligaments, separation of the pelvic symphysis, and dilatation of the cervix, provide for expulsion of the fetus.

Stages

The three stages of parturition are as follows:

1. Uterine contractions (contribute to dilatation of cervix and presentation of fetus)
2. Contractions associated with expulsion of fetus (involve abdominal muscle contraction)
3. Expulsion of placenta

The stages of labor and related events are summarized in Table 13.2.

In monotocous (single-birth) species, the fetus lies on its back during gestation. Just

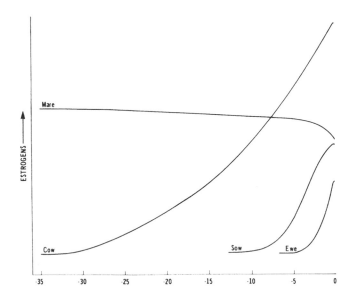

Figure 13.26. Estrogen patterns in the mare, cow, sow, and ewe before parturition. From Edqvist LE, Stabenfeldt GA. Reproductive hormones. In: Kaneko JJ, ed. Clinical biochemistry of domestic animals. 3rd ed. New York: Academic Press, 1980.

TABLE 13.2. Stages of Labor and Related Events in Farm Animals

Stage of Labor	Mechanical Forces	Period	Related Events
I: Dilation of cervix	Regular uterine contractions	Beginning of uterine contractions until cervix is fully dilated and continuous with vagina	Maternal restlessness, elevated pulse and respiratory rates Changes in fetal position and posture
II. Expulsion of fetus*	Strong uterine and abdominal contractions	From complete cervical dilation to end of delivery of fetus	Maternal recumbency and straining; rupture of allantochorion and escape of fluid from vulva; appearance of amnion (water bag) at vulva; rupture of amnion and delivery of fetus
III. Expulsion of placenta	Uterine contractions decrease in amplitude	Following delivery of fetus to expulsion of placenta	Maternal straining ceases; loosening of chorionic villi from maternal crypts; inversion of chorioallantois; straining and expulsion of fetal membranes

*In polytocous species (sow) and twin-bearing species (sheep and goat), this stage cannot be separated from the next stage (III). From Hafez ESE. Reproduction in farm animals. 6th Ed. Philadelphia: Lea & Febiger, 1993.

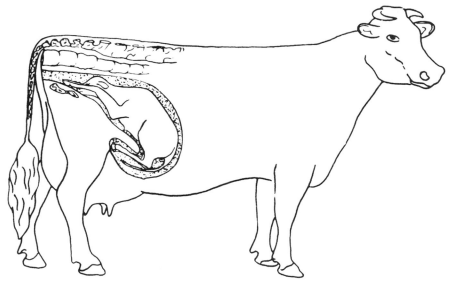

Figure 13.27. Normal presentation for the bovine fetus. From Salisbury GW, et al. Physiology of reproduction and artificial insemination of cattle. Copyright ©1961, 1978 by WH Freeman and Company. Used by permission.

before birth, a position is assumed in the uterus that is characteristic for the species (presentation). Presentation can be initiated by early contractions of the uterus (see previous text). A proper presentation for the bovine fetus is shown in Figure 13.27 . The front feet are pointed toward the cervix, the head is extended and tucked between the feet, and the back of the calf is directed toward the sacral vertebrae. This is known as an anterior presentation. A posterior presentation with the hind feet extended into the pelvic canal is considered normal, but is less common. An example of an abnormal

TABLE 13.3. Average Duration of the Three Stages of Labor in Farm Animals

| Animal | I: Dilation of Cervix | Stage of Labor (h) | |
		II. Expulsion of Fetus(es)	III: Expulsion of Placenta(s)
Mare	1–4	0.2–0.5	1
Cow	2–6	0.5–1.0	6–12
Ewe	2–6	0.5–2.0	0.5–8
Sow	2–12	2.5–3.0	1–4

From Hafez ESE. Reproduction in farm animals, 6th Ed. Philadelphia: Lea & Febiger, 1993.

presentation is one in which there might be an anterior presentation, but with a deviation of the head and neck. Abnormal presentations usually require correction before the fetus can be expelled successfully.

Difficulties are often encountered during parturition, and delays are observed in what are considered normal durations of each stage. Undue delay in providing assistance often aggravates the condition and can injure the mother and cause death to the fetus. "Rules of thumb" for the average duration of the three stages of labor in the mare, cow, ewe, and sow are given in Table 13.3. A difficulty encountered in expulsion of the fetus is referred to as a dystocia.

INVOLUTION OF THE UTERUS

The process by which the uterus returns to its nonpregnant size after parturition is known as involution. The points of attachment of the fetal placenta to the endometrium slough, and the exposed endometrium heals by forming new epithelium. In addition to new epithelial growth, the myometrium contracts and the cells shorten.

COW. Within 6 to 7 days postpartum, the upper two-thirds of the maternal caruncle sloughs into the uterus, becoming part of the fluids discharged. The epithelial cells of the caruncle must be shed for the placenta to be expelled. Within 21 to 35 days all cellular repair has occurred and endometrial gland function is restored. The

caruncles have retracted and cannot be palpated. Normally, estrus is observed in 45 to 60 days postpartum. Suckling by the calf, low energy intake, infections, and heavy lactation delay estrus.

MARE, EWE, AND SOW. Involution in the mare is rapid, but not complete, by the time of "foal heat," which occurs within 6 to 13 days postpartum. Foal heat is usually accompanied by ovulation, and mares bred at this time can become pregnant. Conception rates are lower, however, when breeding occurs during the foal heat.

In the ewe and sow, about 24 to 28 days are needed for complete involution. In the sow, a nonfertile (no ovulation) estrus occurs 3 to 5 days after farrowing. Estrus combined with ovulation is usually inhibited throughout lactation. Sows not nursing their litters during the first week after farrowing have estrus with ovulation within 2 weeks. Weaning of pigs at any time induces estrus with ovulation in 3 to 5 days.

Resumption of estrus in the ewe and mare is consistent with the photoperiod of estrous activity characteristic for these species.

BITCH. The interplacental areas return to normal within a few weeks, but the placental sites require about 12 weeks to involute and heal. Estrus usually does not occur until after the young are weaned.

REPRODUCTION IN THE AVIAN FEMALE

The term oviduct is the anatomical term used to describe the complete tubular

TABLE 13.4. Formation of the Hen's Egg

Oviduct segment	Length* (cm)	Function	Time spent
Infundibulum	8	Pick up of ovulated ova Site of fertilization	15 min
Magnum	33	Secretion of albumin	3 h
Isthmus	10	Secretion of shell membranes	1½ h
Shell gland	12	Addition of fluid to egg (plumping) Stratification of albumen Shell production Secretion of shell pigments (if present)	20 h
Vagina	12	Sperm storage Egg transport	1 min

*Length of the segments differs with size of the hen and changes greatly, depending on relaxation or contraction of the muscular walls. From Burke WH. Avian reproduction. In: Swenson MJ, Reece WO. Dukes' physiology of domestic animals. 11th ed. Ithaca, NY: Avian Cornell University Press, 1993.

genitalia of the avian female. It is highly coiled and extends from the ovary to the cloaca. In the sexually mature chicken, it can be straightened out to a length of 70 to 80 cm. With few exceptions, among the domestic species of birds, only the left ovary and oviduct reach functional development. The left ovary is cranial to the left kidney and is tightly attached to the dorsal body wall, caudal to the left lung, and adhered closely to the caudal vena cava.

The oviduct can be subdivided into five functional regions (Fig. 13.28). Beginning with the ovarian end and extending to the cloaca, they are the infundibulum, magnum, isthmus, uterus (shell gland), and vagina. As described in Chapter 12, the cloaca is a region through which digestive and kidney wastes and genital tract products pass. The function of the infundibulum is to envelop the ovulated oocyte with its yolk and begin its direction through the remaining portions of the oviduct. The infundibulum is also the location where fertilization would occur because it is assumed that sperm would not be able to penetrate the oocyte after it begins to be covered by albumen (egg white). Secretion of albumen occurs in the magnum and it is the longest segment of the oviduct. Albumen surrounds the central yolk mass

and constitutes about two-thirds of the egg's weight. The isthmus secretes the

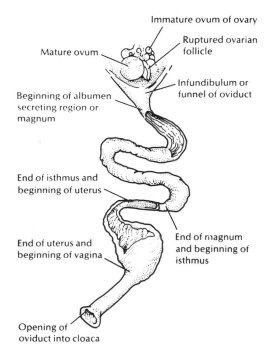

Figure 13.28. The five functional regions of the oviduct of the laying hen. The oviduct is the complete tubular genitalia of the avian female and consists of the infundibulum, magnum, isthmus, uterus, and vagina. From Sturkie PD, Mueller WJ. Reproduction in the female and egg production. In: Sturkie PD, ed. Avian physiology. New York: Springer-Verlag, 1976.

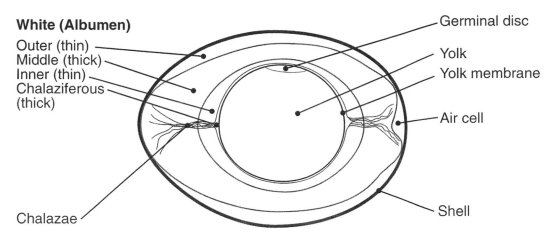

White (Albumen)
Outer (thin)
Middle (thick)
Inner (thin)
Chalaziferous
(thick)

Chalazae

Germinal disc
Yolk
Yolk membrane
Air cell
Shell

Figure 13.29. Midsagittal section of a hen's egg. The chalazae are extensions of the inner albumen layer that holds the yolk and developing embryo in the center so that adhesions of the embryo to the shell membranes do not occur.

fibrous inner and outer shell membranes that enclose the contents of the egg and provide support for deposition of the hard shell. The uterus adds fluid to the developing egg, secretes the hard shell, and adds the cuticle (a proteinaceous layer) to the exterior of the hard shell. The cuticle functions as a blockade against the entrance of bacteria and reduces water loss. The uterus is also the location where pigment is added to the hard shell (e.g., brown eggs). The uterovaginal sphincter, a constricting muscle, is the dividing point between the uterus and vagina. The oviduct terminates with the vagina that is attached to the cloaca. Nothing is added to the egg as it moves through the vagina; its function appears to be the prolonged storage of sperm in its sperm-host glands (additional sperm-host glands of the chicken, but not turkey, located in infundibulum). Storage and maintenance of fertilizing capacity for sperm of chickens is possible for 7 to 14 days and 40 to 50 days for turkeys in these glands. A summary of the hen's egg formation is provided in Table 13.4.

As in mammals at the time of birth, only a small number of the ovarian follicles present at the time of hatching develop to the point of ovulation. The immature avian follicle consists of an oocyte surrounded by granulosa cells and proceeds to the mature follicle that is quite large because of the addition of yolk material. The majority of yolk materials are deposited into the follicle during its rapid growth phase (final 7–11 days before ovulation). Yolk protein and lipid formation occurs in the liver and are transported via the blood to the ovary. Deposition of yolk into the maturing follicle terminates about 24 hours before ovulation. Yellow egg yolk is a complex mixture of water, lipid, protein, and many components in very small amounts, including vitamins and minerals. Inasmuch as there will be no maternal source of nutrition, the yolk is the nutritional source for the developing embryo. Its counterpart in mammals is the yolk sac that exists in vestigial form after birth as Meckel's diverticulum (see previous text). The yellow color of egg yolk is caused by xanthophyll pigments in the diet. It is possible to have light yellow or white egg yolks when xanthophyll is low or lacking in the diet.

A cross section of a hen's egg is shown in Figure 13.29. Extending away from the yolk towards both ends of the egg are twisted strands of protein called the chalazia. They are extensions of the inner albumen layer. It has been suggested that the function of the chalazia is to hold the yolk and developing embryo in the center of the egg so that adhesion of the embryo to the shell membranes does not occur. Most of the shell is secreted during the last 15 hours that the egg spends in the uterus. Its major composition is calcium carbonate. All of the calcium secreted into the uterus during shell formation comes from the blood. Because the amount of calcium in the shell exceeds the total amount of calcium in the blood, a dynamic interchange of skeletal calcium with blood calcium needs to occur. A sizeable amount of each shell's calcium is therefore derived from the bones. Blood and bone calcium is replaced by dietary calcium.

The ovulatory cycle in the domestic hen is about 24 to 26 hours long, and cycles may be repeated day after day without interruption. The period of time from one interruption to the next is called a clutch. In chickens, the clutches can range from 1 to 30 or more eggs. Oocytes not enveloped by the infundibulum are reabsorbed. Eggs that escape from the oviduct after the shell is formed are retained in the abdominal cavity, leading to the condition known as "egg bound".

The act of laying of the egg is known as oviposition. The muscles of the shell gland contract, and the sphincter separating the shell gland from the vagina relaxes. The shell gland contractions coordinate with abdominal muscle contractions (bearing-down reflex) to expel the egg.

Some commercial flocks of egg-laying hens begin to lay at about 22 weeks of age and continue for about a year. In this case, an average production of about 260 eggs/hen per year is typical. Those breeds of chickens that are selected for meat production lay far fewer eggs.

Aside from those breeds selected for egg production, there is a tendency among turkeys and breeds of chickens selected for meat production to exhibit broodiness, an incubation behavior in birds. After a few weeks of laying eggs, there is a desire to incubate them by sitting on them in a nest. When hens become broody, the ovaries regress and egg production ceases. The hormone prolactin causes the ovarian and behavioral changes associated with broodiness.

STUDY AIDS—FEMALE REPRODUCTION

Parts of the Female Reproductive System

1. When conducting a rectal palpation on a cow for the components of the female reproductive system, would one search dorsally (above) or ventrally (below)? What is the relative location of the urinary bladder?
2. Do all domestic animals (intact females) ovulate over the entire surface of the ovary?
3. Compare numbers of spermatozoa and ova that develop from one primary spermatocyte and one primary oocyte, respectively.
4. What is the process of oocyte formation known as?
5. What are primordial follicles? Does their number at birth, aside from those called to become mature oocytes, continue throughout the reproductive life of the female?
6. What function is served by the uterine tubes?
7. What function is served by the uterus?
8. Is the endometrium glandular throughout in all domestic animals (intact females)?
9. What function is served by the glandular secretion of the endometrium?
10. Is the cervix open at all times?
11. What comprises the myometrium and what is its function?
12. What is the major support for the gravid uterus?

13. What is the landmark junction between vagina and vulva? What is the vestibule of the vagina?
14. What is the major blood supply to the uterus? What is fremitus?
15. What function is served by the intertwining (Fig. 13.11) of the uterine artery and vein?

Hormones of Female Reproduction

1. Are diethylstilbestrol and estradiol-17b both estrogens? Are they both steroids?
2. Which female steroid hormone has activities that are performed in concert with estrogens and usually requires previous estrogen priming?
3. Which female steroid hormone prevents contractility of the uterus during pregnancy?
4. What are the main functions of the gonadotropins in the female?
5. Are tonic levels of the gonadotropins in the female increased or decreased by estrogens?
6. What is the role of the hypothalamic-hypophysial portal system in the release of FSH and LH?
7. What is the significance of gradually increasing concentrations of estrogen over a period of time upon LH release?

Ovarian Activity and Follicular Growth

1. How do growing follicles become graafian follicles?
2. What part of the graafian follicle secretes androgens? Do androgens persist as androgens?
3. What hormones cause the formation of a fluid filled space, called an antrum?
4. What functions are served by the pre-ovulatory (24 hours) surge of LH? (Specific functions as listed under "Ovarian Hormone Cycle")?
5. Do all animals ovulate before the end of estrus? What is the difference between spontaneous and reflex ovulation?

6. Does ovulation occur in all developing follicles? Do follicles continue to grow and develop during all phases of the ovarian cycle? What must be a characteristic of follicles for them to ovulate?
7. What changes are involved in the formation of the corpus luteum? How is the corpus luteum maintained?
8. What is the natural luteolytic substance that causes regression of the corpus luteum? Does acute regression of the corpus luteum occur in the bitch and queen?
9. Note the unique delivery system of the natural luteolytic substance in Fig. 13.18.
10. What is a persistent corpus luteum, and what is its most probable cause?

Sexual Receptivity

1. What hormone is required for the initiation of sexual receptivity in all animals?
2. How does progesterone enhance receptivity in some domestic animal species?
3. What domestic animal species require estrogen synergism with progesterone?

Estrous Cycle and Related Factors

1. How is an estrous cycle interval defined?
2. Know the stages of the estrous cycle and their relationship to ovarian activity.
3. Which steroid hormone predominates during the follicular periods?
4. Which stage of the estrous cycle is characterized by sexual receptivity?
5. Review photoperiod influence on cat, horse, sheep, and goat. What does "turn-on" and "turn-off" time relate to?
6. How is nutrition related to puberty and post-parturient resumption of ovarian activity?
7. Note species characteristics associated with their estrous cycles: cow-post-estrus ovulation; ewe-short estrous cycle interval; bitch-vaginal cytologic changes

and classical pseudopregnancy; queen-reflex ovulation, signs of estrus, coital behavior.

Pregnancy

1. Know the length of gestation for each of the domestic species (Table 13.1).
2. What is a sperm reservoir? Where are important ones located?
3. What is capacitation? Name one capacitation change.
4. What is the zona reaction associated with fertilization? Where does fertilization normally occur?
5. What is "uterine milk"?
6. What is implied by implantation?
7. What is placentation? What membranes comprise the fetal placenta?
8. Know the relationship of the placental membranes to each other and to the fetus and mother. Where are the branches of the umbilical arteries and veins located?
9. What is a persistent urachus?
10. Which animals have a cotyledonary placenta? What comprises a placentome?
11. Which steroid hormone predominates during pregnancy? Where is it produced? Do the sources and duration of their production vary among species? When is the corpus luteum source needed by all species?
12. What function is served by pregnant mare serum gonadotropin (PMSG)?
13. What are some signs of pregnancy in the cow as observed by rectal palpation?

Parturition

1. What are some signs of approaching parturition?
2. How is respiratory rate in the sow associated with closeness of farrowing? What happens to body temperature in the bitch just before parturition?
3. What functions are served by estrogen increase just before parturition?
4. What functions are served by $PGF_{2\alpha}$ at the time of parturition?
5. How do oxytocin and presence of feet in the pelvic canal assist parturition?
6. What are the stages of labor?
7. What is meant by presentation of the fetus? How is it initiated?
8. What is the difference between an anterior and a posterior presentation? What is an example of an abnormal presentation?
9. What term is applied to difficulty encountered in expulsion of the fetus?

Involution of the Uterus

1. What is meant by involution? What events characterize involution?
2. What is "foal heat" in the mare?
3. Is post-farrowing estrus (3 to 5 days after farrowing) in the sow fertile or nonfertile?

Reproduction in the Avian Female

1. What is the oviduct in the avian female?
2. Is the avian reproductive tract bilateral? Which side persists?
3. What are the component parts of the oviduct?
4. What are the functions of the infundibulum?
5. What is the function of the magnum?
6. What is the function of the isthmus?
7. What are the functions of the uterus? What is the cuticle and what is its function?
8. What is the function of the vagina?
9. What are sperm-host glands?
10. Where are the yolk proteins and lipids formed?
11. What is the function of the chalazia?
12. What is the immediate source of the calcium needed for hard shell formation?
13. What is the length of an ovulation cycle in the domestic hen? What is a clutch?
14. What is meant by "egg bound" in the avian female?
15. Describe oviposition in the avian female.

SELF-EVALUATION—FEMALE REPRODUCTION

1. A "freemartin" of the bovine species is:
   a. a sterile female calf that develops in same uterus with a normal male twin and shares a common blood supply with the male while in the uterus
   b. same as a. except refers to the male as being sterile
   c. infrequently sterile (reproductively)
   d. a calf with a "free spirit"

2. Which one of the following best describes the action of LH (luteinizing hormone) in the female?
   a. causes lysis or reduction in size of the corpus luteum
   b. increases the blood supply and motility of the uterus
   c. assists in the maturing of an ovarian follicle, its rupture and subsequent development and maintenance of a corpus luteum
   d. stimulates the interstitial cells (Leydig cells) to secrete testosterone

3. Proestrus is characterized by:
   a. sexual receptivity
   b. increasing amounts of relaxin
   c. beginning after regression of the corpus luteum and ending at the onset of estrus
   d. early corpus luteum development

4. Which one of the following would not normally be expected in the sexual cycle of the cow and sow?
   a. proestrus
   b. estrus
   c. metestrus
   d. diestrus
   e. anestrus (long periods of ovarian inactivity)

5. Which one of the following best describes the action of progesterone?
   a. increases libido
   b. increases blood supply and motility of the uterus
   c. increases endometrial development, glandular secretion of the endometrium and decreases motility of the uterus
   d. assists follicular rupture and subsequent development of the corpus luteum

6. Which one of the following is the best example of a seasonally polyestrous animal?
   a. cow
   b. sow
   c. bitch
   d. ewe

7. The theca interna:
   a. is the outer cell layer of the primary and antral follicles
   b. has LH receptors and secretes androgen
   c. has FSH receptors and converts androgen to estrogen
   d. secretes estrogen

8. Intertwining of the ovarian artery with the uterine vein serves:
   a. to cool the ovary
   b. to suspend the ovary
   c. to transport $PGF_{2\alpha}$ from the uterus to the ovary
   d. to transport sperm from the uterus to the ovary

9. Tonic levels of LH and FSH in the female are increased by a decrease in:
   a. estrogen
   b. progesterone
   c. androgen

10. The female steroid hormone that prevents contraction of the uterus during pregnancy is:
    a. estrogen
    b. progesterone
    c. LH

11. What hormone has its concentration increased greatly just before ovulation (preovulatory surge) that assists ovulation and conversion of ruptured follicle to a corpus luteum?
    a. FSH
    b. estrogen

c. LH

d. progesterone

12. An estrous cycle interval is:

    a. diestrus to proestrus

    b. one period of sexual receptivity to the next

    c. the same in all animals

    d. puberty to end of reproductive life

13. The endometrium:

    a. is the muscle layer of the uterus and expels the fetus at the end of gestation

    b. is composed of skeletal muscle

    c. is support system for the uterus

    d. is the lining of the uterus that secretes "uterine milk"

14. Pseudopregnancy is observed most commonly in the:

    a. bitch

    b. mare

    c. doe

    d. queen

15. Which domestic animal ovulates 12 to 14 hours after estrus?

    a. mare

    b. queen

    c. cow

    d. bitch

16. The estrous cycle period that begins after corpus luteum regression and ends at the onset of estrus is:

    a. metestrus

    b. diestrus

    c. proestrus

17. The most predominant steroid hormone at the time of estrus is:

    a. LH

    b. FSH

    c. progesterone

    d. estradiol

    e. LSMFT

18. Which one of the following most closely approximates the gestation period for the sow?

    a. 21 days

    b. 150 days

    c. 16 days

    d. 114 days

19. Difficulty in giving birth to the young is called:

    a. fremitus

    b. libido

    c. dyspnea

    d. dystocia

20. Implantation is achieved when the uterus is dominated by:

    a. relaxin

    b. progesterone

    c. estradiol

    d. diethylstilbestrol

21. Which one of the following approximates the gestation period for the mare:

    a. 21 days

    b. 16 days

    c. 282 days

    d. 336 days

22. Parturition refers to:

    a. the length of the estrous cycle

    b. the length of time for development of the fetus

    c. the act of giving birth to the young

    d. the return of the uterus to normal function and size

23. Which one of the following represents the most intimate attachment of the placenta with uterine tissue?

    a. amnion - allantois

    b. allantois - chorion

    c. amnion

    d. heart - lung preparation

24. The oviduct in the avian female:

    a. extends from the ovary to the horns of the uterus

    b. extends from the ovary to the cloaca

    c. does not include a component known as the uterus

    d. serves only to transport the oocyte

25. The reproductive tract of the avian female is characterized by:

    a. a single left ovary and its oviduct

    b. a single right ovary and its oviduct

    c. a right and left ovary connected to a single oviduct

    d. right and left ovaries and oviducts, both terminating at the cloaca

26. Envelopment of the ovulated oocyte is a function of the:
    a. magnum
    b. isthmus
    c. uterus
    d. infundibulum

27. Fertilization of the oocyte would occur in the:
    a. vagina
    b. uterus
    c. magnum
    d. infundibulum

28. Secretion of albumen takes place in the:
    a. infundibulum
    b. magnum
    c. isthmus
    d. uterus

29. Egg yolk proteins and lipids are formed in the:
    a. ovary
    b. oviduct
    c. liver
    d. cloaca

30. The cuticle functions to:
    a. add hardness to the shell
    b. stabilize the albumen and yolk
    c. reduce bacterial contamination and water loss
    d. glamorize the egg

31. Sperm-host glands are present in the:
    a. cloaca
    b. vagina
    c. uterus
    d. ceca

32. Egg-bound refers to:
    a. the ultimate location of the oocyte
    b. eggs with shells that escape from the oviduct and are in the abdomen
    c. oocytes and yolk not enveloped by the infundibulum
    d. eggs stuck in the cloaca

33. Oviposition refers to:
    a. competition for an oocyte by spermatozoa
    b. the act of laying the egg

c. the location of the oocyte within an egg
d. the position of the female during mating

34. Which plasma cation has the greatest turnover during egg production?
    a. Na^+
    b. K^+
    c. Ca^{2+}
    d. Mg^{2+}

Suggested Readings

Burke WH. Avian reproduction. In: Swenson MJ, Reece WO, eds. Dukes' physiology of domestic animals. 11th ed. Ithaca, NY: Cornell University Press, 1993:728–750.

Dyce KM, Wensing CJG. Essentials of bovine anatomy. Philadelphia: Lea & Febiger, 1971.

Dyce KM, Sack WO, Wensing CJG. Textbook of veterinary anatomy. 2nd ed. Philadelphia: WB Saunders, 1996.

Edqvist LE, Stabenfeldt GA. Reproductive hormones. In: Kaneko JJ, ed. Clinical biochemistry of domestic animals. 3rd ed. San Diego: Academic Press, 1980:513–544.

Frandson RD, Spurgeon TL. Anatomy and physiology of farm animals. 5th ed. Philadelphia: Lea & Febiger, 1992.

Hafez ESE. Reproduction in farm animals. 6th ed. Philadelphia: Lea & Febiger, 1993.

Johnson AL. Reproduction in the female. In: Sturkie PD, ed. Avian physiology. 4th ed. New York: Springer-Verlag, 1986:403–431.

Langley LL, Telford IR, Christensen JB. Dynamic anatomy and physiology. 3rd ed. New York: McGraw-Hill, 1969.

McDonald LE. Veterinary endocrinology and reproduction. 4th ed. Philadelphia: Lea & Febiger, 1989.

Short RV. Role of hormones in sex cycles. In: Austin CR, Short RV, eds. Reproduction in mammals, Book 3. New York: Cambridge University Press, 1972:42–72.

Stabenfeldt GH, Edqvist L. Female reproductive processes. In: Swenson MJ, Reece WO, eds. Dukes' physiology of domestic animals. 11th ed. Ithaca, NY: Cornell University Press, 1993:678–710.

Lactation

Provision of food to the newborn is essential for its survival, so lactation is an important component of the reproductive process. Rapid development of the female mammary glands begins at puberty and functional development (prolactational) is reached during pregnancy. Lactation begins after parturition because of the hormonal changes that occur.

STRUCTURE AND FUNCTION OF FEMALE MAMMARY GLANDS

Mammary Gland of Cows

GENERAL DESCRIPTION. The mammary gland (udder) of the cow has an inguinal location with distinct right and left halves, and each half has a front and hind quarter (Fig. 14.1). Each half is independent from its counterpart in regard to its blood and nerve supply, lymphatic drainage, and suspensory apparatus. A longitudinal furrow marks the ventral separation of the halves. The two quarters of each half are separate in regard to its gland tissue and duct system. All the milk from one teat is produced by the glandular tissue of that quarter. The parenchyma of the mammary gland refers to the epithelial or glandular tissues as opposed to the stroma, which is the connective tissue framework of the mammary gland. The milk-secreting unit of the mammary gland is the alveolus (Fig. 14.2). A number of alveoli converge on ducts that convey milk to a cistern within the gland and finally to a cistern within the teat. Expulsion of milk from the teat occurs through the teat canal, which is kept tightly closed by a muscular sphincter. A number of alveoli grouped together and surrounded by a layer of connective tissue is known as a lobule. A larger connective tissue division surrounds a number of lobules to form a lobe. The secreting units of the mammary gland are thus divided into lobules and lobes.

DUCT SYSTEM. The various ducts converge to form larger ducts that empty into a large basin known as the lactiferous sinus

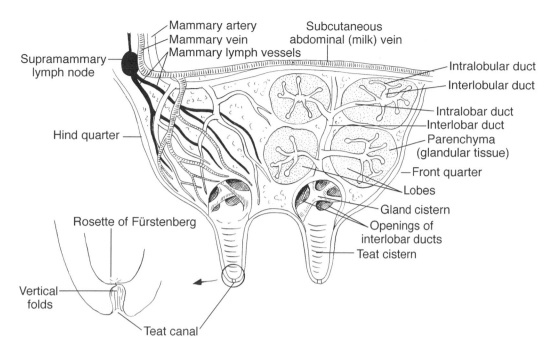

Figure 14.1. Sagittal section of the cow udder through the left half. The four circular areas in the front quarter are schematically shown to illustrate the organization of the glandular tissue and also the various orders of ducts. The lobes are distributed throughout the parenchyma. The lobes are further divided into lobules (not shown). The gland cistern and teat cistern for each quarter are collectively known as the lactiferous sinus. The teat canal magnification shows the vertical folds of the teat canal and also the rosette of Fürstenberg at the upper end.

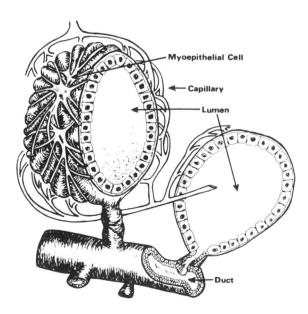

Figure 14.2. Alveolus surrounded by blood vessels and myoepithelial (contractile) cells. Several alveoli in a group form a lobule. Each alveolus converges on an intralobular duct. From Larson BL. Biosynthesis and cellular secretion of milk. In: Larson BL, ed. Lactation. Ames, IA: Iowa State University Press, 1985.

(Fig. 14.1). The ducts are referred to as lobular or lobar, depending on whether they serve lobules or lobes, respectively. Accordingly, intralobular and interlobular refer to ducts within and between lobules, respectively. Interlobular ducts converge on a single intralobar duct; when it emerges from the lobe it becomes an interlobar duct. Interlobar ducts empty into the lactiferous sinus, which is composed of the gland cistern (within the gland) and the teat cistern (within the teat). Dilatations that occur along many of the ducts also store milk, in addition to the lactiferous sinus.

THE TEAT. The part of the mammary gland from which milk is extracted and suckled by the young is called the teat, with one teat for each quarter of the udder. A section of the cow's teat is shown in Figure 14.3. The duct extending from the teat cistern to the teat orifice is the papillary duct (teat canal). It is normally closed by a smooth muscle sphincter that encircles the teat canal (Fig. 14.4). Closure of the teat canal prevents leakage of the milk that accumulates within the lactiferous sinus. The mucosa of the teat canal is marked by vertical ridges which radiate upward from the internal opening forming the rosette of Fürstenberg (Fig. 14.1) which appear as folds of mucosa. The weight of milk in the lactiferous sinus exerts a downward thrust on the folds, thus covering the inner opening to the teat canal and assisting with retention of milk within the udder. External pressure on the teat at milking causes inner expansion of the teat, so that the overlapping folds are withdrawn and milk can escape through the orifice. Inflammation or injury to the rosette can increase its size resulting in partial restriction or blockage

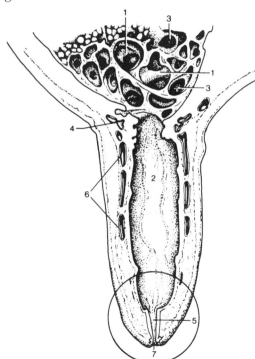

Figure 14.3. Sagittal section through a cow's teat (circled area is shown in Figure 14.4. *1,* gland cistern; *2,* teat cistern (gland cisterns and teat cisterns are collectively known as lactiferous sinuses); *3,* openings of interlobar ducts; *4,* submucosal venous ring; *5,* teat canal; *6,* venous plexus in teat wall; *7,* teat orifice (opening). From Dyce KM, Sack WO, Wensing CJG. Textbook of veterinary anatomy. 2nd ed. Philadelphia: WB Saunders, 1996.

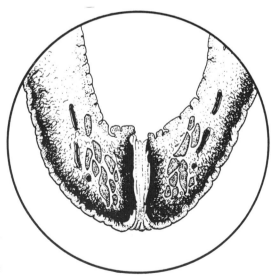

Figure 14.4. Section of the teat (circled area from Figure 14.3) showing the smooth muscle encircling the teat canal (papillary duct). From Dyce KM, Sack WO, Wensing CJG. Textbook of veterinary anatomy. 2nd ed. Philadelphia: WB Saunders, 1996.

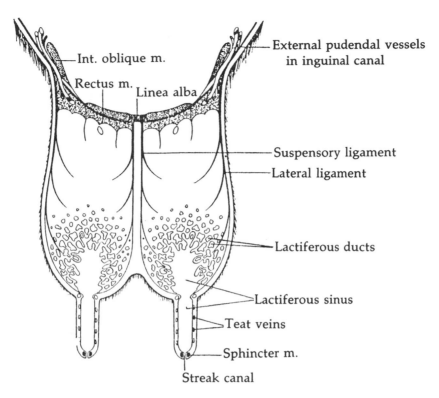

—Int. oblique m.

Rectus m.

Linea alba

External pudendal vessels in inguinal canal

Suspensory ligament

Lateral ligament

Lactiferous ducts

Lactiferous sinus

Teat veins

Sphincter m.

Streak canal

Figure 14.5. Schematic vertical section through the abdominal floor and forequarters of the udder. The structure shown as the suspensory ligament is the medial suspensory ligament and the structure shown as the lateral ligament is the lateral suspensory ligament. Both contribute to the suspensory apparatus. From Dyce KM, Wensing CJG. Essentials of bovine anatomy. Philadelphia: Lea & Febiger, 1971.

of the teat canal. Epithelial cells associated with Fürstenberg's rosette are believed to secrete a bacteriostatic agent. The wall of the empty teat cistern is characterized by numerous longitudinal and circular folds. When the teat is filled with milk these folds are obliterated. The presence of the folds permits expansion of the teat wall without tension. The venous plexus of the teat wall (Fig. 14.3) is believed to be related to maintenance of normal temperature during exposure to cold.

The ease with which milk can be withdrawn from the teat is often determined by the tightness of the sphincter that keeps the teat canal closed. A sphincter that is not tight enough can cause milk to leak from

the teat in the interval between milkings. A loose sphincter also predisposes to mastitis (inflammation of the mammary gland usually resulting from infection by microorganisms).

SUSPENSORY APPARATUS. Support from the longitudinal axis of the body is provided to the udder by the suspensory apparatus, which is composed of medial and lateral suspensory ligaments (Fig. 14.5). The medial suspensory ligament is derived from the elastic fibers (connective tissue) that cover the abdominal wall. It passes down between the two halves of the udder and intimately covers the medial side of each half, passes around the front to about the middle of the cranial quarters, and passes around the back to about the middle of the caudal quarters. The lateral suspensory ligaments are composed of white, fibrous, connective tissue (with little elasticity) derived from the subpelvic tendon. The lateral ligaments cover the lateral side of each half and meet the medial suspensory ligament at the front and back of each half. A number of connective tissue extensions (laminae) are given off from both the medial and lateral suspensory ligaments to enter the mammary gland. The laminae divide each quarter into lobes and lobules. Collectively, the laminae form the stroma (framework) of the mammary gland.

The function of the elastic fibers in the suspensory apparatus becomes apparent when the cow is mature and in production. In addition to providing expansion potential, they allow for absorption of the shock created when the cow walks, and they permit movement of the udder while the cow is lying down.

BLOOD SUPPLY AND VENOUS DRAINAGE. The principal blood supply to each half of the mammary gland is the external pudendal artery (called the mammary artery in the cow) (Fig. 14.1). It passes through the inguinal canal and divides to supply the front and hind quarters on the same side as the artery. The external pudendal vein (mammary vein in the cow) collects blood from the cranial and caudal quarters of the respective side and returns blood through the inguinal ring to the posterior vena cava (Fig. 14.6). The mammary veins are continuous cranially with anastomosing (joining) caudal, superficial, epigastric (subcutaneous abdominal or milk) veins and caudally with anastomosing perineal veins, so that a venous circle is formed at the base of the udder. The milk veins are relatively large, tortuous (winding) veins on the ventrolateral wall that disappear suddenly at a forward location (milk well) to enter the internal thoracic vein. Some believe that

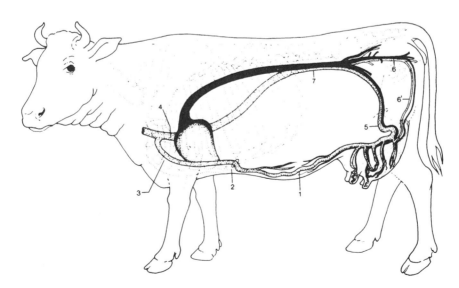

Figure 14.6. Venous drainage of the udder. *1,* Subcutaneous abdominal (milk) vein; *2,* milk "well"; *3,* internal thoracic vein; *4,* cranial vena cava; *5,* external pudendal vein; *6,* internal pudendal vein; *6',* ventral labial vein; *7,* caudal vena cava. From Dyce KM, Sack WO, Wensing CJG. Textbook of veterinary anatomy. Philadelphia: WB Saunders, 1987.

blood can enter the venous circle from the milk veins (a reverse direction). As in other tissues, the interstitial fluid has auxiliary drainage by way of lymphatic vessels with lymph nodes along their length. The major lymph node on each side is the superficial inguinal (mammary or supramammary) lymph node, located near the inguinal ring above the caudal part of the base of the udder (Fig. 14.1). Capillary networks are present, as in other tissues, and for the udder, these surround the alveoli and ducts much as capillaries surround alveoli in the lungs.

MYOEPITHELIAL CELLS. The myoepithelial cells are contractile cells that surround the alveoli and ducts. Because of their location relative to the alveoli, they have been called "basket" cells (Fig. 14.2). When these cells are contracted, they provide compression on the alveoli and ducts and hence cause milk to be directed toward the lactiferous sinus. They contract when the hormone oxytocin circulates and brings about milk let-down.

Mammary Glands of Other Animals

Pigs, Dogs, and Cats

The sow normally has seven pairs of mammary glands (range, four to nine). The teat of the sow has two teat canals and each is continuous with its respective teat cistern, gland cistern, and associated ducts. In the bitch and queen, five pairs of mammary glands are most common and each mammary gland has a mammary papilla, or nipple. The nipples have numerous fine openings (7 to 16) at their distal ends for the ducts of the glands. In the sow, bitch, and queen, the mammary glands are located in two rows parallel to the midline.

SHEEP AND GOATS. The mammary gland has an inguinal location in both the ewe and doe. Each half has only one teat, one teat canal, one teat cistern, and one gland cistern. The sphincter muscles at the tips of the teats are poorly developed and closure is assisted by elastic connective tissue.

HORSE. The horse has an inguinal location for its mammary gland, and each half has only one teat. Each teat has two teat canals and two teat cisterns; each is continuous with a gland cistern that has its own system of ducts and alveoli.

MAMMOGENESIS

Mammogenesis refers to the growth and development of the mammary gland. During embryologic development, a milk (or mammary) line appears on each side of the abdominal wall parallel to the midline (Fig. 14.7). In most animals, mammary glands develop only in the inguinal area of the milk line.

Development in Cattle

At birth, the female calf has teat and gland cisterns that are already somewhat mature in form. The mammary ducts are short and confined to the region of the gland cistern. The stroma is well organized and is interspersed with fat.

The rate of growth of the mammary gland from birth to puberty is the same as for the rest of the body. The mammary gland is a skin gland that responds to female sex hormones. These are present in low concentrations until puberty. At the beginning of puberty, follicle-stimulating hormone (FSH) and luteinizing hormone (LH) are released from the anterior pituitary at cyclic intervals that characterize the estrous cycles. FSH and LH activity cause the ovary to secrete the female sex steroid hormones, estrogens and progestins (primarily estradiol and progesterone). Estradiol is secreted mostly during the follicular phase of the estrous cycle, and progesterone is secreted mostly during the luteal phase. An effective response of the mammary gland to estradiol and progesterone depends on the synergism (working with) provided by the two anterior pituitary hormones, prolactin and somatotropin (STH; growth hormone). During the first several cycles, the growth effected by the synergism of estradiol, progesterone, STH, and prolactin consists of duct lengthening, thickening, and branching. By the age of 18 months, heifers have a system of ducts in the mammary glands. Differentiation of the ducts into alveoli continues with each recurring estrous cycle. The maximum amount of lobule and alveolar growth produced by estrous cycles alone is thought to occur at about 30 to 36 months of age.

When pregnancy begins, the concentrations of estradiol, progesterone, STH, and prolactin increase to cause changes in the uterus that are essential for the survival of the fertilized ovum. Most mammary gland growth occurs during pregnancy in response to the greater hormone concentrations. The adipose is slowly eroded and replaced by ducts, lobule alveoli, blood vessels, lymph vessels, and the connective tissue structures of the suspensory apparatus. Duct and alveolar growth continues throughout gestation.

The source of hormones varies with species. In cattle the placenta is a source of estrogen only. The corpus luteum continues as the major source of progesterone. A placental lactogen (hormone) that contributes to mammogenesis and is similar to STH and prolactin is secreted in several species, and is directed from the fetal placenta to maternal blood. Placental lactogen secretion occurs at midpregnancy and continues until parturition. However, in contrast to other species, secretion of placental lactogen in cattle is most commonly directed to the fetal circulation, and its role in mammary gland development is unknown.

In addition to the pituitary, ovarian, and placental hormones already mentioned as contributors to mammogenesis, other hormones can have a peripheral role, such as adrenal steroids, thyroid hormone, insulin, and relaxin.

Development in Other Animals

In the dog, cat, and sow, mammary glands develop along the entire length of the milk line. In the elephant and primates, mammary glands develop only in the pectoral region.

The placenta becomes a source of both estrogen and progesterone in many species (but not in cattle; see previous text). In sheep and goats, the greatest secretion of placental lactogen coincides with the greatest lobule and alveolar growth of the mammary gland.

LACTOGENESIS AND LACTATION

Stages

Lactogenesis is the process by which mammary alveolar cells acquire the ability to

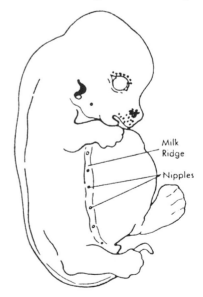

Figure 14.7. A 20-mm pig embryo, showing the milk ridge (milk line) ($\times$ 515). From Frandson RD, Spurgeon TL. Anatomy and physiology of farm animals. 5th ed. Philadelphia: Lea & Febiger, 1992.

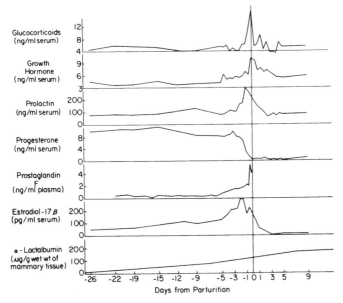

Figure 14.8. Changes in plasma concentration of several hormones found in cows near parturition. From Tucker HA. Endocrine and neural control of the mammary gland. In: Larson BL, ed. Lactation. Ames, IA: Iowa State University Press, 1985.

secrete milk. The first stage includes increases in mammary enzymatic activity and differentiation of cellular organelles that coincides with limited secretion of milk before parturition. The second stage is associated with copious secretion of all milk components shortly before parturition in most species, continuing for several days after parturition.

Hormones and Their Interactions

The hormones involved in the second stage of lactogenesis (onset of copious milk secretion at parturition) include increased secretion of prolactin, adrenocorticotropic hormone (ACTH), and estrogen, and a decrease or virtual absence of progesterone. ACTH stimulates the secretion of glucocorticoids.

Prolactin concentration in cattle does not change appreciably during gestation, but a major increase occurs within 24 to 48 hours before parturition. Other hormones, glucocorticoids, growth hormone, prostaglandins, and estradiol also increase concurrently, whereas the progesterone level declines (Fig. 14.8).

These hormones interact in various ways:

1. Prolactin induces gene expression in mammary tissue for casein synthesis, and glucocorticoids are required for this process.
2. The presence of progesterone prevents the formation of prolactin binding sites in mammary tissue and also saturates the sites where glucocorticoids would bind. The withdrawal of progesterone is thus a prerequisite for lactogenesis.
3. Prostaglandin increase just before parturition causes lysis of the corpus luteum and a consequent decline of the progesterone level.
4. In cattle, the concentration of estrogens begins to increase about 1 month before parturition and reaches a maximum about 2 days before parturition. Lactogenesis is thus enhanced because estrogens stimulate the secretion of prolactin and possibly other hormones from the anterior pituitary.
5. A surge in growth hormone (from the anterior pituitary) occurs just before parturition, perhaps assuming its role

of directing nutrients to the mammary gland for milk synthesis.

Hormonal Maintenance of Lactation

The increase in milk yield in cattle after parturition peaks in 2 to 8 weeks and gradually declines thereafter. To continue with lactation, mammary alveolar cell numbers and alveolar cell activity must be maintained, and the milk produced must be removed regularly. Hormones required for milk synthesis include prolactin, growth hormone, insulin, parathyroid hormone, ACTH, and TSH. The latter two hormones are required for their subsequent stimulation of glucocorticoid and thyroid hormone production, respectively.

Prolactin

Once lactation has been established in cows and goats, the concentration of basal circulating prolactin and the release of prolactin at milking can be reduced to low levels without affecting milk yield. This situation contrasts markedly with that in nonruminants and even in other ruminants, particularly sheep. The increase in prolactin secretion during milking is brought about by stimulation of the udder and teats. No prolactin is released when the udder is denervated.

Growth Hormone

Whereas prolactin is important for milk secretion in nonruminants, growth hormone is more important in the maintenance of ruminant lactation. Growth hormone is galactopoietic (increases milk yield) in cattle and is essential for the maintenance of lactation in the goat. Growth hormone does not directly stimulate the mammary gland, but instead appears to direct nutrients from body tissues toward milk synthesis. It has been shown that plasma growth hormone con-

centration is significantly higher in high-yielding cows than in low-yielding cows, and that a significant reduction occurs when high-yielding cows cease lactating.

Thyroid Hormone

Thyroid hormone is essential for the maintenance of lactation in cattle. Partial removal of the thyroid gland causes a decline in milk production that can be restored by treatment with thyroactive compounds. Treatment of thyroid-intact cattle with thyroactive compounds can increase milk yields that are associated with increases in metabolism at the expense of body fat and protein.

Insulin

Glucose is required for lactose synthesis. Various adaptations favor mammary gland priority in glucose metabolism. In goats and cattle, insulin is not required for glucose transport into the mammary gland alveolar cells or for milk synthesis. Therefore, other tissues do not compete for the available glucose. Also, insulin concentrations are low during early lactation (when milk production is high) and increase as milk production declines. Low insulin concentrations reduce glucose uptake by those tissues that require its presence for transport and permit greater use by those cells that do not (e.g., alveolar epithelium). In cattle and goats, it appears that the pancreas releases less insulin in response to a glucose load. In animals other than cattle and goats, mammary uptake of insulin (associated with uptake of glucose) is maintained throughout lactation and is essential for maintenance of lactation.

Corticosteroids

Intact adrenal glands are essential for the maintenance of lactation in both ruminants and nonruminants. Mineralocorticoid and glucocorticoid components are needed. Plasma corticosteroid concentrations are higher in lactating animals than in nonlactating animals and are higher in high-yielding cows than in low-yielding cows. The exact role of the corticosteroids has not been established but might be correlated with metabolic rate.

Parathyroid Hormone

In view of the relatively high calcium content of milk, it is not surprising that parathyroid hormone is related to the maintenance of lactation. Parathyroid hormone stimulates bone resorption of calcium and the conversion of vitamin D to its active form, 1,25-dihydroxycholecalciferol $(1,25\text{-}(OH)_2D_3)$, which is necessary for the absorption of calcium from the intestine. The concentration of $1,25\text{-}(OH)_2D_3$ in plasma is markedly elevated during lactation.

COMPOSITION OF MILK

Gross Composition

The gross composition of milk refers to the proportions of water, fat, carbohydrate, protein, and mineral it contains. Water content is determined by the loss of weight observed when milk is dried. Fat content is determined by extraction with defined methods. Carbohydrate in milk is usually expressed as lactose equivalent and can include other carbohydrates. Protein content represents all proteins, including enzymes. Milk minerals are usually expressed as ash, which represents the residue remaining after incineration. Tables that show the composition of milk often present only the percentages of fat, protein, lactose, and ash, and they delete water. The aggregate of fat, protein, lactose, and ash is referred to as dry matter or milk solids.

Proteins

The caseins (alpha, beta, gamma, and kappa) constitute the major part of the milk proteins. These protein fractions are insoluble at a pH of 4.6 and comprise what is known as the curd. The other proteins are alpha-lactalbumin, beta-lactoglobulin, blood serum albumin, immunoglobulins, and a proteose-peptone fraction. These other proteins are soluble at pH 4.6 and are referred to as the whey proteins. The immunoglobulins are present in very small amounts, except in colostrum. All the proteins are synthesized in the mammary gland from amino acids except gamma-casein, blood serum albumin, and immunoglobulins (the immunoglobulin fraction of colostrum, however, is synthesized in the mammary gland). The minor proteins, including the enzymes, are present in milk in small amounts.

Carbohydrates

The principal carbohydrate in milk is lactose. It is synthesized in the mammary gland. Lactose is a disaccharide that contains glucose and galactose moieties. It is unique to the mammary gland, but small amounts are found in plasma during lactation. The principal precursor of lactose in the blood is glucose; propionate is also a precursor by way of glucose. Propionate is important in ruminants because of its availability from fermentative processes in the rumen.

Lipids

Milk lipids consist primarily of triglycerides. Other lipids include small amounts of phospholipids, cholesterol, free fatty acids, monoglycerides, and fat-soluble vitamins. Milk fat synthesis in ruminants proceeds mostly from acetic and butyric acids. Acetic acid constitutes about 60% to 70% of the volatile fatty acids from rumen fermentation. A reduction in milk fat concentration occurs when fermentation changes cause a decrease in production of acetic acid.

Minerals

The major minerals in cow's milk are calcium (0.12%), phosphorus (0.10%), sodium (0.05%), potassium (0.15%), and chlorine (0.11%). Other minerals found in trace amounts include magnesium, sulfur, copper, cobalt, iron, iodine, and zinc.

Vitamins

The B vitamins and vitamin K are synthesized by ruminants, and their concentration in milk is not influenced by diet. Vitamin K is also synthesized by the intestine, so its presence in nonruminant milk does not depend on diet. Vitamins A, D, and E are not synthesized in the rumen, so their presence in milk does depend on the diet. The amount of vitamin C in milk is not greatly influenced by diet.

Other Substances

Many drugs pass readily into the milk from the blood. Milk must therefore be withdrawn from the market for a certain period when cows have been treated with specific drugs, particularly antibiotics.

Off-flavors are sometimes detected in milk when cows have eaten certain foods. Fermentation often is a prerequisite to its being detected. Inhalation of volatile components in eructated gas might be the entry route for these off-flavors. The off-flavor component is produced as a result of fermentation in the rumen and, because it is volatile, it becomes part of eructated gas (much of eructated gas is inhaled). The inhaled portion is absorbed readily from the lung, whereas it might not have been absorbed from the rumen.

Species Variation in Composition

The approximate gross composition of milk is presented in Table 14.1 for several domestic animals, whales (marine mammal), and humans. The milk of marine mammals has a high fat content (33.2% in the whale as compared to 3.5% in the Holstein cow). It is believed that this high fat content is a consequence of the concentration necessary to conserve isotonic water. The isotonic water intake of marine mammals is restricted and is limited to that obtained from the fish they eat, so conservation is required. Lactose composition is probably the most constant among species, but still varies considerably. Some have thought that milk with a high protein content is characteristic of species with fast-growing offspring, but this is not a consistent finding. Variations are apparent among breeds within a species (e.g., fat and protein when comparing Holsteins and Guernseys). Differences exist among individuals within a breed and within an individual, depending on the stage of lactation and on whether the milk drawn from the udder is first-drawn or last-drawn. Last-drawn milk in cows has a higher fat percentage. Also, the fat composition in cow's milk is higher during the first 2 weeks after parturition, declines slightly for 3 to 4 months, and gradually decreases thereafter. The fat and protein content of milk is not affected by altering the fat and protein content in the diet.

Colostrum

Colostrum has been variously defined, but it is generally considered to be the initial mammary secretion after parturition. The composition of colostrum is decidedly different from milk composition that is considered normal for the species. The differences apparent in colostrum persist in descending magnitude for 4 to 6 days after parturition.

Colostrum is high in the whey proteins, particularly the immunoglobulins. Passive immunity is transferred to the offspring from the mother by immunoglobulins in

TABLE 14.1. Composition of Milk from Various Species

Species	Component			
	Fat	Protein	Lactose	Ash
Cat	7.1	10.1	4.2	0.5
Cattle				
Ayrshire	4.1	3.6	4.7	0.7
Brown Swiss	4.0	3.6	5.0	0.7
Guernsey	5.0	3.8	4.9	0.7
Holstein	3.5	3.1	4.9	0.7
Jersey	5.5	3.9	4.9	0.7
Shorthorn	3.6	3.3	4.5	0.8
Dog	9.5	9.3	3.1	1.2
Goat	3.5	3.1	4.6	0.8
Horse	1.6	2.4	6.1	0.5
Human	4.3	1.4	6.9	0.2
Mule	1.8	2.0	5.5	0.5
Sheep	10.4	6.8	3.7	0.9
Swine	7.9	5.9	4.9	0.9
Whale	33.2	12.2	1.4	1.4

Modified from Jacobson NL and McGilliard AD: The mammary gland and lactation. In: Dukes' physiology of domestic animals. 10th Ed. Edited by M.J. Swenson. Ithaca, NY: Cornell University Press, 1984.

colostrum. The period during which absorption occurs extends for 1 to 2 days after birth in the pig, horse, cattle, and dog. Under normal circumstances, the period is estimated to be 4 d or less in sheep and goats. Beyond this time, the immunoglobulins are more subject to digestion by proteolytic enzymes. Other significant differences between colostrum and regular milk are its higher concentrations of vitamin A, E, carotene, and riboflavin. Generally, colostrum also contains more protein, ash, and fat and less lactose than regular milk.

MILK REMOVAL AND OTHER CONSIDERATIONS

It was formerly believed that milk secretion occurred during milk removal, and that certain stimulating factors caused this to occur. The intramammary pressure of milk accumulation in the alveoli was thought to create the pressure difference by which milk could be withdrawn from the mammary gland.

It is now known that all the milk removed at a single milking is present in the mammary gland at the time of milking. The pressure increase that directs the milk from the alveoli through the ducts, cisterns, and teat canal is provided by the myoepithelial cells that surround the alveoli and ducts.

Stimulation of the teats or udder results in a reflex secretion of oxytocin from the posterior pituitary gland, which, on reaching the myoepithelial cells, causes them to contract. Often the presence of the calf or other conditioned reflexes can cause the release of oxytocin. The phenomenon associated with contraction of the myoepithelial cells is generally referred to as milk let-down (Fig. 14.9). The milk let-down effect ends in 10 to 15 minutes because of dissipation of the oxytocin. Until milk let-down, the pressure within the mammary gland is relatively low (0 to 8 mm Hg), but it increases to 30 to 50 mm Hg at the beginning of myoepithelial cell contraction.

The secretion of oxytocin for milk let-down is usually associated with tranquil situations, and it can be inhibited by stressful situations. Milk is not let down by tormented or frightened animals.

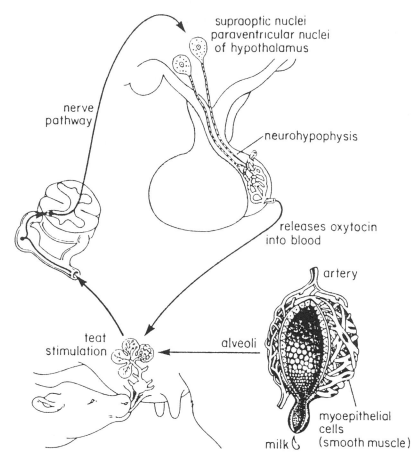

Figure 14.9. Milk let-down. Stimulation of the teats or udder results in a neuroendocrine reflex secretion of oxytocin from the posterior pituitary gland that, on reaching the myoepithelial cells, causes them to contract. From Hafez ESE. Reproduction in farm animals. 6th ed. Philadelphia: Lea & Febiger, 1993.

Milking Interval

It was generally believed that the intervals between milking should be evenly spaced, whether milking occurred twice or three times daily. Although some slight decreases are noted, it is now generally accepted that significant reductions do not occur if the intervals are not evenly spaced. It would seem that regularity of intervals might be a more important factor.

Regression of the Mammary Gland

Lactation does not continue indefinitely, either because animals are "dried off" (milk secretion is not removed) or because the secretion is gradually diminished to an insignificant amount. Several drying off techniques can be used, including the intermittent, incomplete, and abrupt methods. In the intermittent method, the accumulated milk is removed at 2- or 3-day intervals and then stopped. In the incomplete method, milk is only removed partially at the usual regular intervals. The abrupt method is probably most widely used, and milk removal ceases completely. Milk secretion ceases when alveolar pressure increases to a certain point. The usual alveolar and duct accommodation is exceeded and milk secretion ceases. The milk components are enzymatically digested or reabsorbed, the alveolar cells break up, and the gland is infiltrated by phagocytic cells. In a nonpregnant cow that is dried off, insufficient hormones are present to stimulate or maintain mammary growth and the lobules decrease in size, the alveoli collapse, and stromal tissue increases. These changes progress until ultimately the lobules are reduced to a few branching ducts.

In the lactating cow that is pregnant and dried off 2 months before parturition, little regression occurs in the lobule and alveolar tissue. Unless 2 months are allowed for a dry period before the next parturition, milk yield in the subsequent lactation is depressed. Continued lactation apparently interferes with the normal renewal or regeneration of alveolar cells.

STUDY AIDS—LACTATION

Structure and Function of Female Mammary Glands

1. Note the relationship of alveoli, lobules, lobes, ducts, and lactiferous sinus (gland cistern, teat cistern).
2. What is the milk-secreting unit of the mammary gland? Is it part of the parenchyma or stroma?
3. Do teat canal, papillary duct, and streak canal refer to the same thing?
4. What appears to be the function of the rosette of Fürstenberg?
5. What appears to be the function of the venous plexus in the teat wall?
6. What function is served by inward folds of the empty teat wall?
7. What function is served by the sphincter muscle that encircles the streak canal?
8. What function is served by the suspensory apparatus?
9. What is the venous circle of the mammary gland and where is it located?

What is the milk vein? What is the milk "well"?
10. What is the function of the myoepithelial cells?
11. What is the state of mammary gland development in the female at birth?
12. How is mammogenesis affected with successive estrous cycles after puberty?
13. What are the mammary gland changes that occur during pregnancy?
14. What is meant by lactogenesis?
15. Why is progesterone withdrawal a prerequisite for lactogenesis?
16. How is the increase in estrogen concentration before parturition associated with lactogenesis?
17. What is the role of prolactin in lactogenesis?
18. What is accomplished by a growth hormone surge just before parturition?
19. What is the role of growth hormone in the maintenance of lactation in cattle?
20. What comprises the milk solids?
21. What comprises the major part of the milk protein?
22. What is the difference between milk curd and whey?
23. What is the principal carbohydrate in milk?
24. What are the major lipids and minerals in milk?
25. What vitamins are normally found in ruminant milk that are not associated with the diet?
26. How do off-flavors get into ruminant milk?
27. Why does milk from marine mammals have a high concentration of fat?
28. What is colostrum and what are its highlights?
29. What causes intramammary gland pressure increase associated with milk let-down?
30. What is the usual recommendation for "drying off" of a pregnant cow that is lactating with regard to time before parturition?

SELF-EVALUATION—LACTATION

1. Which one of the following hormones causes contraction of the alveolar myoepithelial cells resulting in milk "let-down"?
   a. ADH
   b. relaxin
   c. oxytocin
   d. secretin

2. Which one of the following statements best describes colostrum?
   a. the secretions of the colon
   b. food material mixed with stomach secretions
   c. the last drawn milk at a particular milking which is higher in fat content
   d. the first milk drawn after birth of the young which is high in vitamin A and high in immune globulins

3. Which one of the anterior pituitary hormones is essential for the initiation of milk secretion (lactogenesis)?
   a. oxytocin
   b. estradiol
   c. prolactin
   d. progesterone

4. The teat wall venous plexus in cows is probably related to:
   a. expansion needs when the teat fills
   b. maintenance of normal teat temperature during cold exposure
   c. secretion of bacteriostatic substances
   d. milk secretion

5. Tissue with potential for assisting retention of milk within the udder between milkings coupled with their secretion of a bacteriostatic agent is known as the:
   a. teat (streak) canal
   b. longitudinal and circular folds in the wall of the teat cistern
   c. rosette of Fürstenberg
   d. parenchyma

6. The function of the mammary gland suspensory apparatus is to:
   a. provide upward support
   b. absorb shock when a cow runs or walks and udder is full
   c. allow movement and stretch from elastic element when cow is lying down
   d. all of the above

7. The milk secreting unit of the mammary gland is the:
   a. myoepithelial cell
   b. alveolus
   c. lactiferous sinus
   d. interlobular duct

8. Growth and development of the mammary gland is known as:
   a. mammogenesis
   b. lactogenesis
   c. mammary gland regression
   d. all of the above

9. Most mammary gland growth occurs during:
   a. the follicular and luteal phases of the estrous cycles
   b. pregnancy
   c. lactation

10. Which one of the following hormones must be withdrawn at the time of parturition in the cow for the mammary gland alveolar cells to begin milk secretion?
    a. progesterone
    b. estrogen
    c. prostaglandins
    d. prolactin

11. Estrogen increases in the cow toward the end of gestation. What is the significance of the increase to lactogenesis?
    a. causes lysis of corpus luteum
    b. prevents the formation of prolactin
    c. directs nutrients to the mammary gland for milk synthesis
    d. stimulates the secretion of prolactin and some other hormones from the anterior pituitary

12. Which one of the following hormones is most important for maintenance of lactation in cows?
    a. prolactin
    b. growth hormone

13. What is the relationship of parathyroid hormone to the maintenance of lactation?
    a. increases metabolic rate
    b. assists transport of glucose into alveolar epithelium
    c. increases plasma concentration of calcium
    d. stimulates alveolar protein synthesis
14. The major part of the milk proteins are:
    a. the lactalbumins
    b. the caseins
    c. the lactoglobulins
    d. the immunoglobulins
15. With continued milk secretion, alveolar pressure increases. What happens when alveolar, duct, and sinus accommodation is exceeded?
    a. milk secretion ceases
    b. teat canal sphincter and rosette of Fürstenberg retention potential is overcome and milk leaks to ground
    c. milk is reabsorbed
    d. cows get mean

Suggested Readings

Dyce KM, Sack WO, Wensing CJG. Textbook of veterinary anatomy. 2nd ed. Philadelphia: WB Saunders, 1996.

Frandson RD, Spurgeon TL. Anatomy and physiology of farm animals. 5th ed. Philadelphia: Lea & Febiger, 1992.

Larson BL. Biosynthesis and cellular secretion of milk. In: Larson BL, ed. Lactation. Ames, IA: Iowa State University Press, 1985: 129–163.

Park CS, Jacobson NL. The mammary gland and lactation. In: Swenson MJ, Reece WO, eds. Dukes' physiology of domestic animals. 11th ed. Ithaca, NY: Cornell University Press, 1993:711–727.

Tucker HA. Endocrine and neural control of the mammary gland. In: Larson BL, ed. Lactation. Ames, IA: Iowa State University Press, 1985:39–79.

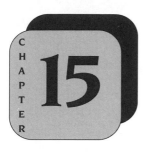

Endocrinology

The endocrine system is considered to be one of the animal body's communication systems, and its products (the hormones) help send messages to other cells. The other communication system is the nervous system, in which nerve networks conduct messages from cells in one part of the body to cells in another part. The nervous system uses physical structures (neurons) to transmit messages (impulses), but the endocrine system uses the body fluids (humors) as its medium to transmit messages (hormones). Because of this, control by the latter system is referred to as humoral control, in contrast to neural control.

The principal function of neural and humoral communication is control or regulation of various body functions. Nerve impulses traveling from the brain to the heart by way of the vagus nerve assist in the control of heart activities. Similarly, thyroid hormone is released from thyroid gland follicles and circulated by the blood and interstitial fluids to all cells of the body to assist in the regulation of metabolic rate.

HORMONES

Hormones have been classically defined as chemical substances produced by specialized ductless glands that are released into the blood and carried to other parts of the body to produce specific regulatory effects. Because of this, many substances that appear to have hormone-like activity are considered to be hormones, but are done so with apprehension because they do not conform to one or more of the criteria in this definition. For example, the prostaglandins are not produced in any one gland of the body, but are produced by most cells of the body. Furthermore, prostaglandins can be transmitted by diffusion in the interstitial fluid rather than by circulation in the blood.

Therefore, it seems best to consider the hormones as chemical regulators and to recognize that they can be produced by cells with a specific location in a particular gland or by cells located diffusely in many parts of the body.

426

Modes of Transmission

The concept of the restriction of hormone transmission to blood circulation only must be abandoned and recognition given to other means of transmission. These means are classified as epicrine, neurocrine, paracrine, endocrine, and exocrine transmission.

EPICRINE TRANSMISSION. In epicrine transmission, hormones pass through gap junctions of adjacent cells without entering extracellular fluid.

NEUROCRINE TRANSMISSION. In neurocrine transmission, hormones diffuse through synaptic clefts between neurons, as do neurotransmitters. Also, the hormone (such as oxytocin) can be synthesized in the neuron cell body, stored in axons (like neurotransmitters), but can be secreted into the blood.

PARACRINE TRANSMISSION. In paracrine transmission, hormones diffuse through interstitial fluid, as do prostaglandins.

ENDOCRINE TRANSMISSION. In endocrine transmission, hormones are transported through the blood circulation. This is typical of most hormones.

EXOCRINE TRANSMISSION. In exocrine transmission, the regulatory agent (hormone) is secreted to the exterior of the body. The lumen of the intestine is considered to be exterior to the body so that hormones secreted into it can affect cell activity more distal to the point of secretion. Some hormones, such as somatostatin, can have exocrine transmission (secretion to intestinal lumen), and subsequently act as inhibitors of many gastrointestinal functions, including intestinal motility and intestinal absorption. Inasmuch as pheromones are chemical communicators, they might be considered to have exocrine transmission because they are received by other animals of the same species (through olfaction) after they have been excreted to the exterior of the body.

Biochemistry

Under the classic definition, hormones are biochemically categorized as amines, peptides, or steroids. The amine hormones include thyroid hormone and the adrenal catecholamines are categorized as epinephrine and norepinephrine. All of the amine hormones are derived from the amino acid tyrosine. The peptide hormones include peptides, polypeptides, and proteins. All the hormones of the hypothalamus and pituitary, as well as insulin and glucagon from the pancreas, are included in the peptide class. The steroid hormones include the adrenocortical and reproductive gland hormones and the active metabolites of vitamin D. Cholesterol is the common precursor of steroid hormones. The prostaglandins (not classic hormones) are derived from arachidonic acid (a fatty acid). More structural detail is provided in this chapter when some hormones of specific endocrine glands or other tissues are discussed.

PITUITARY GLAND

The pituitary gland (hypophysis cerebri) has two distinct parts, the anterior pituitary (adenohypophysis) and the posterior pituitary (neurohypophysis). It is located in a bony recess (sella turcica) at the base of the brain. The divisions, blood supply, and neural connections to the hypothalamus are shown in Figure 15.1. Its location just below the hypothalamus provides for direct delivery of several releasing hormones from the hypothalamus to the anterior pituitary and for direct entry of secretory neurons from the hypothalamus to the posterior pituitary. Assisting the delivery of releasing hormones to the anterior pituitary is a unique arrangement of blood vessels, the hypothalamic-hypophyseal portal system (Fig. 15.1). Similar to other blood portal systems, the venous blood drained from the hypothalamus is redistributed by another capillary system within the anterior pituitary. Shortages of hormones in arterial blood are detected by specific cells within the hypothalamus, which are stimulated to secrete releasing hormones. The releasing hormones produced are distributed by the second capillary bed to their appropriate cells in the anterior pituitary.

Posterior Pituitary

The posterior pituitary is an outgrowth of the hypothalamus (Fig. 15.2A) and contains the terminal axons from two pairs of nuclei (supraoptic and paraventricular) located in the hypothalamus (Fig. 15.2B). The supraoptic and paraventricular nuclei synthesize antidiuretic hormone and oxytocin, respectively, which are transported to the axon terminals where they are stored until released. An action potential, generated by the need for each of the stored hormones, causes the release of the hormone and subsequent absorption into the blood, where it is distributed to the receptor cells.

Anterior Pituitary

The anterior pituitary lies forward from the posterior pituitary and is comprised of three parts, the pars distalis, pars intermedia, and pars tuberalis (Fig. 15.2). The pars distalis is the principal part and has five different cell types that secrete the seven hormones of the anterior pituitary: 1) somatotrope cells, which secrete growth hormone; 2) corticotrope cells, which secrete adrenocorticotropic hormone (ACTH) and beta-lipotropin; 3) mammotrope cells, which secrete prolactin; 4) thyrotrope cells, which secrete thyroid-stimulating hormone; and 5) gonadotrope cells, which secrete follicle-stimulating hormone (FSH) and luteinizing hormone (LH). The pars intermedia has a less certain secretory role. Extracts of the pars intermedia contain melanocyte-stimulating hormone (MSH), associated with the color changes in reptiles, amphibians, and fish that result from the dispersion or concentration of pigment granules in cells known as

Figure 15.1. Schematic representation of the pituitary. **1.** Hypothalamic-hypophyseal portal circulation and the pathway followed by the hypothalamic-hypophysiotropic hormones (releasing and inhibiting) in reaching the anterior pituitary (*left*). **2.** Pathway by which the posterior pituitary hormone oxytocin and ADH (antidiuretic hormone) reach the capillaries of the posterior lobe (*right*). Hormone-containing blood leaves each lobe of the pituitary through a number of hypophyseal veins. The open arrows indicate the direction of blood flow; the closed arrowheads indicate the path taken by the hormones involved. From Cormack DC. Ham's histology. 9th ed. Philadelphia: JB Lippincott, 1987.

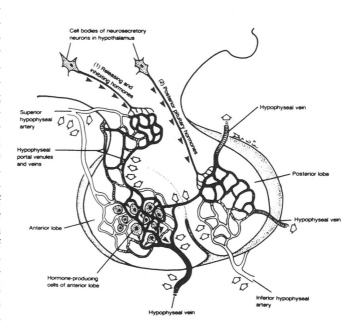

melanophores. Although extracts of mammalian pars intermedia contain MSH, it is not certain whether MSH is secreted, and no function for MSH has been established in homeotherms. The pars tuberalis consists of a layer of cells surrounding the neural stalk for which no specific function has been identified.

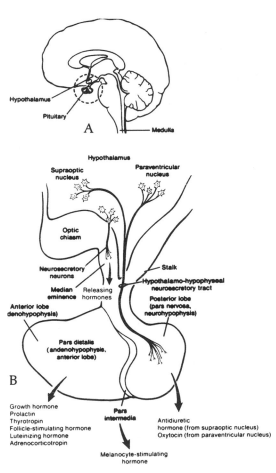

Figure 15.2. Location of the pituitary in the primate brain. **A.** The pituitary is situated at the base of the hypothalamus. **B.** Hypothalamic neurons from the supraoptic and paraventricular nuclei transmit their neurosecretions of antidiuretic hormone and oxytocin, respectively, to the posterior lobe. From Eckert RE, Randall D, Augustine G. Animal physiology: mechanisms and adaptations. 3rd ed. New York: WH Freeman, 1988.

Because of the relatively large number of important hormones associated with the pituitary gland, it is sometimes called the "master gland." Pharmaceutical companies obtain animal pituitary glands from slaughter houses and extract several hormones for commercial and experimental uses. Recovery of the pituitary gland at slaughter is laborious because of its protected location, and yields are low (340 g/100 cattle; 30 g/100 pigs) because of its small size.

Functions of Pituitary Hormones

Anterior Pituitary Hormones

The hormones of the anterior pituitary belong to the peptide class, ranging from polypeptides to large proteins. Differences in structure are noted among species, and replacement therapy from one species to another is not uniformly successful. Sometimes an active core of a hormone is identified that permits its subsequent use after the non-core portion is removed.

GROWTH HORMONE. Growth hormone is also known as somatotropic hormone (STH) because of its stimulating effect on the somatic cells (body cells). It has invariably been referred to as growth hormone because of its stimulation of increase in body size. It causes growth of all tissues of the body that are capable of growth, and it promotes both increased cell size and increased mitosis with development of increased cell numbers. The epiphyseal disks of long bones are particularly sensitive to growth hormone, in which mitotic activity is stimulated and results in lengthening. Growth hormone stimulates the liver to form several small proteins called somatomedins, which then act on cartilage and bone to promote their growth. Bone and cartilage are therefore not stimulated directly by growth hormone, but indirectly by this intermediate compound.

In addition to its general effect of causing growth, STH has several specific metabolic effects. Because of these, it is apparent that STH is needed throughout life and not only during the growth phase. These metabolic effects include 1) increased rate of protein synthesis in all body cells, 2) increased mobilization of fatty acids from fat and increased use of fatty acids for energy, and 3) decreased rate of glucose uptake throughout the body. The preferential use of fats for energy conserves glucose and promotes glycogen storage. Because of glycogen storage, the heart can endure emergency contraction more effectively, whereby glycogen stored in the heart is converted to glucose. Probably most metabolic functions of growth hormone are caused not by its direct effects on the tissues, but by indirect effects through the somatomedins.

An effect of growth hormone in increasing milk yields in the lactating cow has received considerable research interest. The precise cause for the increases is not known, but it might partially be a result of mammary gland growth because milk yield is influenced by the numbers of mammary secretory cells. It is also thought that the increased milk yield might be caused partially by the metabolic effects of STH, which helps to direct more nutrients to the mammary gland.

ADRENOCORTICOTROPIC HORMONE. ACTH causes increased activity of the adrenal cortex. It was formerly thought that ACTH only stimulated the secretion of glucocorticoids by the adrenal cortex, but it is now recognized that mineralocorticoid (aldosterone) secretion is also enhanced. In addition, it has become apparent that ACTH has metabolic effects somewhat similar to those of STH, in which protein synthesis and fatty acid uptake are enhanced and glucose uptake is decreased.

THYROID-STIMULATING HORMONE. Thyroid-stimulating hormone (TSH) stimulates the synthesis of colloid by thyroid gland cells and stimulates the release of thyroid hormone. Associated with these functions are the accumulation of iodine, organic binding of iodine, and formation of thyroxine within the thyroid gland. No extrathyroid activity is apparent for TSH, as for STH and ACTH.

GONADOTROPIC HORMONES AND PROLACTIN. The gonadotropic hormones, follicle-stimulating hormone (FSH) and luteinizing hormone (LH), have specific roles in male and female reproduction, and detailed accounts are provided in Chapters 12 (Male Reproduction) and 13 (Female Reproduction). Specifically, FSH stimulates oogenesis and spermatogenesis in the female and male, respectively. In the female, LH assists ovulation and development of a functioning corpus luteum, and in the male it stimulates the secretion of testosterone. Prolactin helps to initiate and maintain lactation after pregnancy in the female. Also, in the ewe, it is associated with maintenance of the corpus luteum.

BETA-LIPOTROPIN HORMONE. Beta-lipotropin hormone (β-LPH) is secreted by the same cells (corticotrope) that secrete ACTH (see previous text). The physiologic role of β-LPH is still unknown. Products providing pain relief (e.g., endogenous opiates, which are the endorphins and enkephalins) might be derived from β-LPH. Inasmuch as they are associated with ACTH (same secreting cells), the response to stress might include β-LPH secretion and pain relief as a neural response.

Posterior Pituitary Hormones

The hormones of the posterior pituitary are of the peptide class, specifically nonapeptides (they contain nine amino acids). They are formed by nerve cell bodies within hypothalamic nuclei and are transported by axons to terminal positions in the neurohypophysis (posterior pituitary), where they are stored in secretory granules. The posterior pituitary hormones, antidiuretic hormone and oxytocin, are neurosecretions.

ANTIDIURETIC HORMONE. When an animal is given an overload of water, a period of diuresis (increased output of dilute urine) occurs. Diuresis can be prevented by the administration of antidiuretic hormone (ADH), also known as vasopressin. If dehydration occurs (osmoconcentration), osmoreceptors respond to the increased concentration by stimulating greater output of ADH by the axon terminals in the posterior pituitary. The target cells of the secreted ADH are the collecting tubules and the collecting ducts of the kidney. The presence of ADH renders the cells of the collecting tubules and collecting ducts more permeable to water, and more water is absorbed from the tubular fluid so that the plasma osmolality decreases (Na^+ concentration returns to normal) and the urine volume decreases (becomes more concentrated). ADH is therefore important for water conservation by animals. Other stimulators of ADH secretion include reduced blood volume, trauma, pain, and anxiety.

OXYTOCIN. The functional activity of oxytocin is related to the reproductive processes, which include lactation. Oxytocin is released from the posterior pituitary as a result of neuroendocrine reflexes. The act of suckling or similar teat stimulation causes release of oxytocin and subsequent milk letdown. Similarly, an estrogen-dominated myometrium, such as is found at ovulation and at parturition, is more responsive to oxytocin, and greater contraction of the uterus results. Oxytocin release at these times is associated with appropriate stimuli and subsequent myometrial contraction, which assists in the transport of sperm to the oviduct at copulation and in the expulsion of the fetus at parturition.

THYROID GLAND

In most mammals, the thyroid gland is located on the trachea, just caudal to the larynx. In cattle it consists of two laterally placed, somewhat flattened, lobes joined by an isthmus (Fig. 15.3). The lateral lobes have a less substantial isthmus in the horse and no isthmus in the dog and cat. Pigs have a compact thyroid form with a large median lobe (instead of an isthmus) in addition to the lateral lobes. The thyroid gland is composed of numerous folli-

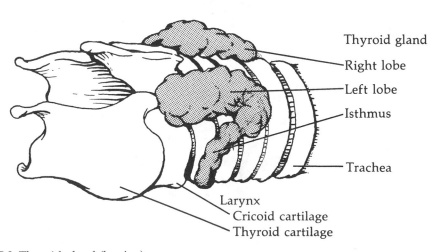

Figure 15.3. Thyroid gland (bovine).

cles (Fig. 15.4) lined by simple epithelial cells and filled with a fluid known as colloid. The surface area of the lining epithelium is increased by villi that project into the follicle.

Thyroid Hormones

The thyroid hormones belong to the amine classification of hormones—they are derived from the amino acid tyrosine. A further characteristic of the thyroid hormones is that they contain iodine. Iodine is bound organically in the thyroid gland in four forms (Fig. 15.5). The thyroid hormones, thyroxine (T_4), and 3,5,3'-triiodothyronine (T_3), are combinations of two molecules of diiodotyrosine, as in T_4, or one molecule of monoiodotyrosine with one molecule of diiodotyrosine, as in T_3. In both cases the combination results in the loss of one water molecule and an amino acid residue, glycine. Iodine trapping and iodination are unique features of the thyroid gland that are assisted by TSH.

Biochemistry of T3 and T4 Formation

Thyroglobulin is a large glycoprotein molecule secreted into the follicle by the lining cells. Thyroglobulin has a molecular weight of about 680,000. It contains many tyrosine molecules; when iodinated, they consist of both monoiodotyrosine and diiodotyrosine. Tyrosine coupling occurs while the tyrosine residues are still attached to the thyroglobulin molecule. The lining cells of the follicles provide the enzymes required for coupling to form T_3 and T_4. The coupled tyrosines, still attached to the thyroglobulin molecule, are stored after synthesis within the follicle.

Release and Transport of T3 and T4

The thyroglobulin molecule, with enclosed T_3 and T_4, is not released into the blood from the thyroid follicles. Extensions from the follicle cells enclose parts of colloid, so that colloid becomes a vesicle within the cell (endocytosis). Lysosomes release proteolytic enzymes that separate T_3 and T_4 from thyroglobulin and permit their absorption from the base of the cells. The monoiodotyrosine and diiodotyrosine freed similarly by digestion are not absorbed, but are deiodinated, and both the iodine and tyrosine are recycled into new thyroglobulin. About 90% of thyroid hormone released is T_4.

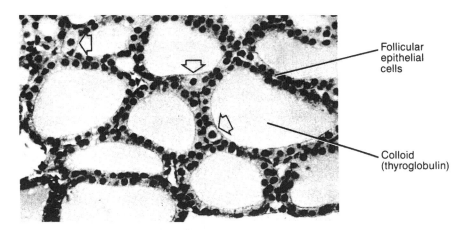

Follicular epithelial cells

Colloid (thyroglobulin)

Figure 15.4. Photomicrograph of the canine thyroid gland (lower power). The arrows indicate parafollicular cells (C cells); the remainder are follicular cells. From Cormack DC. Ham's histology. 9th ed. Philadelphia: JB Lippincott, 1987.

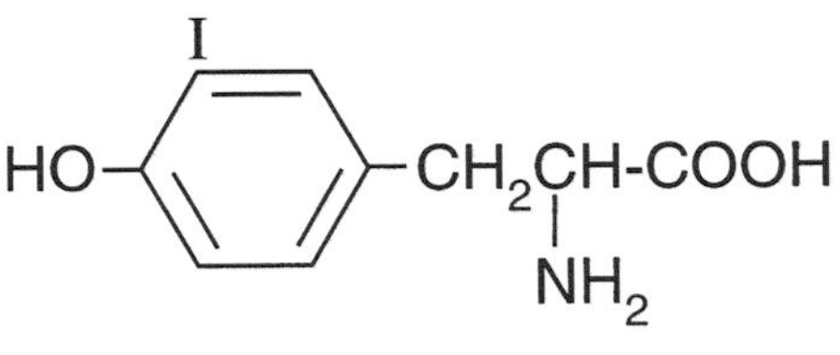

MONOIODOTYROSINE

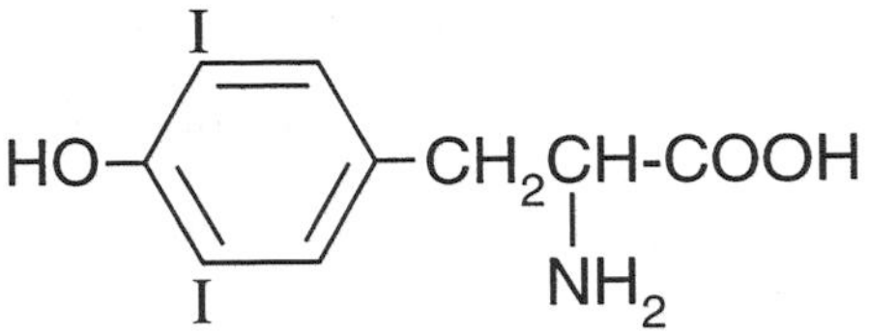

DIIODOTYROSINE

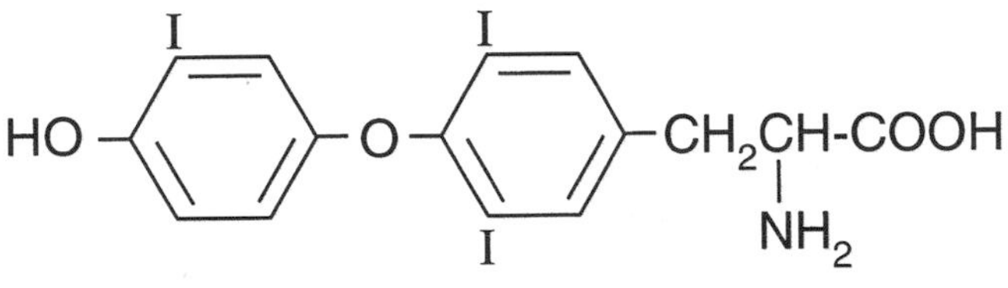

3,5,3' TRIIODOTHYRONINE

Figure 15.5. Structural formulas of the iodinated amino acids monoiodotyrosine and diiodotyrosine and the compounds formed by their coupling. The coupling of monoiodotyrosine and diiodotyrosine with loss of H_2O and glycine produces 2,5,3'-triiodotyrosine, known as T_3. The coupling of two molecules of diiodotyrosine with loss of H_2O and glycine produces thyroxine, known as T_4.

T_3 and T_4 are combined immediately with plasma proteins for transport in the blood. The major plasma protein is termed thyroxine-binding globulin (TBG). This protein has a high affinity for the thyroid hormones, but a greater affinity for T_4 than for T_3. All the T_4 and T_3 are bound, but because of the greater affinity of TBG for T_4 than for T_3, more T_3 is released to tissue cells than T_4. Once within the tissue cells, T_3 is more potent than T_4, but its duration of action is shorter. Thus, short-term and long-term demands by cells can be met effectively by the different release and potency characteristics associated with T_4 and T_3.

Functions

The most well-known function of thyroid hormones is their ability to raise internal heat, thereby increasing the rate of oxygen consumption. Thyroid hormones stimulate the metabolic activities of most tissues of the body except for the brain, lungs, retina, testes, and spleen. The ability to increase metabolic activity and oxygen consumption is partly a result of the stimulation or activation of some key enzymes, including alpha-glycerophosphate dehydrogenase, hexokinase, diphosphoglycerate mutase, and cytochromes b and c. The lipolytic effect of epinephrine is also markedly potentiated by thyroid hormones. The specific role of thyroid hormones in increasing internal heat production has not been elucidated definitively, but it has been suggested that the increased heat is secondary to increased protein synthesis stimulated by thyroid hormones.

Regulation of Secretion

To provide consistent quantities of thyroid hormones, feedback control mechanisms are provided through the hypothalamus and anterior pituitary. Decreased levels of thyroid hormones result in the secretion of thyrotropin-releasing hormone (TRH) into the hypothalamic-hypophyseal portal system. The thyrotrope cells of the anterior pituitary (adenohypophysis) are thereby stimulated by TRH to secrete TSH. TSH secretion is followed by increased thyroid gland activity, including the release of T_3 and T_4 from the thyroglobulin molecule, their absorption into the blood, and transport to cells. A constant level consistent with normal metabolism is ensured by this feedback mechanism. The rate of TSH secretion increases above normal by the exposure of animals to cold environments. The response is mediated by the cooling of the anterior hypothalamus, resulting in an increase in metabolic rate and an attendant increase in heat production. Excitement and anxiety result in a decreased output of thyroid hormones because the stimulation of the sympathetic nervous system by these states causes an increase in epinephrine and norepinephrine output, resulting in an increase in metabolic rate and heat production.

Thyroid Deficiency and Antithyroid Compounds

The typical form of thyroid hormone deficiency results from an iodine deficiency and consequent inability of the thyroid gland to produce T_3 and T_4. The lack of circulating hormones causes the usual feedback mechanisms, so that TSH is produced, and the resulting stimulation of the thyroid gland causes thyroglobulin accumulation without effective output of T_3 and T_4. The thyroid gland enlarges because of colloid accumulation, a condition known as goiter. Thyroid gland enlargement can be caused by hypothyroidism (e.g., iodine deficiency) or hyperthyroidism (e.g., increased thyroxine demands, tumor). Goiter caused by iodine deficiency is rarely seen in the domestic animals, and other causes of thyroid dysfunction are relatively uncommon in sheep, cattle, and swine. The clinical signs of hypothyroidism and hyperthyroidism, however, are common in dogs and cats. Lack of activity (lethargy), hair loss, dry and dull hair, cold sensitivity, and anemia are common clinical signs of hypothyroidism. Fatigue, weight loss, hunger, nervousness, and sensitivity to heat are associated with hyperthyroidism.

Natural substances have been identified that cause goiter by inhibiting thyroid function, called goitrogens. Because thyroid function is inhibited, thyroxine is not produced in sufficient amounts and TSH continues to be secreted, resulting in thyroglobulin accumulation. One such goitrogen, goitrin, is produced in the intestinal tract after the ingestion of a progoitrin contained in cruciferous plants (e.g., cabbage, rutabaga, turnip). Thiocyanate, another goitrogen, is also contained in some plants, and plant goitrogens are important causes of animal goiter in some parts of the world. Goitrin and related compounds cause goiter by interfering with the organic binding of iodine, but thiocyanate interferes with iodine trapping by the thyroid gland. In the latter case, the effects can be overcome by feeding excess iodine. Antithyroid compounds are used for the treatment of hyperthyroidism; these include thiourea, thiouracil, the sulfonamides, and chlorpromazine. The use of antithyroid compounds to promote weight gain has not produced satisfactory results.

Calcitonin

Calcitonin is a hormone of the thyroid gland secreted by parafollicular or C cells (Fig. 15.4) that are also present in the walls of thyroid gland follicles. Calcitonin is a polypeptide of 32 amino acids (MW 3000).

The stimulation for secretion of calcitonin is hypercalcemia and, to a lesser extent, hypermagnesemia. Calcitonin inhibits osteoclastic bone resorption and thereby attempts to lower the plasma Ca^{2+} concentration. Calcitonin also inhibits phosphate resorption and enhances calcium loss in the kidney. Calcitonin is antagonistic to the action of another hormone associated with calcium homeostasis, parathyroid hormone (see later section). The latter hormone protects against low plasma concentrations of Ca^{2+}.

PARATHYROID GLAND

The parathyroid glands are located near or embedded within the thyroid gland. In domestic animals it consists of one (pig) or two (dog, cat, ruminants, horse) pairs of beanlike organs. The parathyroids are sometimes so close to the thyroid gland that differentiation is difficult.

Parathyroid Hormone and Calcium Ion Regulation

Parathyroid hormone (PTH) is a polypeptide with a molecular weight of 9500 that contains a chain of 84 amino acids.

A low plasma Ca^{2+} concentration stimulates secretion of PTH from the parathyroid gland, whereas hypercalcemia inhibits PTH secretion. A less effective stimulator of PTH secretion is hypomagnesemia.

Calcium and phosphorus are absorbed from bone under the influence of PTH by two processes. The most rapid means by which PTH increases the plasma Ca^{2+} concentration is called osteolysis; it involves osteoblasts and osteocytes. These cells are normally involved in calcium and phosphorus deposition, but in osteolysis they are involved in absorption. PTH inhibits osteoblast synthesis of new bone but increases osteoblast-initiated recruitment of osteocytes to transport calcium and

phosphorus from the bone fluid to the extracellular fluid. In this instance, absorption of Ca^{2+} and phosphorus occurs without loss of bone matrix. However, PTH also increases osteoblast-initiated recruitment of osteoclasts (bone dissolvers). In contrast to osteolysis, osteoclastic activity causes loss of bone matrix and, over a period of time, excavations are visible. Osteolysis is considered to be the rapid phase of calcium and phosphate absorption and activation of osteoclasts is considered to be the slow phase of bone absorption and calcium phosphate release.

Action of PTH on the Kidneys

PTH elevates plasma Ca^{2+} concentration, but its action would be ineffective if a change did not occur in the kidneys to increase Ca^{2+} absorption from tubular fluid. This change is brought about by PTH. At the same time, phosphate reabsorption by the kidney diminishes (Fig. 15.6). This change is also effected by PTH, and the calcium:phosphorus ratio of ~2:1 in plasma is maintained.

PTH and 1,25-Dihydroxycholecalciferol Formation

Parathyroid hormone greatly enhances both calcium and phosphate absorption from the intestines by increasing the rate of formation of 1,25-dihydroxycholecalciferol, (1,25-$[OH]_2D_3$), the active form of vitamin D. The original forms of vitamin D are converted through a succession of reactions in the liver and kidney. The first conversions occur in the liver and the final conversion of 25-dihydroxycholecalciferol to 1,25-$(OH)_2D_3$ occurs in the kidney under the influence of PTH (Fig. 15.7). In the intestinal epithelium, 1,25-$(OH_2)D_3$ causes the formation of a calcium-binding protein that functions at the brush border to transport calcium into the cell cytoplasm. Calcium-binding protein remains

Figure 15.6. Steps in the restoration of decreased plasma calcium concentration toward normal through the actions of parathyroid hormone and vitamin D. Its active form is 1,25-(OH)$_2$ D$_3$. From Vander AJ, Sherman JH, Luciano DS. Human physiology: the mechanisms of body function. 4th ed. New York: McGraw-Hill, 1985.

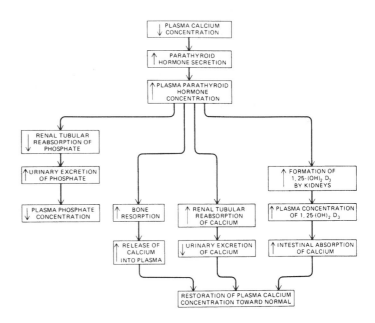

Figure 15.7. Metabolism of vitamin D to its active form 1,25-(OH)$_2$D$_3$. Parathyroid hormone activates the kidney enzyme that mediates the final step. The principal function of activated vitamin D is stimulation of the intestinal absorption of calcium. From Vander AJ, Sherman JH, Luciano DS. Human physiology: the mechanisms of body function. 4th ed. New York: McGraw-Hill, 1985.

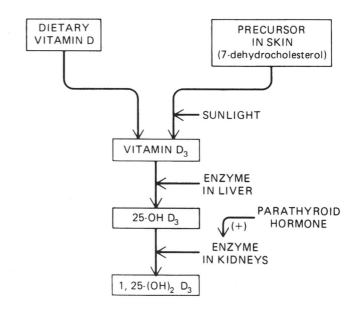

in the cells for several weeks, providing a prolonged effect on calcium absorption.

Enhancement of intestinal phosphate absorption might result from the direct effect of 1,25-(OH)$_2$D$_3$, but it could be a secondary result of the hormone's action on calcium absorption, in which calcium acts as a transport mediator for phosphate.

ADRENAL GLANDS

The adrenal glands are small, paired structures that lie immediately cranial to the kidneys and are close to the junction of the renal vein with the posterior vena cava (Fig. 15.8). A sagittal section of the adrenal gland (Fig. 15.9) reveals an outer cortex and

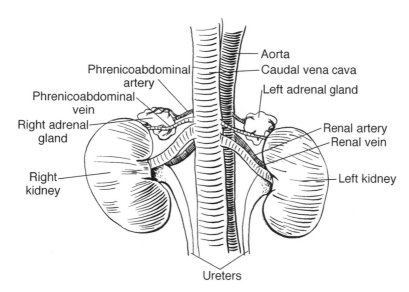

Figure 15.8. The canine adrenal glands (ventral view). Their blood supply and venous drainage is by way of branches from the phrenicoabdominal arteries and veins.

an inner medulla. The adrenal cortex has three distinct cell types arranged in zones from the outside to the inside—the zona glomerulosa, zona fasciculata, and zona reticularis. The adrenal medulla is homogeneous in structure and contains secretory granules. Its nerve supply is by way of preganglionic sympathetic neurons. The cells of the medulla are thought to be modified postganglionic sympathetic nerve cell bodies.

Hormones of the Adrenal Cortex

The hormones of the adrenal cortex are steroids formed mainly from cholesterol. The membrane of the adrenal cortex has receptors for low-density lipoproteins (rich in cholesterol) and, after their attachment, these are absorbed by endocytosis. Seven adrenocortical hormones (corticosteroids) are recognized as secretions of the adrenal cortex. Four of these—corticosterone, cortisol, cortisone, and 11-dehydrocorticosterone—are termed glucocorticoids. The other three—11-deoxycorticosterone, 17-hydroxy-11-deoxycorticosterone, and aldosterone—are called mineralocorticoids. The

structural formulas of the two principal adrenocortical steroids (aldosterone and cortisol) are presented in Figure 15.10.

Functions of the Glucocorticoids

The glucocorticoids have a principal role in carbohydrate metabolism in that they enhance gluconeogenesis. The noncarbohydrate source from which new glucose is synthesized is mostly protein, but a definite effect on fat metabolism is also recognized. Two other hormones, glucagon and epinephrine, increase blood glucose levels by glycolysis of liver glycogen. The glucocorticoids, however, appear to be necessary for glycolysis effected by glucagon and epinephrine. The gluconeogenic effect of the glucocorticoids is the basis for their use in the treatment of bovine ketosis.

The glucocorticoids are associated with water diuresis. Not only do they inhibit ADH secretion and thus interfere with the effect of ADH on the collecting tubules and collecting ducts, but they also increase the glomerular filtration rate. Because of the diuresis, sodium loss is common after glucocorticoid therapy, even though the gluco-

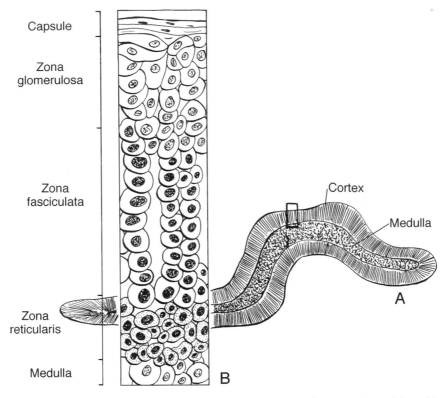

Figure 15.9. Diagrammatic representation of the adrenal gland. **A**. Cross-section of the adrenal gland showing the contrasting appearance of the cortex and medulla. **B**. Magnification of boxed-in area in **A** that shows the different cell types associated with the three zones of the cortex.

Figure 15.10. Structural formulas of the principal adrenocortical hormones.

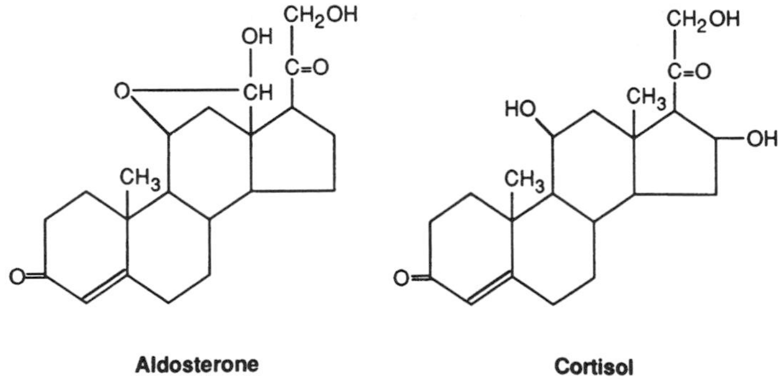

Aldosterone   **Cortisol**

corticoids possess considerable sodium retentive activity.

A common therapeutic use of the glucocorticoids is related to their anti-inflammatory activity, and they are included in ophthalmic preparations, otic (ear) drops, and skin ointments. Injection of glucocorticoids into inflamed articulations or bursae provides temporary relief, and their systemic use is sometimes useful in the alleviation of some allergic responses. Prolonged systemic use often is associated with exaggeration of other physiologic functions of the glucocorticoids, such as sodium retention related to their having some mineralocorticoid activity (retention of Na^+ and H_2O). More potent pharmacologic preparations can minimize these side effects but do not eliminate them altogether.

Functions of the Mineralocorticoids

The principal function of the mineralocorticoids can be illustrated by aldosterone and its action on the kidney to enhance sodium reabsorption and potassium excretion. The mineralocorticoids are also effective in promoting membrane transport in sweat glands, salivary glands, intestinal mucosa, and between the intracellular and extracellular fluid compartments. Just as glucocorticoids have some mineralocorticoid activity, the mineralocorticoids have some glucocorticoid activity. These secondary activities are most apparent when therapeutic uses are made of these compounds and the amounts used are in excess of normal endogenous amounts.

Regulation of Glucocorticoid Secretion

The glucocorticoids are secreted by the zona fasciculata of the adrenal cortex. Their secretion is regulated by ACTH from the anterior pituitary. Free plasma cortisol (not protein-bound) concentrations influence ACTH secretion—low levels stimulate ACTH release and subsequent secretion of glucocorticoids from the zona fascicularis. Stimuli such as stress can also cause ACTH secretion that raises glucocorticoid concentrations above normal levels. An example of an adrenal response to adaptation can be seen with the overcrowding of domestic chickens whereby excess ACTH secretion results in adrenal hypertrophy because of greater output of glucocorticoids. The same phenomenon is observed in wild mammals whose population density increases.

Regulation of Mineralocorticoid Secretion

Three processes are usually considered to be the means by which aldosterone secretion from the zona glomerulosa increases: 1) renin-angiotensin system; 2) increased plasma concentration of potassium (hyperkalemia); and 3) ACTH stimulation. In the renin-angiotensin system, renin is secreted by juxtaglomerular cells in the kidney in response to their decreased perfusion by blood. Renin acts on a circulating blood globulin, angiotensinogen, to form angiotensin I. Angiotensin I is converted by the vascular endothelium of the lung to angiotensin II, which is the stimulus for the secretion of aldosterone from the zona glomerulosa. The result of this stimulation is promotion of Na^+ reabsorption and consequent retention of water, which expands blood volume and thus reestablishes normal blood pressure (low blood pressure was the cause for renin secretion).

The secretion of aldosterone in response to hyperkalemia provides a means for controlling the critical plasma concentration of potassium. Aldosterone secretion promotes Na^+ reabsorption with simultaneous K^+ excretion. This action of aldosterone occurs in the distal tubule, collecting tubule, and collecting duct. At other places in the nephron, K^+ is reabsorbed. Even though Na^+ is reabsorbed in the process of K^+ excretion, the Na^+ concentration in the plasma is not regulated by aldosterone. The plasma Na^+ concentration decreases can cause aldosterone secretion, but the decreases necessary for stimulation are of greater magnitude than the effective increases of K^+ that cause aldosterone secretion.

The role of ACTH in promoting aldosterone secretion has less significance. The increase in ACTH associated with stress causes some increased output of aldosterone and might augment the output produced by other means, such as angiotensin II.

Hormones of the Adrenal Medulla

The hormones of the adrenal medulla belong to the amine chemical class and are known as epinephrine (adrenalin) and nor-

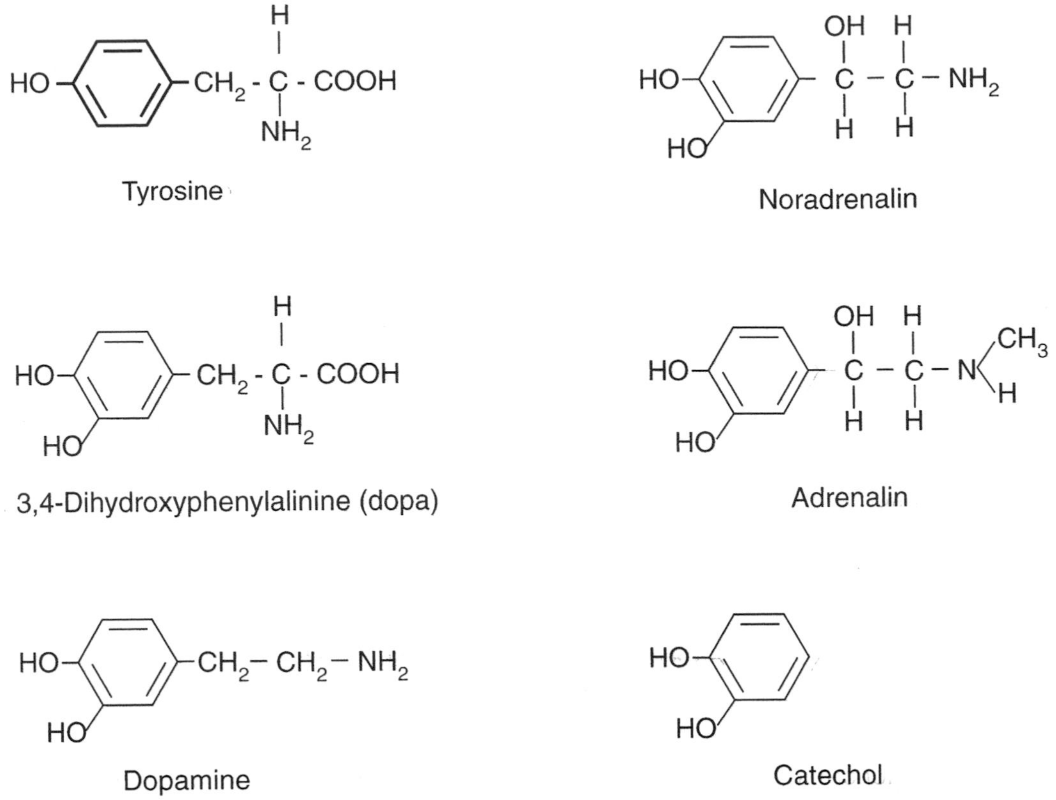

Tyrosine

3,4-Dihydroxyphenylalinine (dopa)

Dopamine

Noradrenalin

Adrenalin

Catechol

Figure 15.11. Structural formulas of catecholamine hormones. They are formed from the amino acid tyrosine and are derivatives of catechol. The abbreviation "dopa" is derived from the German name of this compound, dioxyphenylalamine.

epinephrine (noradrenaline). They are referred to as catecholamines and are derived from the amino acid tyrosine. The catecholamine hormones (including epinephrine and norepinephrine) are shown in Figure 15.11. Epinephrine is secreted only by the adrenal medulla, but norepinephrine is also secreted by postganglionic sympathetic neurons. More epinephrine is secreted by the adrenal medulla than norepinephrine. The inactivation of the catecholamines is rapid—the half-life of epinephrine is about 20 to 40 seconds.

It appears that the adrenal medullary secretion is a continuous process and it increases dramatically during an emergency. The continuous secretion enables the maintenance of a state of readiness or tone, and the larger outpouring provides for an immediate response to emergencies.

The actions of epinephrine and norepinephrine are similar and differences are expressed depending on the receptors, which can have a preference for epinephrine or norepinephrine. The two adrenergic receptors are alpha and beta receptors. Alpha receptors are stimulatory (except those in intestinal smooth muscle, where they are inhibitory) and beta receptors are inhibitory (except those in cardiac muscle, where they are stimulatory). Epinephrine and norepinephrine stimulate both receptors, but the alpha effect of norepinephrine is more potent than that of epinephrine, and epinephrine has a more potent action than norepinephrine on the beta receptors.

In addition to the "fight-fright-flight" reactions associated with the catecholamines, they have pronounced metabolic effects. These are associated with the increased activity caused by catecholamines and include hyperglycemia, increased calorigenesis, lipolysis, and an elevated blood lactate concentration. The hyperglycemia results from enhanced liver glycogenolysis, and the increased blood lactate level is caused by stimulation of muscle glycogenolysis. The calorigenic effect results from the increased muscle activity and an increase in lactic acid oxidation in the liver.

PANCREATIC GLAND

The pancreas has both exocrine and endocrine functions. The exocrine functions are those associated with digestion and include digestive enzyme and bicarbonate secretion.

Hormones of the Pancreas

The hormones of the pancreas are insulin, glucagon, somatostatin, and pancreatic polypeptide. They are secreted by specific cells located in islets scattered throughout the pancreas. Four major types of cells are found in the islets, each responsible for the secretion of one hormone. The cells are identified as alpha cells (glucagon), beta cells (insulin), delta cells (somatostatin), and F cells (pancreatic polypeptide). The pancreatic hormones are polypeptides.

INSULIN. The tissues differ in regard to their sensitivity to insulin. Whereas the liver, muscle, adipose tissue, and leukocytes respond readily to insulin, the brain, kidney, intestines, and erythrocytes show little response. The principal effect of insulin on carbohydrate metabolism in those tissues sensitive to insulin (except the liver) is to allow the transport of glucose across the cell membrane. In these tissues, insulin enhances facilitated diffusion. In the liver, insulin enhances glucose uptake by stimulating enzymes in the liver cells that assist in the production of glycogen and lipogenesis and by inhibiting enzymes that catalyze glycogenolysis. Generally, insulin promotes fat deposition and protein synthesis. The result of insulin activity is lowering of the blood glucose concentration.

GLUCAGON. The result of glucagon activity is elevation of the blood glucose concentration. This is achieved by the activation of adenylcyclase in liver cells, which in turn stimulates phosphorylase and results in the breakdown of glycogen. In addition, glucagon increases gluconeogenesis, increases metabolic rate, and stimulates lipolysis. Another action of glucagon is stimulation of the secretion of insulin (so that the new glucose can diffuse into cells) and of somatostatin.

SOMATOSTATIN. Somatostatin usually appears to act as an inhibitory agent to slow the output of nutrients into the circulation and to moderate the metabolic effects of insulin, glucagon, and growth hormone. In this regard, somatostatin inhibits the secretion of insulin and glucagon. Also, as a moderator, it inhibits the secretion of gastrin, secretin, cholecystokinin, pancreatic exocrine secretion, and gastric acid. Somatostatin also moderates gastrointestinal motility and the absorption of glucose.

PANCREATIC POLYPEPTIDE. Pancreatic polypeptide secretion is stimulated by the ingestion of protein, by exercise, and by fasting. No definite function has been established for pancreatic polypeptide.

Control of Insulin and Glucagon Secretion

The secretion of insulin and glucagon is controlled directly by the blood glucose concentration. Because of the dual control (insulin decreases, glucagon increases) of glucose concentration, blood levels show little variation.

Important stimulatory effects on insulin secretion are caused by the gastrointestinal hormones, gastrin, secretin, cholecystokinin, and other hormones. The gastrointestinal hormones are secreted in response to food ingestion and actually cause insulin to be secreted before glucose absorption. Insulin secretion is also stimulated by pancreatic glucagon (see previous text).

Glucagon secretion is stimulated by hypoglycemia, gastrin, cholecystokinin, and stress and is inhibited by glucose, secretin, insulin, and somatostatin. Somatostatin release is enhanced by almost every factor that increases insulin secretion.

PROSTAGLANDINS AND THEIR FUNCTIONS

The prostaglandins were first isolated from accessory sex gland fluids and were termed prostaglandins because of their association with the prostate gland. It is now recognized that they are secreted by almost all body tissues and, indeed, the prostate gland association is too narrow a definition.

The prostaglandins are derived from arachidonic acid. Their structure and synthesis are shown in Figure 15.12. The prostaglandins are usually short-acting. Some forms never appear in the blood (so some have not been classified as hormones) and others are degraded after they circulate throughout the liver and lungs.

The functions of prostaglandins have been studied most in regard to their role in the reproductive process. Prostaglandin $F_{2\alpha}$ ($PGF_{2\alpha}$) is the natural luteolytic agent that terminates the luteal phase of the estrous cycle and allows for the initiation of a new estrous cycle in the absence of fertilization. $PGF_{2\alpha}$ is also particularly potent in terminating early pregnancy.

The prostaglandins promote inflammation. The anti-inflammatory activity of aspirin (and perhaps of other drugs) is a result of its ability to inhibit the synthesis of prostaglandin G_2 (PGG_2) from arachidonic acid. The anti-inflammatory action of the glucocorticoids might also be caused by interference with prostaglandin synthesis. Other functions of some prostaglandins include inhibition of gastric secretion and relaxation of bronchial smooth muscle. One prostaglandin (prostacyclin, PGI_2) that is produced in the endothelium of blood vessels inhibits platelet aggregation (essential for blood coagulation), and a prostaglandin derivative (thromboxane A_2) favors platelet aggregation.

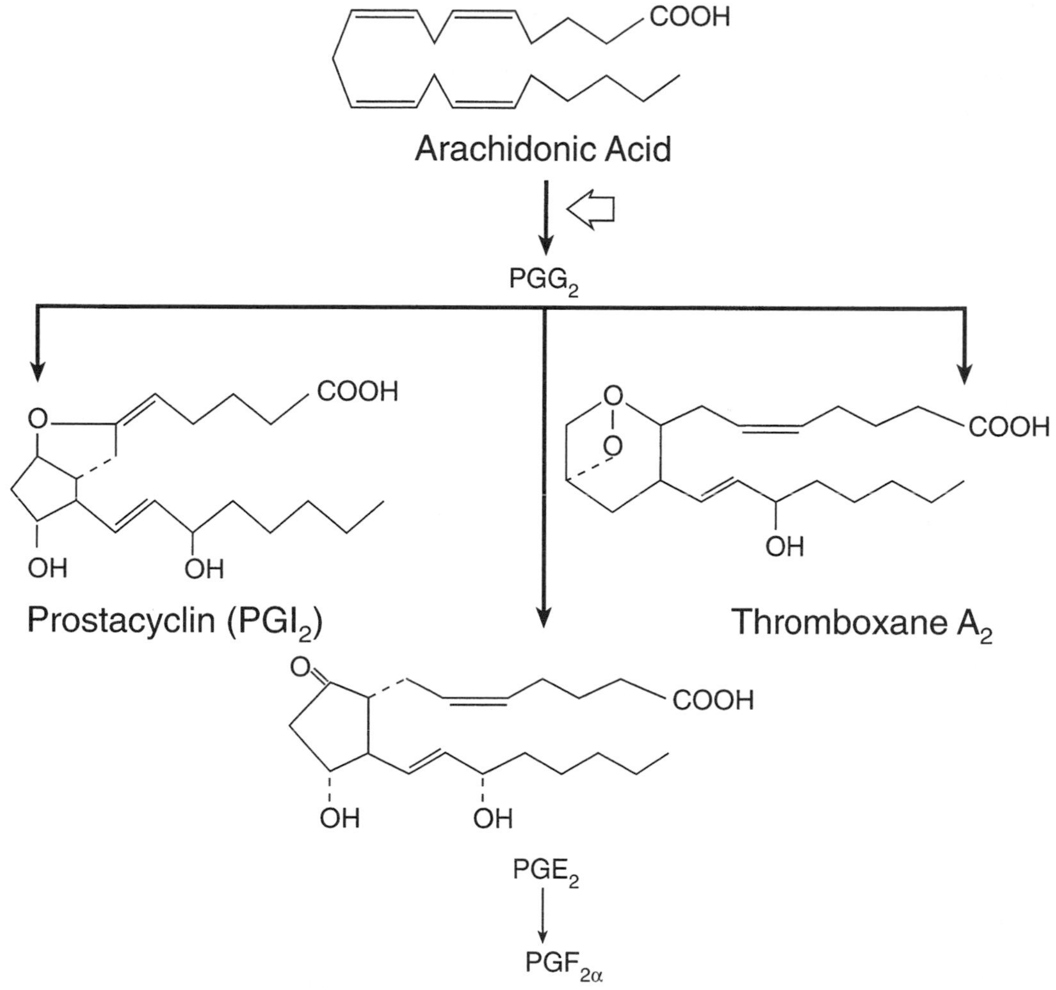

Figure 15.12. Three major pathways of prostaglandin synthesis. The open arrow indicates the site of aspirin inhibition. Thromboxane A_2 is biochemically related to the prostaglandins and is formed from them as shown. Thromboxane A_2 promotes the platelet release reaction associated with blood coagulation. Therefore, aspirin retards blood coagulation.

STUDY AIDS—ENDOCRINOLOGY

Hormones

1. Are all hormones transported by blood? How does endocrine transmission differ from exocrine transmission?
2. What is an amine hormone? What is a peptide hormone? What is a steroid hormone? Finally, what is the biochemical derivation of the prostaglandins?
3. What is the common precursor of the steroid hormones?

Pituitary

1. What is the hypothalamic-hypophyseal portal system? What is its function?
2. What are the abbreviated names of the anterior pituitary hormones?
3. Briefly list the functions of each of the anterior pituitary hormones. Is STH needed throughout life or only during the growth phase?
4. What is meant by posterior pituitary hormones being known as neurosecretions?
5. Briefly list the functions for the posterior pituitary hormones.

Thyroid Gland

1. What is the substance called that fills the thyroid follicles?
2. Sketch the thyroxine molecule and note the presence of iodine. How does T_3 differ from T_4?
3. What is thyroglobulin? How are T_3 and T_4 stored in the thyroid gland after their formation? Describe the release and absorption of T_3 and T_4 from the thyroid follicles.
4. What fraction of thyroid hormone release from the thyroid gland is T_4?

5. Describe the plasma transport, release, and cell utilization characteristics of T_3 and T_4.
6. What is the most well-known function of the thyroid hormones?
7. Note how low levels of thyroid hormones cause the secretion of the thyroid hormones.
8. What is calcitonin? Where is it secreted? Is it secreted in response to hypercalcemia or hypocalcemia? What, then, is its function?

Parathyroid Gland

1. What is parathyroid hormone? Where is it secreted? What are the stimuli to PTH secretion? Is plasma Ca^{2+} concentration increased after PTH secretion?
2. What are the mechanisms whereby PTH increases absorption of Ca^{2+} from bone?
3. How does PTH influence the kidney so that the plasma Ca^{2+} increase from bone absorption is not lost by kidney excretion?
4. What is the active form of vitamin D? Where is it formed? Is PTH involved in its formation?
5. Where does the active form of vitamin D exert its influence? What is its effect?
6. Study Figures 15.6 and 15.7 for summaries of PTH and vitamin D activity and formation of the active form of vitamin D, respectively.

Adrenal Glands

1. Where are the adrenal glands located?
2. What are the two principal hormones of the adrenal cortex? What is their biochemical classification?
3. What is the role of the glucocorticoids in carbohydrate metabolism? What is the main noncarbohydrate source of new glucose formation?
4. Do glucocorticoids have some mineralocorticoid activity?
5. What is the principal function of the mineralocorticoids? Do they possess some glucocorticoid activity?

6. What regulates the secretion of the glucocorticoids?
7. What are the processes whereby aldosterone secretion increases?
8. What are the hormones of the adrenal medulla?
9. What is the biochemical classification for epinephrine and norepinephrine? Are they also considered catecholamines?
10. What division of the autonomic nervous system secretes norepinephrine? Is it a postganglionic or preganglionic secretion?

Pancreatic Gland

1. Delineate the endocrine and exocrine functions of the pancreas.
2. What are the four pancreatic hormones? Briefly describe the functions of each (providing that they are known).
3. What are the pancreatic islets?
4. Does insulin activity increase or decrease blood glucose concentration?
5. How does glucagon elevate blood glucose?

Prostaglandins

1. How did the prostaglandins get their name?
2. What is the range of tissues associated with prostaglandin production?
3. Do prostaglandins promote or inhibit inflammation?
4. Do prostaglandins promote or inhibit blood coagulation?
5. Could aspirin use interfere with inflammation and blood coagulation?

SELF-EVALUATION— ENDOCRINOLOGY

1. The action of which one of the following would provide for gluconeogenesis (production of new glucose)?
   a. growth hormone
   b. norepinephrine
   c. aldosterone
   d. adrenocorticotropic hormone
2. Thyroxine (T_4) and T_3 are produced:
   a. in the thyroid follicle
   b. in the epithelial cells which line the thyroid follicles
   c. in the anterior pituitary
   d. in the blood after the components have been secreted by the thyroid epithelial cells
3. Iodine is a part of which one of the following hormones?
   a. growth hormone
   b. hydrocortisone
   c. parathyroid hormone
   d. thyroxine
4. Parathyroid hormone increases the absorption of calcium from the intestinal tract by its action on:
   a. intestinal epithelial cells
   b. bone cells
   c. the kidney to activate Vitamin D
   d. cholesterol to form Vitamin D
5. Cholesterol and arachidonic acid are the respective precursors of:
   a. amino and peptide hormones
   b. steroid and prostaglandin hormones
   c. prostaglandin and steroid hormones
   d. peptide and amine hormones
6. The anterior pituitary hormone that causes growth of all body tissues that are capable of growth and that also has several metabolic effects is:
   a. somatotropic hormone
   b. adrenocorticotropic hormone
   c. thyroid-stimulating hormone
   d. gonadotropic hormone
7. Which one of the following hormones is a neurosecretion of the posterior pituitary?
   a. adrenocorticotropic hormone
   b. antidiuretic hormone
   c. epinephrine
   d. somatotropic hormone

8. The hormone that directly influences water reabsorption by the kidneys is:
   a. oxytocin
   b. aldosterone
   c. antidiuretic hormone
   d. insulin

9. Which one of the following hormones is released in response to cooling of the anterior hypothalamus?
   a. antidiuretic hormone
   b. insulin
   c. T_4 and T_3 (thyroid hormones)
   d. aldosterone

10. Plasma $[Ca^{2+}]$ is decreased by:
    a. calcitonin
    b. parathyroid hormone
    c. 1-25-dihydroxycholecalciferol
    d .cortisol

11. The mineralocorticoids influence the plasma concentrations of:
    a. calcium and phosphorus
    b. sodium and potassium
    c. calcium and sodium
    d. potassium and calcium

12. Epinephrine and norepinephrine appear to be continuous secretions of the adrenal medulla with dramatic increases during an emergency.
    a. true
    b. false

13. What pancreatic function is associated with the secretion of insulin, glucagon, somatostatin, and pancreatic polypeptide?
    a. endocrine
    b. exocrine

14. Blood glucose concentration is decreased by the secretion of:
    a. glucagon
    b. pancreatic polypeptide
    c. insulin
    d. lucocorticoids

15. Aspirin use is associated with its ability to be anti-inflammatory and also to inhibit platelet aggregation that enhances blood coagulation. These characteristics are mediated through:
    a. specific prostaglandins
    b. glucocorticoids
    c. a thyroid hormone
    d. beta-lipotropin hormone

Suggested Readings

Cormack DH. Ham's histology. 9th ed. Philadelphia: JB Lippincott, 1987.

Dickson WM. Endocrine glands. In: Swenson MJ, Reece WO, eds. Dukes' physiology of domestic animals. 11th ed. Ithaca, NY: Cornell University Press, 1993:629–664.

Griffin JE, Ojeda SR, eds. Textbook of endocrine physiology. New York: Oxford University Press, 1988.

Hullinger RL. The endocrine system. In: Evans HE, ed. Miller's anatomy of the dog. 3rd ed. Philadelphia: WB Saunders, 1993: 559–585.

McDonald LE. Veterinary endocrinology and reproduction. 4th ed. Philadelphia: Lea & Febiger, 1989.

Turner CD, Bagnara JT. General endocrinology. 6th ed. Philadelphia: WB Saunders, 1976.

Vander AJ, Sherman JH, Luciano DS. Human physiology: the mechanisms of body function. 6th ed. New York: McGraw-Hill, 1994.

Answer Key

NERVOUS SYSTEM

1. b	6. b	11. d	16. d	21. b	26. b	31. b	36. a
2. c	7. c	12. a	17. b	22. c	27. c	32. c	37. c
3. c	8. a	13. c	18. a	23. c	28. d	33. d	38. c
4. b	9. b	14. a	19. a	24. b	29. b	34. b	39. b
5. a	10. a	15. c	20. a	25. a	30. b	35. a	

THE SENSORY ORGANS

1. a	6. b	11. a	16. c	21. d	26. a	31. a	36. a
2. a	7. a	12. c	17. d	22. d	27. c	32. a	37. d
3. c	8. b	13. b	18. a	23. b	28. b	33. b	
4. a	9. b	14. b	19. b	24. c	29. a	34. a	
5. c	10. b	15. c	20. a	25. d	30. c	35. c	

MUSCLE

1. a	4. c	7. a	10. c	13. d	16. a
2. a	5. b	8. a	11. d	14. b	17. b
3. b	6. c	9. d	12. a	15. c	18. c

BONES, JOINTS, AND SYNOVIAL FLUID

1. b	5. b	9. d	13. b	17. a	21. c	25. c
2. c	6. d	10. b	14. a	18. c	22. a	26. b
3. b	7. c	11. a	15. b	19. a	23. c	
4. c	8. c	12. c	16. d	20. c	24. b	

BODY WATER

1. c	3. c	5. b	7. b
2. b	4. b	6. c	8. a

BLOOD AND ITS FUNCTIONS

1. c	5. c	9. c	13. b	17. b	21. a	25. c	29. a
2. a	6. c	10. d	14. a	18. b	22. c	26. d	30. b
3. d	7. c	11. c	15. b	19. b	23. a	27. a	31. a
4. b	8. b	12. c	16. d	20. b	24. b	28. c	

THE CARDIOVASCULAR SYSTEM

1. a	5. d	9. b	13. c	17. a
2. c	6. c	10. a	14. b	18. b
3. c	7. a	11. b	15. e	19. c
4. a	8. d	12. a	16. c	20. b

RESPIRATION

1. c	6. a	11. b	16. a	21. b	26. c	31. b
2. c	7. a	12. a	17. b	22. c	27. c	32. a
3. b	8. a	13. b	18. c	23. a	28. b	
4. b	9. c	14. a	19. b	24. c	29. c	
5. b	10. a	15. b	20. c	25. a	30. a	

THE KIDNEYS

1. b	6. b	11. c	16. b	21. b	26. c
2. c	7. c	12. c	17. c	22. a	27. b
3. b	8. c	13. a	18. d	23. b	28. c
4. d	9. c	14. a	19. a	24. b	29. c
5. c	10. c	15. a	20. a	25. b	30. b

DIGESTION AND ABSORPTION

1. a	10. c	19. b	28. c	37. c	46. b	55. a	64. b
2. c	11. d	20. d	29. b	38. a	47. b	56. a	65. c
3. a	12. b	21. c	30. d	39. c	48. a	57. a	66. c
4. c	13. d	22. c	31. c	40. c	49. d	58. a	67. a
5. a	14. b	23. d	32. a	41. b	50. a	59. b	68. b
6. b	15. d	24. c	33. d	42. c	51. b	60. a	69. b

7. b	16. a	25. b	34. b	43. a	52. c	61. a	70. b
8. d	17. c	26. d	35. b	44. b	53. c	62. a	
9. c	18. a	27. a	36. c	45. a	54. c	63. b	

BODY HEAT AND TEMPERATURE REGULATION

| 1. b | 3. c | 5. b | 7. d | 9. b |
| 2. b | 4. b | 6. d | 8. a | 10. b |

MALE REPRODUCTION

1. b	4. c	7. d	10. b	13. c	16. b	19. c
2. c	5. d	8. c	11. a	14. b	17. c	20. c
3. a	6. a	9. a	12. c	15. c	18. b	

FEMALE REPRODUCTION

1. a	7. b	13. d	19. d	25. a	31. b
2. c	8. c	14. a	20. b	26. d	32. b
3. c	9. b	15. c	21. d	27. d	33. b
4. e	10. b	16. c	22. c	28. b	34. c
5. c	11. c	17. d	23. b	29. c	
6. d	12. b	18. d	24. b	30. c	

LACTATION

1. c	4. b	7. b	10. a	13. c
2. d	5. c	8. a	11. d	14. b
3. c	6. d	9. b	12. b	15. a

ENDOCRINOLOGY

1. d	4. c	7. b	10. a	13. a
2. a	5. b	8. c	11. b	14. c
3. d	6. a	9. c	12. a	15. a

Index

Italic pages indicate figures; pages with t indicate tables.